Also by Anne Harrington

The Cure Within: A History of Mind-Body Medicine

Reenchanted Science: Holism in German Culture from Wilhelm II to Hitler

Medicine, Mind, and the Double Brain

The Placebo Effect: An Interdisciplinary Exploration (editor)

MIND
FIXERS

Psychiatry's Troubled Search
for the Biology of Mental Illness

Anne Harrington

W. W. NORTON & COMPANY
Independent Publishers Since 1923

For information about permission to reproduce selections from this book, write to
Permissions, W. W. Norton & Company, Inc., 500 Fifth Avenue, New York, NY 10110

For information about special discounts for bulk purchases, please contact
W. W. Norton Special Sales at specialsales@wwnorton.com or 800-233-4830

Manufacturing by Lake Book Manufacturing
Book design by Daniel Lagin
Production manager: Lauren Abbate

Library of Congress Cataloging-in-Publication Data

Names: Harrington, Anne, 1960– author.
Title: Mind fixers : psychiatry's troubled search for the biology of mental illness /
    Anne Harrington.
Description: First edition. | New York : W. W. Norton & Company, [2019] | Includes
    bibliographical references and index.
Identifiers: LCCN 2018053059 | ISBN 9780393071221 (hardcover)
Subjects: LCSH: Mental illness—Physiological aspects. | Neuropsychiatry.
Classification: LCC RC455.4.B5 H37 2019 | DDC 616.89—dc23
LC record available at https://lccn.loc.gov/2018053059

ISBN 978-0-393-35806-3 pbk.

W. W. Norton & Company, Inc., 500 Fifth Avenue, New York, N.Y. 10110
www.wwnorton.com

W. W. Norton & Company Ltd., 15 Carlisle Street, London W1D 3BS

1 2 3 4 5 6 7 8 9 0

*To my students, whose questions first inspired me
to write this book. To my husband, John, my toughest
critic and most loyal advocate. To my son, Jamie,
because he makes me remember how much of the best
parts of life happen outside a library and office.*

CONTENTS

Part III: **Unfinished Stories**

ACKNOWLEDGMENTS

The ideas for this book were first incubated in a large general education undergraduate lecture class I have taught for some years at Harvard University. I am indebted in ways I can never fully document to the hundreds of students who accompanied me on the evolving journey of that course and my own thinking. They shared insights, questions, and stories of their own, made me question my own assumptions, and in some cases were a first audience for some of the arguments laid out in this book.

For early research assistance (when I imagined completing a rather different final project), I am indebted to former students Kevin Stoller, Brittany Benjamin, and Lauren Libby. For archival materials, I thank the staff of the Oskar Diethelm Library at the DeWitt Wallace Institute for the History of Psychiatry at Weill Cornell Medical College in New York City, the Schlesinger Library at Radcliffe Institute for Advanced Study, the Center for the History of Medicine at the Countway Library of Harvard Medical School, and the many dedicated professionals who have in recent years made so much rich archival material available for scholars to access online.

For feedback on the revised project in its early stages, I am grateful to my editor, Amy Cherry, to my agent, Katinka Matson, and to colleagues at the Newhouse Center for the Humanities at Wellesley College, the Max

Planck Institute for the History of Science in Berlin, and the Freiburg University Institute for Advanced Studies in Freiburg. For these early sojourns in Germany, I am grateful for funding support from the MPI and the Humboldt Foundation Alumna Return Program.

Tim Hawley provided line edits on the first rough drafts of chapters, tightening the prose and asking pointed questions. I feel very lucky to have had him in my corner. For generous conceptual feedback on the manuscript as a whole, I am particularly grateful to Elizabeth Lunbeck, Steven Hyman, and John Durant.

Dr. Yvan Prkachin provided exemplary assistance managing all the permissions and images associated with this publication. A talented young historian of neuroscience himself, he also was a trusted sounding board in the final months of preparation.

Over the years, the thinking reflected in this book has benefited from encounters, conversations, and more formal interviews with scientists, clinicians, parents, and patients. While it is impossible to adequately thank them all, I would particularly like to acknowledge Steven Hyman, Thomas Insel, Alan Stone, Elyn Saks, Kay Redfield Jamison, Barbara Leadholm, Peggy Senturia (who helped me reach out to other mothers who lived with mental illness in their families through the formative 1970s), and Linda Schneider.

For support and nurturing intellectual community, especially in the final months of work on this book, I am indebted to the Freiburg Institute for Advanced Studies (FRIAS) at the University of Freiburg. I also gratefully acknowledge funding in this period from the People Programme (Marie Curie Actions) of the European Union's Seventh Framework Programme (FP7/2007–2013) under REA grant agreement n° [609305].

INTRODUCTION

Our Biological Enthusiasms

IN 1978 THE HISTORIAN AND SOCIAL CRITIC MARTIN GROSS APPEARED on the television show *Firing Line* to talk about his scathing new book, *The Psychological Society*. Scorning the current infatuation of psychiatry with psychoanalytic practices, he prophesied that "within the next ten years... psychiatry will come out of the dark ages, will drop all the nonsense and expertise about human behavior of which they know absolutely nothing that my grandmother didn't know, if they know that much, and will turn to medicine." His interlocutors were more than a little skeptical and even amused by his passion. One of them, the newspaper publisher and editor Sylvan Meyer, asked ironically how Gross thought that "a major body of science that's been in business for a fairly long time could be disposed of so quickly."[1]

It was Gross, though, who had the last laugh, and he did not have to wait ten years, or even five, to have it. Just two years after he sounded off on *Firing Line*, the *Los Angeles Times* reported on a meeting of the American Psychiatric Association and the major changes in process:

Ten years ago, the typical psychiatrist was still something of a Freudian facsimile, an aloof figure guiding his troubled patients—on the couch—through the mazes of their unconscious. . . .

No more.... The typical "shrink" of the '80s is more likely to view "craziness" as a combination of genetic, developmental and environmental stress factors coming together. And the excitement in the field centers on advances in brain biochemistry and neuro-anatomy; convention seminars on such subjects as "the psycho-pharmacology of depression" now draw standing-room only crowds.[2]

A year later, in 1981, two prominent psychiatrists predicted in *Psychology Today* the coming of a post-Freudian world, one where patients with emotional problems were treated, not with mere talk, but in a proper medical fashion—with "drugs [that] ... normalize a deep abnormality close to underlying causes."[3] And a year after that, the *Washington Post* told readers that everything they believed about mental disorders was on the verge of fundamental change: "During the past decade—barely a blink of the eye in the history of scientific research—scientists have unlocked the doors to understanding the body's most complicated and baffling organ: the brain.... It is as if a small trail painstakingly carved through a jungle over the course of centuries had been, within the space of 10 years, turned into a superhighway."[4]

By 1984, the Pulitzer Prize–winning science journalist Jon Franklin felt able to drop all pretense of deference toward the alleged opposition and to mock psychoanalysis as "the bumbling and sometimes humorous step-child of modern science." The future of psychiatry, he said, lay not with the old talk therapists and analysts but with a new generation of clinician-scientists he called "the mind-fixers": "research psychiatrists ... working quietly in laboratories, dissecting the brains of mice and men and teasing out the chemical formulas that unlock the secrets of the mind."[5]

That same year the psychiatrist Nancy Andreasen released a book whose title seemed to say it all: *The Broken Brain: The Biological Revolution in Psychiatry.* In it, she told her readers that "psychiatry is in the process of undergoing a revolutionary change, and realigning itself with the main-stream biological traditions of medicine." Everyone should celebrate this fact, she said, not least because once the public at large realized that mental illnesses were diseases like any other, the mentally ill—long stigmatized and misunderstood—could finally be understood simply "as human beings who deserve as much sensitivity and love as people who suffer from cancer, muscular dystrophy, or heart disease."[6] No one should mourn the passing of the psychoanalytic era, she said, because the new biological perspectives were opening the door not only to more effective treatments but to a more humane and compassionate approach to mental illness.

By 1988—a mere ten years after Gross had been gently mocked on *Firing Line*—psychiatry's transformation into a biological discipline seemed complete. That fall the psychiatrist Samuel Guze gave a lecture at London's Maudsley Hospital provocatively titled: "Biological Psychiatry: Is There Any Other Kind?" His answer was implied in the title: of course not. Psychiatry was a branch of medicine, and all medicine was "applied biology," end of story. "I believe," he concluded, "that continuing debate about the biological basis of psychiatry is derived much more from philosophical, ideological and political concerns than from scientific ones."[7]

All this added up to nothing less than a palace revolution in American psychiatry, an astonishingly rapid, 180-degree turnaround in understanding and approaches to ailments of the mind. Why did it happen? What caused an entire profession to reorient itself so quickly and so completely?

For the psychiatrists who heralded these developments in the 1980s, the answers seemed clear. In the late nineteenth century, they believed, the field of psychiatry—especially in German-speaking Europe—had actually been on the right track. Under the leadership of Theodor Meynert and Emil Kraepelin, it had pursued a robust biological research program. Unfortunately, the Freudians had come along, turned everyone's heads, and led the field into a scientific wasteland for more than half a century. Finally, however, exciting new developments in neuroscience, genetics, and psychopharmacology had changed things. Irrefutable evidence that mental disorders were brain diseases had emboldened a new generation of biological psychiatrists to overthrow the Freudians and to bring back the brain as the primary object of psychiatric research, diagnosis, and treatment. It was a simple explanatory story, one with clear heroes and villains, and above all a satisfyingly happy ending.[8]

The only trouble with this story is that it is wrong—not just slightly wrong but wrong in every particular. The nineteenth-century brain psychiatrists were not early versions of the 1980s biological revolutionaries, save perhaps for the fact that they wore longer waistcoats and had more facial hair. Their project did not fall victim to the siren call of psychoanalysis. It failed on its own terms. The Freudian psychiatrists came into positions of significant power only after World War II (not before), and they did so not because they were briefly able to persuade enough people to buy into their nonsense, but because they appeared to have grasped the mental health challenges of the postwar era better than the biologists had. (Some shrewd public relations work helped create that perception.) In the late 1970s and '80s, a "biological revolution" was indeed declared, and people did point to various developments in biological research and pharmacology to justify the call for a changing of the guard. But these extraordinarily rapid changes did not happen because new science triumphed over ossified dogmatism. In fact, the developments to which people pointed most frequently were in many cases decades old.

Put another way, American psychiatry's 1980s biological revolution was what people in my field call an "actor's category."[9] We confuse ourselves if we try invoking it to make analytic sense of developments in this period, simply because the period was not marked by any revolutionary new understandings of the biology of mental illness. If, though, we understand that it was instead a vision of psychiatry's identity and destiny that was summoned rhetorically into existence in the 1980s, then we can start asking questions about why it was summoned, and all the ways in which it became a critically important mindset and belief system under which all sorts of stakeholders carried out—and still carry out—their business.

We can also understand why it left behind such an unsatisfactory legacy. For make no mistake: today one is hard-pressed to find anyone knowledgeable who believes that the so-called biological revolution of the 1980s made good on most or even any of its therapeutic and scientific promises. Criticism of the enterprise has escalated sharply in recent decades. It is now increasingly clear to the general public that it overreached, overpromised, overdiagnosed, overmedicated, and compromised its principles.

In 2013 the NIMH's then-director, Thomas Insel, called the field out in the starkest of terms. Thirty years after the biological psychiatrists declared victory, he noted, *all* of psychiatry's diagnostic categories were still based, not on any biological markers of disease, but merely "on a consensus about clusters of clinical symptoms." In the rest of medicine, he said scathingly, this would be "equivalent to creating diagnostic systems based on the nature of chest pain or the quality of fever."[10] Put another way, there seemed to be little if any sound biology undergirding the psychiatric enterprise.

Also in 2013, Insel's colleague, Steven Hyman—another former NIMH director—sounded the alarm about the abandonment of the field by the pharmaceutical industry. In spite of all the 1980s declarations of revolutionary science driving change, Hyman noted, psychiatry had actually had no good new ideas about molecular targets for diagnoses and treatments *since the 1950s*. As a consequence, "the underlying science remains immature and . . . therapeutic development in psychiatry is simply too difficult and too risky."[11]

It is clear that we need a new story. This book is an effort to offer one, to take a deep dive into our long effort to understand the biological basis of mental illness and above all why it has been so troubled. Except for Chapter 1, my geographical focus is primarily American, because I believe the current confusion, frustrated hopes, and anger over the state of biological psychiatry in this country cry out most urgently for historical perspective and illumination.

I have organized the story into three parts. Part I offers a synthetic narrative of the century-long persistent—if also repeatedly frustrated— effort on the part of especially American psychiatry to define a biological mission for itself. The story is not particularly comfortable. A thread of institutionalized racism and gender bias runs through large parts of it. Late nineteenth-century figures who are celebrated today as forerunners of the "biological revolution" turn out to have had an understanding of biology that was highly stigmatizing. For a long time, they saw patients under their care as more valuable after they were dead (when their brains could be examined) than while they lived. Moreover, their project came to an end not because it fell victim to the siren call of psychoanalysis but because it failed, by common consensus, to deliver any unambiguous or lasting insights. In the United States, biological psychiatry then underwent a distinctly pragmatic turn, pursuing an array of hard-nosed projects, from shock to sterilization to surgery. For four or more decades, biological and nonbiological approaches coexisted in American psychiatry, somewhat uneasily but largely peaceably, a detente that was partly enabled by the leadership of the today-almost-forgotten "psychobiologist" Adolf Meyer.

Only when a new generation of Freudian psychiatrists stepped into positions of leadership after World War II did tensions grow. These so-called Freudians (many of whom had actually strayed quite far from classical teachings) did indeed seem to be calling the shots—and in these years, they seemed like the real revolutionaries, people who had the future in their bones. They were often patronizing toward their biological colleagues, portraying them as behind the times and sequestered in decaying mental hospitals. At the same time, they boldly reframed psychiatry, not just as one medical specialty among many but as a means of meeting the social challenges of the postwar world. In doing so, they increasingly claimed to hold the keys to understanding so much human behavior that in the end they exempted virtually nothing and no one from their clinical gaze.

In a development filled with irony, however, the years of Freudian dominance also witnessed virtually all the scientific and treatment developments to which the biological psychiatrists would later point as evidence that they should be in charge. All the major categories of drugs still used today in psychiatry were discovered then—to be sure, largely through serendipity and opportunism. There was important early research on the functioning of neurotransmitters as chemical messengers within the brain. There was influential genetic research. All this happened, yet the Freudians stayed in power. On fundamental issues, no minds were changed that did not want to be changed.

What finally catalyzed change was not some new piece of decisive science but a sense of professional crisis. By the 1970s, a range of rebels and critics had emerged who, in different ways, had grievances with the Freudian old guard. They accused the Freudians of collusion with immoral political causes, of racism and sexism, of blaming and abandoning families, and of bringing the field as a whole to the brink of professional suicide through grandiosity and systematic lack of rigor. The situation was so bad, clinicians pointed out, that large segments of the public were no longer even sure that mental illness existed!

Members of the biological faction sensed an opportunity to present themselves as a party of rigor, common sense, and compassion. They pointed to psychiatry's past commitments to biology. *Of course* mental illnesses were real. *Of course* biology mattered! Nevertheless, their call to "biologize" was not bound to any particular biological finding—it was rather justified by a basket of potential or candidate findings, any element of which was subject to change. This was because what they were really fighting for was less any specific explanation of mental illness than the *idea that mental disorders were medical disorders*. By the late 1970s, an initially quite marginal project to reform American psychiatry's diagnostic manual became a device for regime change.

Part I of this book ends there, but it leaves unanswered the question of how a reform in diagnostic practices alone could have served as the basis for a *biological* revolution. What were these candidate findings held up by the biological psychiatrists to support their new claims to authority and how did they come to be? How persuasive were they? Where did they come from? There must have been more to it, and there was. Part II therefore offers a second pass through psychiatry's struggle to discover a biological basis of mental illness, seen this time through the lens of three specific diseases: schizophrenia, depression, and bipolar disorder (manic-depression). Each story is quite distinct. The science in play was different for each, and different events catalyzed the drive both to biologize and to squelch rival perspectives. Drugs were important in different ways. Families and the public mattered in different ways. Patients had different kinds of experiences. In other words, one argument of this book is that the history of psychiatry's efforts to understand mental illness biologically is a pluralistic one. It cannot be told in a simple, linear way.

Part III brings the story home by exploring how the optimistic biological psychiatry of the 1980s began to unravel in the 1990s and especially in the new millennium. I argue that this happened, not just because the gap between hype and the state of scientific understanding was too great to bridge (though it was), but also because of a critical error that the original revolutionaries had made. Instead of reflecting on the extent to which the Freudians had lost credibility by insisting that they could be experts on everything, the new generation of biological revolutionaries repeated their mistake: they declared themselves the *new* experts on everything. No one suggested that it might be prudent to decide which forms of mental suffering were best served by a medical model, and which might be better served in some other way. Revolutionaries don't cede ground.

Like the Freudians they replaced, the new revolutionaries eventually paid a price for their ambition and arrogance. To tell that story, I look first at the ways psychiatrists leveraged their new biological identity to push back against psychologists and social workers seeking professional privileges like prescribing rights. Because they were medically trained, the argument went, only psychiatrists possessed the requisite knowledge to safely give patients drugs. (Ironically, under the Freudian regime, psychiatrists had insisted that only they possessed the requisite medical knowledge to safely offer patients *psychoanalysis*.) I then look at the ways many psychiatrists, having tethered so much of their identity to drugs and prescribing rights, sold their services to drug companies. I track how the drug companies themselves, from the 1990s on, responded to the lack of new scientific ideas about drug development by brilliantly marketing old drugs for new purposes. From there, I look at the rise of an increasingly multivoiced chorus of public critics of the new biological psychiatry, and how it swelled into a force no less virulent than the one that helped undermine the Freudian leadership in the 1970s. Finally, I look at the emergence of a sense of internal crisis in psychiatry, as drug companies began to abandon the field, as the diagnostic manual in which the field had invested so much fell into disrepute, and as key thought leaders spoke out publicly about the malaise in which the field found itself.

I have written this book because I believe history matters. We perhaps don't need history to see that psychiatry today is not a stable enterprise marked by a consensus about mission, but rather a fraught one, where rhetoric still far outstrips substance, where trust is fragile, and where the path forward is unclear. But we do need history to understand how we came to be where we are now and therefore what might need to happen next. Heroic origin stories and polemical counterstories may give us momentary emotional satisfaction by inviting us to despise cartoonish renderings of our perceived rivals and enemies. The price we all pay, though, is tunnel vision, mutual recrimination, and stalemate. For the sake not just of the science but of all the suffering people whom the science should be serving, it is time for us all to learn and to tell better, more honest stories.

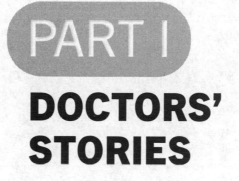

PART I

DOCTORS' STORIES

CHAPTER 1

Betting on Anatomy

MOST PSYCHIATRISTS WHO CAME OF AGE IN THE 1980s OR LATER "know" that the nineteenth-century German psychiatrist Emil Kraepelin —arm in arm with colleagues like Wilhelm Griesinger, Theodor Meynert, and Karl Westphal—laid the foundations upon which modern American biological psychiatry was later built. Many today think this because the textbooks they read during their training told them so. One of the most articulate early advocates of this historical claim, however, was the psychiatrist Nancy Andreasen, who developed it in her 1984 book, *The Broken Brain*. "The modern biologically oriented psychiatrist is truly the descendent of Emil Kraepelin," she told her readers. After all, Kraepelin's "Department of Psychiatry in Munich was composed of clinicians, neuroanatomists, and neuropathologists."[1]

Since then it has become commonplace to say, not only that modern American biological psychiatrists owe a great debt to their nineteenth-century German scientific brethren, but also that the importance of their work became clear only recently, because Americans were so long in the thrall of the Freudians. Thus in his 2009 *Encyclopedia of Schizophrenia*, the historian and clinical psychologist Richard Noll lamented "the tragic years of psychoanalysis" before declaring that "it took major advances in medical

technology, specifically the computer revolution and the rise of new techniques in neuroimaging, genetics research, and psychopharmacology to
swing the pendulum back to Kraepelin's search for the biological causes
of the psychotic disorders." A widely used 2010 textbook on biological
psychiatry similarly opened by paying homage to the accomplishments of
nineteenth-century biological workers like Kraepelin, then lamented the
"eclipse of progress" caused by the rise of "psychological theorizing" with
its "disastrous effects" on scientific progress. "It was not until the second
half of the 20th century," the authors concluded, "that biological approaches
to psychiatry flowered again . . . plac[ing] psychiatry once again securely as
a medical discipline."[2]

The late nineteenth century was indeed a time of intense research on
and theorizing about the biological basis of mental disorders. Some of the
clinicians involved in that work recorded observations and had insights that
may of course still be of interest.[3] But these men were also most emphatically not us. Their way of thinking biologically was not the same as ours.
They were preoccupied with the brain's solid tissue—with anatomy. They
had no understanding of the biochemical approaches that so animate our
agendas. Their understanding of heredity was marked by dark concerns
about racial decline. They were fatalistic about the possibility of recovery
from mental illness. They did not see the search for treatment as a priority. They freely dissected their patients' brains and generally did not worry
about obtaining consent. All in all, we would find much of what they did
and believed quite alien, and in some cases even repugnant.

Nevertheless, we do need to understand the late nineteenth-century
effort to find the biological basis of mental disorder—not just to understand
all the ways in which the men who pursued it were not early versions of ourselves, but also because it failed. The much-vaunted Kraepelin himself was
clear about this fact, and we need to become clear about it too, because it
mattered for what happened next. The men who pursued this project "bet"
on anatomy and lost. For decades, their failure cast a long shadow over
American psychiatry. On the one side, some clinicians, including a number of neurologists, responded by turning to nonbiological understandings of mental disorders, including psychoanalytic ones. On the other side,
the remaining biological wing of psychiatry was left in a state of disarray

and increasingly pursued a hodgepodge of theories and projects, many of which, in hindsight, look both ill-considered and incautious.

DEGENERATION

Nineteenth-century psychiatry's original hopeful embrace of biological research was catalyzed by an earlier failure: that of a newly invented institution called the lunatic asylum. Originally, the lunatic asylum's mission was simply to offer the mentally ill a reasonably humane form of incarceration, an alternative to the horrors of the old madhouses, jails, and poor houses. Increasingly, however, the view took hold that there was something distinctly therapeutic about spending time in one of these places: that institutionalization was itself a form of treatment. The architecture, the grounds, the ward system, the system of rewards and punishments, the daily rhythm of work and recreation, the firm but fair way in which the staff managed the patients—all contributed, it was said, to the recovery of sanity.[4]

In 1856 the British asylum director John Conolly gave a rosy picture of the therapeutic asylum in action: "A man of rank comes in, ragged and dirty, and unshaven and with the pallor of a dungeon upon him; wild in aspect, and as if crazed beyond recovery. He has passed months in a lonely apartment, looking out on a dead wall; generally fastened in a chair." Once in the hospital, the kindly staff ensured that his situation changed. "Liberty to walk at all hours of the cheerful day in gardens or fields, and care and attention, metamorphose him into the well dressed and well-bred gentleman he used to be."[5] Humane treatment toward the mentally ill turned out to be not just the right thing to do on moral grounds. It also turned out to be good medicine.

Buoyed by a sense of optimism and humanitarian conviction, men such as Conolly assumed professional titles (superintendent, director, medical officer), set up their own societies, founded journals, and honed narratives of triumph. They were buoyed along by the passage of laws across western Europe and the United States that mandated the construction of new public asylums and guaranteed the right of access to all who needed them. And as they carried out their mission, they were confident they were on the right side of history.

Until they weren't. By the 1870s or so, we hear less and less talk about how therapeutic it was to spend time in a lunatic asylum. The system did not seem to be working. The often-harsh reality of institutional life too often seemed to lag behind the ideal. There were always too many patients. There never seemed to be enough money or trained staff. Newspapers continually published reports of scandals, corruption, unexplained deaths, and the occasional dramatic murder. And perhaps most discouraging of all, patients did not seem to be getting well.

On the contrary, even though asylums now dotted the landscape in both Europe and the United States, insanity seemed to be on the rise. Institutions built to house five hundred patients now accommodated as many as fifteen hundred. "The increase in the number of the insane has been exceptionally rapid in the last decade," the *Boston Medical and Surgical Journal* observed uneasily in 1885. Five years later a prominent American asylum superintendent, Dr. Pliny Earle, agreed: "All the known data ... very clearly lead to the inference that insanity in the United States is increasing, not merely absolutely in correspondence with the increase of population, but relatively as compared with the number of inhabitants." And three years after that, the Irish mental health administrator William Joseph Corbet summed up the consensus: "Account for it how we may, as time progresses, the stream of insanity broadens and deepens continually. The great central fact stares us in the face, it cannot be hidden, no effort of obscurantism can conceal it."[6]

Why was this happening? Even today there is no consensus. Some historians have suggested that the asylum created its own expanding clientele: once these institutions existed, people perceived them as a go-to solution for forms of behavior that might previously have been hidden away or handled in some other way.[7] Other scholars have offered an epidemiological explanation. We know, for example, that the late nineteenth century saw a sharp increase in cases of syphilis, and that syphilis in its late stages can result in general paralysis of the insane (GPI), a condition in which motor syndromes are accompanied by manic-like symptoms, grandiose fantasies, and dementia. Research into the clinical records of various asylums in Europe and the United States shows that the number of patients in the asylum system diagnosed with GPI increased significantly in the late nineteenth century: in some institutions, they made up 10 to 20 percent of the total intake.[8]

Back then, however, a different understanding took hold, based on the simple claim that some people were biologically unsuited to handle the pressures of modern life. The challenges of life in an advancing, fast-paced society did not spur them onward and upward but instead unmasked their inadequacies, addled their nervous systems, and in some cases literally derailed their minds. To make matters worse, many of these defective people then passed their tainted biology on to their offspring, putting each generation at greater risk of mental disorder than the one before. As the British asylum doctor Henry Maudsley gloomily put it in 1867, "an increase of insanity is a penalty which an increase of our present civilization necessarily pays."[9] The term usually used to describe this way of thinking was degeneration.[10] On one level, degeneration was a way of grappling with the unsettling implications of a biological theory of human origins that we still know well today, but tend to think about differently than did many people in the past: evolution. There were a number of theories of evolution—not just Darwin's—competing for the allegiance of late nineteenth-century European scientists and intellectuals. And in ways that we largely no longer accept, virtually all of these theories taught that the overall thrust of evolution was a progressive one, in which life ascended from more primitive forms to more complex ones.

That claim then was often tempered by another one: that the gains of evolution were unstable; they could be reversed. As one early Darwinian put the matter in these years: "If it was possible to evolve, it was also possible to devolve . . . complex organisms could devolve into simpler forms or animals."[11] This included human beings. Could this alleged fact explain the upsurge everyone was seeing in mental derangement? Some thought so, and often thought so in a way that embedded this conclusion within a much more comprehensive and also extremely pessimistic diagnosis of retrograde forces in society generally. For some time, social commentators had been struck by the fact that, even as European and American societies were plainly making so many strides forward, they were also apparently being held back by rising rates of violent crime, suicide, intractable poverty, drunkenness, sexual "vice," and—not least—mental illness, or "lunacy." Degeneration could explain all this. Because all forms of mental illness and derangement supposedly sprang from common biological roots, the same degenerative processes might produce a madman in one family line, a criminal in another, and a prostitute, a hysteric, an epileptic, a political anarchist, or a crazy artist in yet another. Badness was not a thing apart from madness but rather a kind of madness of its own. This explains why, in an 1899 lecture, Emil Kraepelin—a degenerationist like most of his contemporaries—could blame inherited forms of mental derangement for "sexual crimes and arson" as well as "dangerous assaults, thefts, and impostures."[12]

It also explains why, during the 1882 trial of President James A. Garfield's assassin, Charles Guiteau, an American neurologist, Edward Charles Spitzka, insisted that Guiteau was no more responsible for his crime than a madman was responsible for his delusions. Guiteau was a moral monster, but it wasn't his fault—he had been born with a "congenital malformation of the brain." By way of evidence, Spitzka pointed to physical signs of Guiteau's inborn depravity: his asymmetrical facial features, his lopsided smile, and the fact that, when he stuck out his tongue, it deviated to the left.[13]

The idea that signs of certain kinds of degeneracy might be etched into people's faces had been argued especially by the Italian criminologist Cesare Lombroso. Beware, Lombroso had warned, of those among you with protruding ears, large jaws, inward-sloping foreheads, asymmetrical faces, a fondness for tattooing, and a propensity to be left-handed. The brains of such people, he explained, often showed structural anomalies otherwise seen only in apes and "savages" (by which he meant people from non-European parts of the world, like Africa).[14] Such people were likely to commit savage crimes because they had been born savage. In the end, Spitzka's defense was not enough to save Guiteau from the gallows, but his views on Guiteau's strange brain continued to intrigue all the same—so much that it was acquired for the purposes of study by the Mütter Museum in Philadelphia. Parts of it are still on display today.[15]

ANATOMICAL AMBITIONS

The rise of degeneration theory left the purpose of the mental asylum in a state of limbo. If it was no longer a therapeutic institution—because its directors and superintendents no longer believed that most mental illness was curable—then was it good for anything beyond acting as a warehouse for the rising numbers of incurably ill?

Yes, came one answer. The whole field of asylum medicine could find a new lease on life by reorienting itself away from treatment and toward research. All the incurably ill patients currently living in asylum were ripe for study. Their diseased brains were crying out for investigation.

The people talking this way, however, were not the asylum directors and superintendents but a group of medical specialists who called themselves neurologists. Neurologists were the new kids on the block—they had come of age only in the 1850s. Many had originally trained in anatomy, physiology, or internal medicine but then focused on disorders caused by damage or disease to the brain and nervous system—paralyses, palsies, and epilepsy. Because most people with such disorders were beyond any hope of real cure, neurologists also, from the beginning, emphasized the pure scientific interest of their work.

And they quickly chalked up some significant scientific successes. By the mid-1860s, they had "localized" the seat of articulate speech in the brain's frontal lobes, by observing that certain speech-impaired people, when examined after death, consistently showed a pattern of localized damage in a particular area of their frontal lobes.[16] This work led to an explosion of further investigations into the relationship between specific forms of brain damage and specific kinds of mental defects. By the end of the 1870s, this so-called "brain localization" project was in full swing. Generations of medical students learned to observe and test patients for evidence of different kinds of breakdown, all while waiting for them to die so the clinical findings could be correlated with autopsy findings.[17]

As neurologists basked in their apparent successes, some began to look at the lunatic asylums, filled with patients who were suffering from incurable disorders but whom no one was studying anatomically. They asked why not?, then why not us? After all, "in every case of mental disease," one must "recognize a morbid action of" the brain, as the German neurologist Wilhelm Griesinger announced on the first page of his acclaimed textbook.[18] Given this, it followed that the current generation of asylum directors must be completely unsuited to look after the mentally ill because they knew nothing about the brain.[19]

In 1878 the New York neurologist Edward Spitzka (who would later testify on behalf of the assassin Guiteau) encouraged a group of his American colleagues to reflect on the absurdity of their situation. As neurologists, they were deprived of access to all the interesting case materials held in the asylums. At the same time, the asylum superintendents—the men who were keeping them out—had no interest in their "scientific duty" and instead were mostly concerned "over the prizes gained by their hogs and strawberries from the asylum farms at agricultural fairs."

> Judging by the average asylum reports, we are inclined to believe that certain superintendents are experts in gardening and farming ... in roofing ... drain-pipe laying ..., engineering ... in short, experts at everything except the diagnosis, pathology and treatment of insanity.[20]

John Gray, superintendent of the prestigious Utica State Hospital in upstate New York, led the counterattack. To the American neurologists, Gray embodied the arrogance and fat-cat complacency (he actually weighed some three hundred pounds) of the moribund profession they were trying to oust, but Gray gave as good as he got. As editor of the *American Journal of Insanity*, he made full use of his visible public platform to attack. "Criminal!," "atheist!," "moral monster!" were only some of the accusations he slung back at the neurologists. "Shallow pretenders!" "Ignorant indifferentists!" were some of the answering insults.[21]

Upping the ante, the New York neurologists reached out to various reform-minded laypeople and told them that the asylum superintendents' incompetence actually posed a danger to patients' health and well-being. Finally in 1880, a New York State Senate investigative committee agreed to hold hearings. The neurologists testified to the flagrant incompetence of their rivals, while the asylum superintendents defended their record. In the end, nothing was done. The asylum superintendents all stayed in power. The outraged neurologists accused them of cronyism. The asylum superintendents promptly created a rule denying any neurologist admission to their professional society.

In Europe, especially in the German-speaking countries, it was a different story. There we see new journals being established to advance the new biologically oriented approach. We see the creation of new kinds of psychiatric research clinics, where interesting patients could be studied, prior to being sent off to a rural asylum for long-term care. The understanding was that, when the time came, the brains of these same patients would be shipped back to the clinic for additional study. We also see research-minded anatomists becoming directors of large psychiatric hospitals, which they outfitted with autopsy theaters and dissection laboratories. We see the establishment of collections of human brains for research and teaching purposes—so-called brain banks.[22]

True, these changes did not come without some resistance and push-back. In 1869 the Austrian neurologist Theodor Meynert complained—much as the American neurologists would do—about asylum superintendents who cared more about the interiors of their buildings than the "inner structure of the brain."[23] For his part, Ludwig Schlager—director of the Imperial Asylum in Vienna—accused anatomists like Meynert of caring only about brain tissue and not about the needs of the mentally ill. "The well-being of the insane would truly be in a sorrowful condition," he said, "if reform . . . were dependent upon the slow and painful progress made in the fields of neuroanatomy and research of the brain's structure and function."[24] Nevertheless Schlager, despite his concerted efforts, was unable to block Meynert's advancement to a full professorship with his own institute. The future of German-speaking psychiatry seemed increasingly clear: the brain now came first.

So widely was this understood that in Switzerland, a series of prominent German anatomists were appointed to the directorship of a large psychiatric hospital outside Zurich (the Burghölzli), even though none of them understood a word their patients said because none of them spoke the local Swiss dialect.[25] The fact that this was not seen as an impediment to their ability to carry out their duties is hugely telling. In other institutions, where anatomists sometimes did interact with patients, the conversations tended to be highly directive and designed to advance teaching and research goals. As the historian Katja Guenther has shown, some patients responded by being chatty, some flattered the doctor, some got angry with the students and assistants taking notes, and some were subtly mocking. One patient, asked "Are you being treated well?" slyly replied, "I cannot answer this, I am keeping the result to myself."[26]

DATA FROM CORPSES

The resolutely brain-oriented focus of these neuroanatomists may, to be sure, strike us today as rather coldhearted. Indeed, in his 1971 biographical novel of Sigmund Freud, Irving Stone imagined critics of Theodor Meynert attacking him for his single-minded focus on anatomical research. "To Meynert," Stone imagined the critics saying, "the only good lunatic is a dead lunatic. He can't wait until they die to get their brains for dissection."[27]

It is unclear, however, how widespread such feelings actually were in the late nineteenth century. Many saw honor and even a kind of romance in the figure of the brain researcher awaiting patiently the demise of his scientifically intriguing patients. Sigmund Freud, in his 1893 obituary of the great French neurologist Jean-Martin Charcot, explained how Charcot had long employed a servant who suffered from a tremor disorder, even though "in the course of the years she cost him a small fortune in dishes and plates." Charcot had done it, Freud explained, because the tremor interested him, and he wanted, after her death, to be able to study its anatomical basis. And he got his wish. "When at last she died," Freud wrote admiringly, "he was able to demonstrate from her case that *paralysie choréiforme* was the clinical expression of multiple cerebro-spinal sclerosis."[28]

Far from seeing themselves as callous, these clinicians actually envisioned their work as fundamentally humane and progressive. Transforming hospitals into research centers was part and parcel of a larger modernizing strategy that left behind what they considered to be a previous reliance on harsh, antiquarian practices: physically restraining unruly patients, putting them in special seclusion rooms, and so on. After all, as Wilhelm Griesinger had put it in the 1860s, these patients might be beyond hope of cure, but they were not "living machines" and had the right to live in dignity, within their means.[29]

Indeed, in the years following the rise of brain psychiatry, at least some patients seem to have experienced less "management" and more personal freedom than before. The neuroanatomist and asylum director Bernhard von Gudden, for example, was committed to a policy of "no restraint" in the hospitals he supervised over the years (in Werneck, Zurich, and Munich), and he regularly allowed his patients to travel into town without an escort, a practice that led to occasional run-ins with the local police.[30] This permissive approach may or may not have improved the patients' quality of life; a colleague of Gudden, Auguste-Henri Forel, later wrote, "I learnt enormously while with Gudden, but above all how not to direct asylum, for his tendency to let [allow] everything resulted in indescribable disorder."[31] Moreover, Gudden's laissez-faire approach to patient management may ultimately have led to his own demise. In 1886 he and one of his most important private patients, the "mad king" Ludwig II of Bavaria, took an evening stroll together to a lake, with no attendants present. A few hours later the corpses of both men were recovered from the water. To this day, it remains unclear what happened that evening.[32]

That said, at least some patients may have felt somewhat unnerved living in a modernized research hospital outfitted with autopsy theaters, dissecting chambers, and brain banks. In his 1903 memoir of his treatment in a psychiatric hospital in Leipzig, the brilliant but severely psychotic Daniel Paul Schreber comments, "God does not really understand the living human being and has no need to understand him, because ... he deals only with corpses."[33] This rather strange comment makes considerably more sense when one realizes that the hospital where Schreber was confined was run by the brain psychiatrist Paul Flechsig, who was passionately committed to "collecting data from corpses" in order to advance knowledge of mental illness.[34] Schreber also believed that Flechsig—to whom he attributed godlike powers—had invaded his "nerves" in order to "murder" his "soul." And in fact, Flechsig had repeatedly insisted that modern brain science had shown that the "soul" was nothing more than a system of "nerves."[35]

All of this research unfolded, moreover, in a time that lacked any notion of informed consent along the lines that we largely take for granted today. This was true especially for charity patients, living at the state's expense. Well into the twentieth century, in fact, the directors of state-funded prisons, workhouses, and lunatic asylums legally owned the bodies of any people who died on their premises. They had the right to dissect those bodies themselves, and they also had the right to sell them to medical schools for teaching purposes. Dissection of the institutionalized poor could generally only be avoided if relatives filed a formal objection or claimed the body within forty-eight hours of death; however, relatives could only do this if they were informed of that death in a timely manner (and there was generally little incentive for doing this). We may find this quite chilling, but the medical heads of asylums and other institutions for pauper patients considered it simply fair. During life, these patients had all their needs attended to; it was only right that, upon their deaths, they give something back.[36]

"BRAIN MYTHOLOGY"

In the end, it all led to more or less nothing. Despite the long, tedious hours anatomists spent peering through microscopes at brain slices and searching for patterns of abnormality, no consistent anatomical markers for specific mental disorders were found.[37] But unwilling to admit defeat, they plowed on, their arguments becoming ever more hand-waving and speculative.[38] In the early twentieth century, the psychiatrist Karl Jaspers summed up the general consensus about all this effort. He called it "brain mythology."[39] As he explained, "These anatomical constructions . . . became quite fantastic. . . . Unrelated things were forcibly related, e.g., cortical cells were related to memory, nerve fibres to associations of ideas. Such somatic constructions have no real basis."[40]

Buried in criticisms like this was another one: that the brain anatomists had failed so miserably because they focused on the brain at the expense of the mind. As chance would have it, during the years when they had been hard at work in their dissecting chambers, the new field of experimental psychology had been coming of age. Led by the Leipzig psychologist Wilhelm Wundt and others, experimental psychology used methods of introspection—"observing" and reporting on the contents of a person's inner experience—to better understand the structure and working of consciousness.

The brain psychiatrists generally disregarded or took a scornful view of such work. As early as 1868, Theodor Meynert had smugly dismissed the effort by quoting the philosopher Hermann Lotze: "Our soul knows nothing . . . of our body . . . whose interior it neither sees nor understands without outside help."[41] Having once decided that efforts to study the mind were useless, he never seems to have budged. The philosopher Alois Höfler once buttonholed Meynert at a salon gathering and made the case for introspection as an indispensable method for studying the mind. As he recalled, the anatomist responded archly, "But I ask you then: isn't then this psychology [based on introspection] basically nothing other than a new kind of religious teaching?"[42]

One who saw things distinctly differently was the psychiatrist Emil Kraepelin—the very man who, in the 1980s, would be portrayed as the true founder of biological psychiatry and foil to that arch-mentalist Sigmund Freud. Kraepelin was indeed hostile to psychoanalysis, but emphatically not because he cared only about biology and was uninterested in the scientific study of the mind. Quite the contrary, his objection was to Freud's focus on sexuality and his unscientific investigating methods.[43]

Having worked under Wilhelm Wundt, he considered himself one of his students and lamented "the often astonishing ignorance" of so many of his biologically oriented colleagues in psychiatry when it came to "psychological things." Yes, he admitted, the highly speculative psychological thinking of the early nineteenth century had not had much to offer psychiatry. But the rise of experimental psychology had dramatically changed the situation:

> Over the course of the last decade, psychology has become a natural science like any other and therefore it has a legitimate right to expect that its achievements receive the same respect and recognition as other auxiliary disciplines that we use to construct our scientific house.[44]

Not only did Kraepelin believe that it was important to study the mind directly; he was also keenly aware of the abysmal failures of the anatomical research enterprise pursued by Theodor Meynert and others. The "results of postmortem examinations continue to leave us entirely in the lurch," he complained as early as 1886. The reasons, he felt, were obvious: the neuroanatomists were studying brains taken from the corpses of patients who had suffered from unknown diseases. None of them had been properly diagnosed, because most of his colleagues didn't believe that diagnostics in psychiatry was very important. All the different psychotic syndromes, many insisted, were just different manifestations of the same progressive brain disease, so why create distinctions that were ultimately artificial and arbitrary? One of the most influential advocates of the idea that there was only one psychosis (expressing itself in different ways) was Wilhelm Griesinger—perhaps ironically, an influential early champion of the project to root psychiatric research in neuroanatomical methods.[45]

Kraepelin, breaking with all that, believed that psychiatry, like every other branch of medicine, must identify specific diseases before it could do anything else. His colleagues needed to stop focusing on the brains of dead patients and start focusing on the symptoms of living ones. They needed to observe what the patients did and said and seemed to experience—not because the cause of disease lay in the patients' inner world, in the ways Freudians believed, but because that was how diseases got to be known. Clinical observation, Kraepelin said, needed to come before any kind of biological research.

To this end, Kraepelin undertook a series of rich descriptive studies of the varieties of mental illness; attempting, as objectively as possible, to describe the mental states of patients he saw on the wards:

> The patients . . . see mice, ants, the hound of hell, scythes, and axes. They hear cocks crowing, shooting, birds chirping, spirits knockings, bees humming, murmurings, screaming, scolding, voices from the cellar. . . . The voices say "filthy things," "all conceivable confused stuff, just fancy pictures"; they speak about what the patient does . . . They say: "That man must be beheaded, hanged," "Swine, wicked wretch, you will be done for." . . .
>
> [The patients'] surroundings appear changed to them; faces are double, dark; their own faces look black in the mirror; they see a blaze of light, white fumes, "opium-morphia-chloroform vapour." [People] look like "phantoms" . . . the physician is "only a sort of image" of the devil. The chairs are moving. . . . The patient hears a murmuring and a whispering, a roar, the crackling of hell.[46]

Vivid descriptions like these would become a model for generations of clinicians. The problem with them, though, Kraepelin finally and reluctantly concluded, was that it was impossible to clearly distinguish between categories of psychosis simply by comparing symptoms at any point in time.

"BIG DATA" PSYCHIATRY

And so he shifted gears. What was necessary, he decided, was a different approach, focused not just on description but on course and prognosis. How often did a patient's symptoms change over time, and in what way? How often did patients get better? How often did patients die as mentally ill as when they were first admitted? Modern medicine had shown that the only way to understand a true disease was to track it over time: document its course, its fluctuations, its changing symptoms, and finally its outcome. Psychiatry would now also need to learn this lesson.[47]

In 1891 Kraepelin had accepted a professorship in Heidelberg, where he was able to marshal sufficient resources to systematically track the disease courses of patients in asylums, not just in Heidelberg but across the Baden-Württemberg region. He sent the families of discharged patients forms to fill out, much like those used by nineteenth-century census-takers. What was more, he did it all on an unprecedented scale; it was truly a "big data" project for its time.[48]

And it led to a moment of elegant simplicity. There were only two major kinds of psychoses, Kraepelin concluded. The first, dementia praecox (which roughly corresponds to what we today call schizophrenia) was a chronic disorder marked by a range of defects of perception and reasoning, whose symptoms inevitably worsened over time (see Chapter 5). The second, manic-depression, was a disorder that mostly affected mood and was marked by periods of remission and sometimes full recovery (see Chapter 7). The biggest difference between manic-depression and dementia praecox, Kraepelin thought, was not that the one affected "cognition" and the other affected "mood." In the acute phase of both diseases, patients manifested states of agitated delirium that were sometimes virtually indistinguishable from each other. No, the most important difference between the two disorders lay in their different prognoses. Patients with dementia praecox were not going to get better—and they were going to get worse. Patients with manic-depression, in contrast, could look forward to their condition possibly stabilizing or even improving.[49]

No one had ever talked before in such a comprehensive, longitudinal way about diagnostics. By 1899, when this impassioned, workaholic psychiatrist laid out his most refined version of his theory, it was clear that the field was going to have to reckon with him. To be sure, he attracted many critics, but he also attracted a growing number of defenders. The distinctions he offered were too useful to dismiss. European and American psychiatry did not become "Kraepelinian" in any straightforward way, certainly not right away, but Kraepelin succeeded in shifting the conversation about what psychiatry needed in order to put itself on a sound medical basis.[50] And it did not involve a call for more research on the anatomical basis of mental disorder, on the brain, or on any physiological process at all.

ANATOMICAL FANTASIES

Meanwhile in France, another effort to pursue anatomical research on institutionalized mental patients would result in a huge blowup—with repercussions that would linger well into the twentieth century. The story here is well-known but no less powerful for all that. It features the Parisian neurologist Jean-Martin Charcot, who in the 1850s and '60s had made a reputation as a stunningly talented neurological researcher. Among other things, he had successfully elucidated the defining features of both multiple sclerosis and tabes dorsalis (a degeneration of sensory nerve function that, medicine would later realize, was caused by syphilis). A highly visual person, Charcot became famous for his capacity to look beyond individual cases to see the "essence" of a disease, by looking at multiple cases and overseeing dissections of multiple associated brains. First he sought to identify the common patterns of symptoms shown by all the patients; then after they died, he related that pattern to a common structural abnormality in their brains. This so-called "clinico-anatomic" method was designed to ensure that he would not be led astray by inevitable individual variations in disease presentation.[51]

In the 1860s, with his reputation at a peak, Charcot was appointed to an enormous municipal hospital in Paris, the Salpêtrière. Its 5,000 patients were divided into two sections: one comprised nearly 2,000 indigent elderly women, patients with incurable cancers, and the blind; the other consisted of more than 3,000 intellectually disabled, mentally ill, and epileptic patients. Assigned to help direct the latter section, Charcot decided to study hysteria, a disorder associated with emotional lability and mental "fits" but that also presented with physical symptoms like paralysis, loss of sensation, and convulsions. Because both epilepsy and hysteria were associated with convulsions, hospital administrators had recently decided to rehouse their hysterics and epileptics in the same wards.

But did the existence of convulsions in both disorders mean that epilepsy and hysteria had a common origin, or were they two distinct diseases with one common symptom? Charcot wanted to know, and having never failed before in his efforts to differentiate disorders, he did not expect to fail. He thus began observing, comparing, and dissecting brains, all with the goal of revealing the secrets of hysteria.

The project quickly ran into problems on one critical front. When he attempted to relate what he was finding in his clinical observations to data from the brain dissections, he was not successful. The postmortem microscopic observations of the brains of hysterical patients showed no consistent abnormalities. In fact, many did not look structurally abnormal at all.[52]

The great neurologist was not discouraged. Eventually better microscopes and new techniques, he decided, would reveal the defects that surely lay hidden in the brains of the hysterical patients. Meanwhile investigations into patients' family histories were strongly suggesting that hysteria was a product of inherited degenerate biology. At the same time, patterns in patients' presenting symptoms were coming into focus. Order was emerging out of chaos. For example, Charcot identified two kinds of hysterical symptoms: (1) permanent physical defects (hemiparalysis, tunnel vision, partial loss of sensation), which (in a deliberate anticlerical jab) he called "stigmata," and (2) periodic fits (convulsive crises) that came on sometimes spontaneously, and sometimes when a patient was startled, emotionally distressed, or frightened. The crises also followed a clear sequence of distinct stages. Neurology might not yet know the specific brain areas involved, he said, but at least the field was beginning to figure out the laws and logic of the disease.

To allow for more precise study of all these findings, Charcot assigned his assistant Paul Richer to the task of sketching pictures of patients in various conditions and stages.[53] This work was helpful as far as it went, but Charcot worried about the ability of a line drawing to capture all the subtle aspects of the disease. He therefore turned to the new technology of photography to do the same work of visual recording but more precisely. Charcot's photography director, Albert Londe, bragged at the time that the photographic plate was "the true retina of the scientist."[54] People could see wrongly or misunderstand what they were seeing, but the camera simply recorded what was there. It therefore provided the objective evidence Charcot needed to prove that hysteria followed consistent patterns that would in due course be related to consistent brain defects.

To further ensure precision and consistency, Charcot also employed another technology, one he had recently helped to rehabilitate: hypnosis. Charcot's understanding of hypnosis was quite different from our own. It had nothing to do with "suggestion" or anything mental at all. Rather, it was a technique for physically manipulating the nervous systems of susceptible (hysterical) patients. As such, it allowed researchers to create specific hysterical symptoms at will and then to maintain them as long as needed for investigatory purposes. In this way, Charcot believed, hypnosis transformed the study of hysteria from an observational science to an experimental one.[55]

Charcot explained his program on hysteria to his colleagues in the early 1880s, and as everyone knew, he had never been wrong about such things before. Interest grew. His public lectures, involving dramatic demonstrations, became the talk of the town. By the mid-1880s, he was known as "Napoleon of the neuroses," the man who had conquered hysteria. He seemed at the top of his game.

Things then began going wrong. A physician from the French city of Nancy, Hippolyte Bernheim, publicly insisted that he could use hypnosis to reproduce all of Charcot's allegedly objective symptoms of hysteria in his own patients, then, still using hypnosis, make them change or disappear. Charcot, Bernheim said, had not *discovered* anything about hysteria at all.

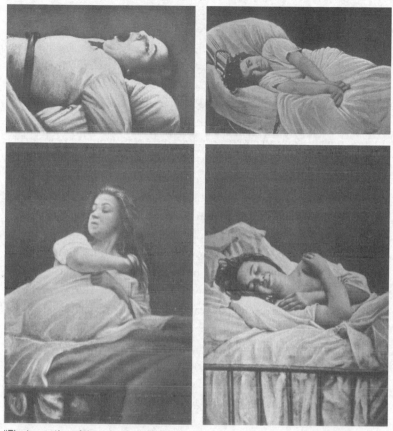

"The true retina of the scientist": Photographs of Charcot's hysterical patients taken for research purposes. Plates from Désiré-Magloire Bourneville et Paul Regnard, *Iconographie photographique de la Salpêtrière (service de M. Charcot)*, first edition (Paris: Publications du Progrès Médical, 1878). Images from the Osler Library of the History of Medicine, McGill University.

He had instead inadvertently created the symptoms he believed himself to have discovered; he had engaged in an elaborate theater of illusions that had nothing to do with the brain and nervous system and everything to do with patients' suggestibility (a concept Bernheim championed) and Charcot's charismatic influence over them.[56]

Charcot and his colleagues tried to brush off Bernheim's criticisms. In 1888 Charcot even mocked them in a public lecture: some people were claiming that the kind of hysteria he was showing them existed only in his own hospital, he said, "as if I have created this condition by my own will-power." It would indeed be "a marvel," he joked, if scientists could create their own objects of inquiry according to their "whims" and "fantasies." But the critics were chasing a whim of their own. "In fact," Charcot concluded, "all I am is a photographer. I describe what I see."[57]

By the spring of 1885, however, the tide was turning against him. Doubts about his approach were growing, and as fate would have it, during this period, Charcot welcomed a visitor from Vienna. A young neurologist (and former student of the neuroanatomist Meynert), Sigmund Freud, had received a small grant to spend several months in Paris that spring expressly to learn about hysteria from Charcot.

On many fronts, Freud was deeply impressed with Charcot, gushing in a letter to his fiancée Martha, "I sometimes come out of his lectures as from Notre Dame, with an entirely new idea about perfection."[58] But he also found himself intrigued by the new critique that hysteria was not an objective physiological disorder but rather a product of "suggestion." Hoping to make his own mark on the debate, he proposed to Charcot a study that would clarify the similarities and differences between organic and hysterical paralyses.

The outcome was a stunner. Freud's article, "Some Points for a Comparative Study of Organic and Hysterical Motor Paralyses," opened up an entirely new way of thinking about hysteria—one that went beyond both Bernheim's concept of "suggestion" and Charcot's attempt to understand hysteria in conventional neuroanatomical terms. Not published until 1893, it indicated that hysterical ailments were profoundly different from organic ailments caused by stroke or injury. A hysteric with a paralysis of the leg, for example, would drag the limb behind her, while someone with true organic paralysis would make a circumduction with her hip. This was significant because the hysteric's way of walking *didn't make any anatomical sense*—paralysis of the leg resulting from brain damage almost invariably spared the hip area. Patients, however, did not know that. Hysteria, Freud concluded, therefore consisted of symptoms that reflected a folk or popular understanding of anatomy and physiology. Or in his famous words, it "behaves as though anatomy does not exist or as though it had no knowledge of it."[59]

Freud was not alone in realizing this point. A rising young star in Charcot's own department, Pierre Janet, pointed out the same thing in his 1892 medical dissertation, a year prior to Freud's delayed publication:

> The hysteric person who paralyzes her hand seems not to know that the immobility of her fingers is due in reality to a muscular disturbance in her forearm. She stops her anesthesia at the wrist, as would the vulgar who, in their ignorance, say that if the hand does not move, it is because the hand is diseased. Now this popular conception of the limbs is formed by old ideas we have about our limbs, which we all keep in spite of our anatomic notions. So these hysteric anesthesias have something mental, intellectual, in them.[60]

Janet and Freud would later clash over who had first understood the psychological mechanisms underlying hysteria, but the key issue is that they both recognized, in their different ways, that the anatomical approach to hysteria was crumbling. By the end of the 1880s, Charcot himself had pretty much quietly abandoned it and instead begun to emphasize the role of emotional trauma and self-suggestion in the etiology of hysteria.[61] Janet then broadened the conversation—especially after Charcot's death in 1893—by saying that normally the symptoms of hysteria were not produced passively by shock and "suggestion." Outside the experimental setting of a hospital, they were actively created by toxic "fixed ideas" in a patient's mind that were "dissociated" from conscious awareness. These "fixed ideas" did not wholly disappear but expressed themselves in meaningful bodily symptoms. Symptoms were not just signs of brain defect; they could also act as a quasi-secret language which normally was used to confess the traumatic memories that the conscious mind was not willing to confront.

Janet at this point found a new use for hypnosis: to transform his patients' "fixed ideas" into sanitized (and fictionalized) "memories" they could live with. In his view, compassionately manipulating how patients remembered past traumatic events was justified if it allowed them to move forward with their lives in the present.

Working in Vienna and initially out of the limelight, Freud and his colleague Josef Breuer also began to believe that hysteria was the body's way of expressing "forgotten" (he would later say "repressed") memories. In contrast to Janet, however, they argued that the road to recovery lay not in changing traumatic memories, but in recalling, reexperiencing, and ultimately making peace with them.

Either way, both Freud and Janet were transforming investigations into hysteria into practices that had nothing to do with anatomy or the brain; practices that were more confessional than medical, more focused on biographical detective work than on conventional medical diagnostics. In his contribution to the 1895 book *Studies on Hysteria*, Freud reflected on how far his thinking had moved since his training as a neuropathologist:

> Like other neuropathologists, I was trained to employ local diagnoses and electro-prognosis, and it still strikes me as strange that the case histories I write should read like short stories and that, as one might say, they lack the serious stamp of science. I must console myself with the reflection that the nature of the subject is evidently responsible for this, rather than any preference of my own. The fact is that local diagnosis and electrical reactions lead nowhere in the study of hysteria, whereas a detailed description of mental processes such as we are accustomed to find in the works of imaginative writers enables me, with the use of a few psychological formulas, to obtain at least some kind of insight into the course of that affection. . . . [There is] . . . an intimate connection between the story of the patient's sufferings and the symptoms of his illness.[62]

By the late 1890s, Freud was making a far more specific and audacious claim: that in any specific case of hysteria, when the analyst traced back the symptoms to their biographical roots, he *always* found a specific memory of forced sexual activity in childhood with an adult, often a parent. He called this "sexual seduction." (We would today call it sexual abuse.)[63]

By 1897, however, Freud had changed his mind. He had been wrong, he now said, in believing that his patients' reports of sexual seduction were memories of things that had really happened. They were not, but they were also not lies. Instead, they were something else altogether: remembered fantasies of sexual encounters from childhood. As he later explained, little boys, by and large, didn't really have sex with their mothers, or little girls with their fathers, but they did begin, sometime around age six, to develop forbidden erotic feelings for their parent of the opposite sex. Because such feelings were taboo, most people buried them in their unconscious, where they usually remained for a lifetime. In cases of hysteria, however, something happened to stir memories of those childhood erotic fantasies: patients then believed they were remembering real events because, Freud explained, the unconscious mind could not distinguish between fantasy and true events.[64]

In 1914, with his followers increasing in number and dissent growing in the ranks, Freud sought to define the field he was creating—he called it psychoanalysis—by publishing a polemical "history of the psychoanalytic movement." Its aim, above all, was to identify himself as the sole founder of his system and to marginalize the doubters and skeptics. He also doubled down on his insistence that sexual fantasies always lay at the root of what were now increasingly called "neurotic" symptoms.[65]

In 1914 war broke out in Europe, with consequences that would ultimately cast doubt on the claim that all neuroses were caused by sexual fantasies, and in ways far more effective than any objections mustered by Freud's critics. The Great War, later called World War I, was unlike any that either soldiers or military planners had ever known.[66] It was the first war to make military use of airplanes and other flying machines; the first to use tanks, submarines, and chemical gas in battle; and the first to employ heavy artillery on the field. It was also the first war to send thousands of young soldiers for months at a time into trenches stretching across hundreds of miles, into which shells could land at any time. On the Western Front, extending from the North Sea to the Swiss frontier, the trenches became notorious for their regular massive bombardments by heavy artillery, for the rats that lived in them and gorged on corpses, and for the miles of barbed wire that soldiers had to cut through—often under fire—before the line could advance.

When military physicians examined some of the soldiers who had spent time in this hellish environment, they encountered a range of odd disabilities. Some soldiers had trouble seeing, hearing, smelling, tasting.

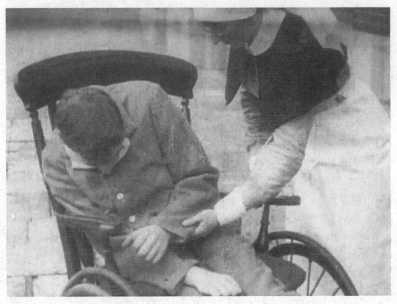

Still from the 1917 film *War Neurosis*, showing shell-shocked soldiers (in this case, one suffering from hysterical paralysis), recorded at Seale Hayne and the Victorian Netley Hospitals in England. Wellcome Collections, London.

Others had trouble walking or talking. Still others had developed strange twitches, paralyses, and convulsions. And still others suffered from memory loss or shook uncontrollably all day long.

What they all had in common was that none of them had been obviously injured in any way; nor did any of them suffer from any evident organic disease. The term *shell shock* was used to label these cases, originating in an early theory proposed by the English physician Charles Myers that all these soldiers' symptoms might have their source in shocks to the nervous system brought about by proximity to artillery explosions. But when soldiers who had never been close to artillery and had never even seen combat also began developing strange physical symptoms, it became clear that a different kind of explanation was needed.

One possible explanation was that what afflicted these men was precisely the same thing that afflicted malingerers everywhere: nothing. These men with their strange symptoms, some insisted, really suffered not from a medical condition at all but from a shameful cowardice. After the war, one high-ranking British officer—Lieutenant-Colonel Viscount John Gort—testified to the War Office that there was a clear difference between genuine "nervous breakdown" and "shell shock." Shell shock, he said,

> like measles, is so infectious that you cannot afford to run risks with it. . . . It must be looked upon as a form of disgrace to the soldier. A certain class of men are all right out of the line, but the minute they know they are to go back they start getting "shell shock." . . . Officers must be taught much more about man mastership in the same way as horse mastership. . . . It is all to a great extent a question of discipline and drill.[67]

In some camps, shaming, taunting, and inflicting pain were used to goad soldiers back to fighting fitness. In other instances, the ultimate deterrent was employed: court martial and death by firing squad.

Some military physicians who had seen these men, however, were not persuaded that the situation was so simple. Even if these unfortunate young men's symptoms had no physiological cause, they nevertheless did have a real cause—just one that was mental in origin. Most physicians were reluctant to use the word *hysteria*—still associated with women and weakness—but judging from the writings of the time, almost everyone realized that this is what they were facing, and in epidemic proportions. The roots of this male hysteria lay, though, not in taboo sexual fantasies but in taboo experiences of overwhelming fear, sometimes exacerbated by guilt and a sense of failure.

The war ended before the larger questions raised about the relationship between shell shock, hysteria, and theories of psychoanalysis could really be resolved. It also left behind a great mass of human suffering, caused by the inability of countless soldiers to make peace with the intolerable. In some ways, the war poets of this era understood their situation best:

> *These are men whose minds the Dead have ravished.*
> *Memory fingers in their hair of murders*
> *Multitudinous murders they once witnessed.*[68]

BUGS IN THE BRAIN

By the time the war had ended, the original European brain psychiatry program, focused on anatomical research, was barely hanging on, reduced to insisting desperately on its continued relevance.[69] As it struggled, though, something happened that unexpectedly put biology—if not anatomy—back on the map.

To understand how, we need to familiarize ourselves with a disorder first described by French asylum doctors a century earlier, known as general paralysis or paresis of the insane (GPI). This illness presented with a striking tangle of motor and mental symptoms. On the motor side, patients typically developed first an unsteady gait and problems with speech, then a progressive paralysis that eventually left them without any capacity for voluntary movement, including swallowing and bowel control. Symptoms on the mental side typically began with agitated behaviors that were grandiose, disinhibited, and socially inappropriate. Patients then became ever more disorganized in their thinking, finally succumbing to an all-encompassing dementia. The disorder always ended in physical collapse and death.

In the mid-nineteenth century, as asylums filled with such patients, many asylum doctors found themselves strangely fascinated. We can tell because the nineteenth-century medical literature is sprinkled with rich word pictures of their grandiose and grotesque antics. A typical one was offered by an English asylum doctor in 1859:

> He is full of all manner of schemes . . . and talks of the wealth he fancies his projects have brought him. . . . The whirl of the spirits increases. . . . Arrived at this pitch, everything becomes invested with immensity, grandeur, or beauty. Common pebbles are transformed into gems. . . . [Thereafter] incessantly talking and restless, violent and destructive, tearing everything tearable to shreds. . . . He lies on his bed . . . or on the padded floor of his room in a dream of happiness and splendour, which contrasts horribly with his hollow features and emaciated, squalid body. Happily death is at hand—exhaustion or paralytic coma soon closes the scene.[70]

In the eyes of many clinicians, a disease trajectory like this made GPI a classic exemplar of a degenerative condition. The fact that the case histories of so many of the patients pointed to a previous life of vice, drinking, and fast living in the big cities further reinforced this assumption. There was one problem with this way of conceiving GPI, though. Degenerative conditions were assumed to cluster within the badly bred and lower classes. GPI, however, struck the lowly and the great, the poor and the well-to-do alike. In 1890 George Savage—superintendent of Bethlehem Hospital from 1879 to 1889—admitted that it had even struck and killed some of his friends, a fact that shook him: "as years pass on, it seems to appeal to us more personally as one and another of our friends or patriots fall out of rank, victims to this malady."[71]

By the 1890s, more and more clinicians were also pointing out something else: that many of the middle-aged and older patients with GPI they saw had previously been treated for syphilis, or the "great pox" (contrasted with smallpox). This was a disorder that people had long known was transmitted through sexual contact, and that had been on the rise in recent decades—a development that was often blamed on the rise of prostitution in the big cities. The disease typically begins with fever, genital sores, and rash. Before effective treatments were developed, a latency period of weeks or months would lead to a second stage characterized by the spread of pocks on the face and body, often with accompanying severe joint and muscle pains. The pocks in turn often degenerated into open ulcers and lesions, some of which would eat into the bone. In some cases, people's noses basically collapsed—a symptom so common that it led to a market for artificial noses and stimulated new developments in plastic surgery.

There were long-standing treatments for syphilis, especially concoctions involving mercury. Patients took mercury in pill form, rubbed it as a cream into their skin, or even injected it into various bodily cavities like the nose or genitals. It did not cure quickly (if it cured at all) and produced chronic side effects of its own, but doctors prescribed it and patients used it because there was nothing better available and many believed that, if used regularly and diligently, it helped. "*A night with Venus, a lifetime with mercury*," as the saying at the time went.[72]

Maybe, though, many of the patients who believed that mercury had

helped clear up their symptoms were not cured after all. Given the frequency with which GPI patients had syphilis in their histories, some people asked a question that, at the time, seemed strange: Was it possible that
GPI was a previously unrecognized late-stage symptom of syphilis? How
would one find out? In 1897 a neurologist in Baden-Baden, Richard von
Krafft-Ebing, oversaw an experiment to test for a possible causal link.
Krafft-Ebing's assistant, Josef Adolf Hirschl, injected pus from the sores
of known syphilitics into the blood of nine GPI patients. The two men
knew that syphilis could be contracted only once, so if the men under their
care now developed the early symptoms (fever, rash, genital sores), that
meant they had never had syphilis before. If they failed to develop syphilis, it meant that they had been previously infected. Over the next several
months, none of them developed any symptoms, and so Krafft-Ebing and
Hirschl concluded that the patients must previously have been infected
with the disease.[73]

Even at the time, this little experiment was seen as ethically fraught
(many readers of this book probably feel some degree of outrage), but its
outcome was widely understood as a milestone in the effort to understand
GPI's causes. One problem, however, remained: How could an illness that
began with genital sores and fever later lead to mental disorder and paralysis? Ultimately, the most persuasive answer would come from the still-new
paradigm in medicine known as germ theory.

Germ theory, associated with Louis Pasteur in France and Robert
Koch in Germany, held that a whole range of deadly and poorly understood disorders—from cholera to tuberculosis and rabies—were caused
neither by bad heredity nor by bad smells or bad air (all common beliefs
at the time), but by the presence of dangerous microorganisms (bacteria)
in the human body. Biologists had been generally aware of the existence of
these microorganisms for centuries but not their relationship to disease.
Germ theory turned the study of bacteria into a medical matter. It insisted
that specific diseases were caused by specific bacteria. If one drank water
contaminated with the bacterium *Vibrio cholerae*, for example, one would
fall ill with cholera, but not with some other disease. All this is obvious
now, but it was far from obvious then.

In 1905 the German biologist Fritz Schaudinn brought syphilis into the general paradigm of germ theory. Using a microscope, he and his colleague Erich Hoffman examined pus from the sores of known syphilitics and saw that it teemed with a previously unknown, spiral-shaped bacterium later called *Treponema pallidum*. Eight years later the Japanese bacteriologist Hideyo Noguchi and his American colleague, J. W. Moore, discovered *Treponema pallidum* in the *brains* of a number of patients who had died following the classic course of GPI. The evidence was shocking: "The spirochaetae were found in all layers of the cortex with the exception of the outer, or neuroglia layer. . . . In all instances they seemed to have wandered into the nerve tissue."[74]

The conclusion seemed clear: GPI was a form of syphilis in which the bacteria colonized the brain. It was an *infectious* disease. For the first time, psychiatry had discovered a specific biological cause for a common mental illness. If it could be done once, some people began to say, maybe it could be done again.

CHAPTER 2

Biology in Disarray

NEUROLOGISTS DEFECT

The discovery that GPI was a form of neurosyphilis and had infectious origins was widely recognized as a scientific triumph. Nevertheless, it was not obviously extendable to all other disorders. And as Europe's classical neuroanatomical program slowly crumpled, the consensus regarding how best to move forward generally with a biological agenda in psychiatry broke down. In the United States, different groups struck out in a range of directions. And ironically enough, the group that had previously led the charge to biologize mental disorders ended up partially defecting from that quest altogether: the neurologists.

How could this be? American neurologists had once coveted nothing more than an anatomical research program like the one their European colleagues had won. They had fought tooth and nail for access to lunatic asylums, but having lost that battle—and because the American medical school system was too weak for most of them to find academic positions—many of them then settled into private practice as so-called "nerve doctors." And that shift in their professional focus changed the game for them.

Nerve doctoring in the late nineteenth century was a way for neurologists to trade on their neurological expertise, but in order to treat a very specific kind of patient. This patient typically suffered not from any recognized neurological disease or injury but from diffuse symptoms caused by what were delicately called "bad nerves." These symptoms might include headache, exhaustion, tremors, joint pain, upset stomach, insomnia, and waves of heat and cold. Paralyses, sensory disturbances and motor tics might also be present, but of the sort widely recognized by nerve doctors as hysterical in nature. When Sigmund Freud first hung out his shingle in Vienna, it was as a nerve doctor; that was how he came to be treating the hysterical patients who ultimately inspired him to invent psychoanalysis.[1] In the United States, by the 1870s, patients who visited nerve doctors were more likely to be diagnosed not with hysteria but with a disorder called neurasthenia. Invented by the neurologist George Beard, it was supposed to be marked by a state of (literal) "nervous exhaustion," a breakdown in the overall functioning of a person's "nerves."[2]

"Nervous" and "neurasthenic" patients visited nerve doctors both to be assured that they were not crazy (and so were not potential candidates for the lunatic asylum) and to be cured of their woes. Nerve doctors offered them both assurance and treatment. Gentle electrical stimulation— designed to rev up tired nerves—was standard; so were various regimes involving massage, sedatives, water, rest, and exercise.

The thing was, the symptoms of many of these patients were odd. They *looked* on the surface as if they had a neurological basis, but in practice they did not act the way they should if they were *really* neurological. They often fluctuated with the patient's changing emotional state. In particular, if a physician encouraged or scolded a patient, the symptoms sometimes disappeared (usually temporarily). Thus, as early as 1876, George Beard admitted to his colleagues at the newly founded American Neurological Association that mental factors—especially "expectation"—seemed to be involved in many of the cases he saw in his private practice. He had attempted to cure patients of "rheumatism, neuralgia, sleeplessness, and various forms of chronic disease," not by using the neurologists' standard somatic treatments, but simply by telling them that he expected them to get well on "a certain day or hour, or even a specific minute in some cases." Many patients duly experienced significant relief. Given this, Beard suggested to his colleagues, why not integrate "expectation"—a kind of talking cure—into their repertoire of therapies?[3]

Listening to Beard's talk, the neurologist William Hammond declared himself outraged: "If the doctrine advanced by Dr. Beard was to be accepted," he announced dramatically, he should feel like "throwing his diploma away and joining the theologians." He hoped, he concluded indignantly, that Beard's views on these matters "would not go to the public with the endorsement of the Society."[4]

Twenty-five years later, no one was expressing outrage anymore. The evidence for the importance of mental factors in so-called nervous disorders had become just too compelling. And the practical need to develop effective therapeutics for such nervous patients had become too great.

In the United States, at least two intervening developments had helped solidify that new consensus. During the last quarter of the nineteenth-century, train travel was increasingly common but still risky, and accidents were not rare. Passengers injured in such accidents often demanded compensation from the railroad companies for their debilitating symptoms: back pain, trembling, exhaustion, numb extremities, headache, anxiety, insomnia, and memory defects. So common was this package of complaints that it became the basis of a new syndrome known as "railway spine" or (sometimes) "railway brain."

Strangely, though, symptoms of railway spine often tended to emerge only after a significant delay. Even stranger, they often resolved after the victim had been awarded compensation. Did injured people actually suffer from real, if perhaps microscopic and impermanent, physical injuries, such as hemorrhage or compression? Were they con artists looking for a payout from the railroad companies? Or was railway spine yet another face of that great imitator of physical disease, hysteria? By the 1890s, the smart money was on the last interpretation.[5]

Even as the debate over railway spine continued apace, American neurologists scrambled to respond to another threat, this one from religion. The second half of the nineteenth century had seen the rise of a number of Christian "mind cure" movements: Christian Science (the most authoritarian and the best known today), Unity Science, Divine Science, and more. The basic premise animating all these movements was that believing something is so makes it so. People could be healed if they were able, truly and deeply, to believe that they would be healed.

Many of these movements' new churches went so far as to offer their members techniques for cultivating such belief: affirmation exercises, prayer, chanting, and visualization. And in 1900 the prominent Harvard psychologist William James bluntly told his colleagues that they could not afford to ignore the remarkable results: "The blind have been made to see, the halt to walk; lifelong invalids have had their health restored.... One hears of the 'Gospel of Relaxation,' of the 'Don't Worry Movement,' of people who repeat to themselves, 'Youth, health, vigor!'"[6]

The American medical profession took note. American neurologists took particular note since it was widely assumed that mind cures would be most effective in alleviating the symptoms of so-called "nervous disorders." The neurologists were therefore at particular risk of losing business to the "quacks." To reduce that risk, a consensus grew that they needed to become experts on the range of mental techniques—suggestion therapy, hypnosis, affirmation therapy, and more—that were increasingly being shown to influence the body. By the late nineteenth century, the general term used to refer to all these techniques was *psychotherapy*.[7] And for better or worse, these techniques were now of intense interest to the neurologists, because they were of intense interest to their patients. As the New York neurologist C. L. Dana summed up the situation: "The question is not whether we should use psychotherapeutics, hypnotism or suggestion; we as neurologists are confronted with the fact than an enormous number of mentally sick people are running around and getting their psychotherapeutics from the wrong well."[8]

By the turn of the century, and for the sake of their livelihoods, increasing numbers of American neurologists thus turned their attention from brain anatomical projects to focus instead on "psychotherapeutics," especially the new understandings of these practices coming out of France. They took note of Charcot's work in the 1880s and '90s, showing that hysteria could be triggered not only by degenerate physiology but also by emotional "trauma." (Charcot had himself been influenced by the railway spine debates.) They studied the work of Bernheim and others on the medical uses of "suggestion" and hypnosis. The French thinker they respected the most, however, was the psychologist Pierre Janet who, in a series of lectures at Harvard University in 1906 (published in English soon afterward), argued that hysteria was not an organic disorder at all but rather a splitting or doubling of consciousness.[9] It occurred when traumatized patients split off their memories of upsetting or frightening events and expressed them in the form of physical symptoms—sensory motor disturbances, visual problems, gastric problems, and more. Hypnosis provided a way to access and engage with those split-off parts of the hysterical mind and find out the true reasons for the patient's symptoms.[10]

This was the larger backdrop to an event that would later come to seem highly significant. In 1909 the American psychologist G. Stanley Hall invited the then little-known Viennese neurologist Sigmund Freud and his Swiss colleague, Carl Gustav Jung, to give a series of lectures about their approach to psychotherapy at Clark University in Worcester, Massachusetts.[11] After much hesitation, Freud accepted; it would be his first and only visit to the United States, a country that, according to at least one biographer, he later called a "gigantic mistake."[12]

It was a gratifying visit for Freud all the same, even if he might have wished for more sophisticated admirers with European sensibilities. In five lectures (delivered in German without notes), he laid out his theory of psychoanalysis. He began by explaining that "hysterical patients suffer from reminiscences. Their symptoms are the remnants and the memory symbols of certain (traumatic) experiences." He clarified how he saw the relationship between his ideas and those of Charcot and especially Janet. He then introduced the concept of the "unconscious" and defined it as a part of the mind that contained "repressed" traumatic memories. He described his talking method for making such memories conscious again, noting that it did not involve hypnosis. He talked about dreams as a "royal road" to the unconscious and ways to analyze them for their insights. Finally (aware that he would face skepticism), he discussed his most radical insight: that virtually all so-called neurotic disorders have roots in repressed sexual "impressions." He made clear that this was a discovery and not one that he particularly welcomed. And he further described the implications of his discovery for both psychotherapeutic work and general understandings of childhood development and human motivation.[13]

The Clark experience was indubitably good not just for Freud personally but also for the development of psychoanalysis in the United States. Freud solidified for himself several significant American converts: Smith Ely Jelliffe, William Alanson White, and especially James Jackson Putnam, who a few years later, in 1911, became the first president of the newly established American Psychoanalytic Association. All these men were originally trained as neurologists. Putnam had even trained in London with John Hughlings Jackson, one of Europe's most influential and theoretically sophisticated neurologists during the heyday of the neuroanatomical approach.[14]

Nerve doctoring, though, had fundamentally changed what it meant to be a neurologist. A bit like Freud himself, Freud's new American followers had come up against the practical limitations of conventional neurology. They needed new ideas.[15] Thus after the Clark meeting, arrangements were made for Freud's Clark lectures to be published in English (he had been persuaded by his hosts to write them down), along with others of his key works.[16] Freudian ideas began to circulate—and it was a small group of determined American neurologists, above all, who ensured that they did.[17]

In contrast, many of America's psychiatrists or alienists—still caring for the chronically ill in asylums—were originally among the most resistant to Freudian ideas. At their 1914 annual meeting, the alienist Charles Burr gave a scathing lecture, attacking psychoanalysis as a "filthy examination into the past sexual life" of patients. He declared Freud's dream theory as lacking in plausible acceptable evidence and noted that nothing generally observed in patients in hospitals supported his ideas.[18] Most of Burr's audience seems to have taken his side. The few exceptions stand out. One of them, William Alanson White, insisted that Burr had not fairly presented the ideas of psychoanalysis, and he called on his colleagues to give them a fair shake.

As superintendent of St. Elizabeths Hospital in Washington, D.C., White was also prepared to put his money where his mouth was: he would soon turn St. Elizabeths into an important early center for psychoanalytic psychotherapy—at least, for white patients. In this Jim Crow era, most African-American patients at St. Elizabeths (and there were many—25 percent of first admissions were African American) were excluded from participating, on the grounds that they were too impulsive, juvenile, and lacking in sufficient self-control to benefit. Many of the staff indeed seem to have regarded their black patients as (in the words of one staff member) "strangers within our gates." Denied psychoanalytic treatment, they instead became part of a larger project in "comparative psychiatry" at St. Elizabeths, in which their mental conditions were compared to and contrasted with those of white patients.[19]

MEYER CHAMPIONS "FACTS"

Another person who attended the 1909 Clark meeting where Freud and Jung spoke was the Swiss-American neurologist Adolf Meyer. Even before Freud's visit, Meyer had welcomed the potential of psychoanalysis to offer a corrective to tired biological materialism. "Freud has opened the eyes of the physician to an extension of human biology," he declared approvingly as early as 1906.[20] And in his own lecture at Clark, Meyer made a point of praising the fresh perspectives brought by Freud and Jung, especially their "ingenious interpretations" that allowed clinicians to make sense of "otherwise perplexing products of morbid fancy."[21] Nevertheless, Meyer had his own understanding of mental illness and was no fan of Freud's dogmatism (as he saw it) or his unhealthy preoccupation with sexuality (as he perceived it).

We need to care about Meyer's (ambivalent) views on psychoanalysis because, for more than thirty years, he was an almost overwhelmingly influential force in American psychiatry. As his colleague and sometime rival Elmer Southard conceded as early as 1919, "no greater power to change our minds about the problems of psychiatry has been at work in the interior of the psychiatric profession in America than the personality of Adolf Meyer." Southard could not then resist adding a barbed joke: "I don't know that we could abide two of him. But in our present status we must be glad there was one of him."[22]

To bring the story of Meyer into focus, we must go back to the start of the twentieth century, when American asylum superintendents—a generation after being savaged by neurologists for being more interested in their gardens than in medical research—finally decided it was time to take their medical identity seriously. In 1892 they changed the name of their professional organization from the Association of Medical Superintendents of American Institutions for the Insane, to the American Medico-Psychological Association. They stopped calling themselves "superintendents" and began to call themselves "alienists," to call attention to their medical expertise. (In 1921 they would rename their organization the American Psychiatric Association, and they would all become known as psychiatrists. The term *alienist* is still used occasionally to refer to an expert in forensic psychiatry).

Some of these men also decided that they were finally ready to embrace a research mission focused on the brain. To that end, one reformer, John Chapin, director of the Willard Insane Asylum in New York, reached out to a prominent neurologist for help. In 1894 the American Medico-Psychological Association was preparing to celebrate its fiftieth anniversary. In anticipation, Chapin asked the American neurologist Silas Weir Mitchell to be the keynote speaker. Mitchell accepted but warned his host that he likely would have some strong words to share—he was not going to offer simple pleasantries and congratulations. Chapin consulted with his colleagues and responded to Mitchell that this was no problem: they all wanted to hear what he had to say.

Things then unfolded more or less as Chapin must have expected. In his speech, Mitchell did not mince words: asylum medicine, he said, had isolated itself from the rest of medicine. It lacked a research mission and had failed miserably to advance understanding of mental illness. Why? Mitchell asked.

> What is the matter? You have immense opportunities, and, seriously, we ask you experts, what have you taught us of these 91,000 insane whom you see or treat? . . . Where are your annual reports of scientific study, of the psychology and pathology of your patients? . . . We commonly get as your contribution to science, odd little statements, reports of a case or two, a few useless pages of isolated post-mortem

records, and these sandwiched among incomprehensible statistics and farm balance sheets.[23]

It looked on the face of it like a scene from the 1870s, when neurologists flung insults at benighted and ignorant superintendents. But this was no attack by a neurologist seeking to humiliate and perhaps oust a group of rivals; it was an invited critique that had been actively masterminded by a reform-minded alienist.[24] A decade earlier Chapin had narrowly failed to persuade the city of Philadelphia to invest in what would have been the first German-style psychiatric research and training institute in America, complete with laboratories, an army of young researchers, and formal clinical teaching. Despite that failure, Chapin remained a restless advocate for reform.[25] He and other reform-minded alienists needed and wanted neurologists like Mitchell to shake things up.[26] It is telling that Chapin and others responded to Mitchell's harsh critique by promptly making him an honorary member of their association. It is equally telling that the alienists would continue to discuss Mitchell's speech for at least the next fifty years—often defensively, to be sure, but also with a tinge of pride. It became part of their lore, part of their coming-of-age story.[27]

And Mitchell's dinner speech seems to have had immediate practical ripple effects as well. In 1895, a year later, a hospital in New York established a German-style biological research center. The mission of the Pathological Institute of New York was to pursue "studies on abnormal mental life and their neural concomitants." For a brief period, Chapin's reformist vision seemed on the verge of being realized.

Then problems set in. The institute's first director, neuropathologist Ira Van Gieson, quarreled with the asylum doctors with whom he was meant to collaborate. An anatomist's anatomist, he was seen to care only for his "specimens." In 1901 he was forced to resign. The institute's whole faculty then resigned in protest and issued a formal "Protest of the Friends of the Present Management of the N.Y. Pathological Institute." One of its signatories was none other than Weir Mitchell.

At this point, the institute recruited the Swiss-born American neurologist Adolf Meyer to take over its directorship. He came with apparently impeccable credentials in the best German-speaking traditions of neuropathology. Ironically, though, by the time he accepted the position, he no longer believed in the classical neuroanatomical research agenda. A bit like Kraepelin (who came to be an important influence on him), he had come to feel that psychiatry needed to learn how to describe and make sense of its clinical material before it tried to do more.

This conclusion was partly born of bitter experience. On arriving in the United States from Switzerland in 1892, Meyer had been unable to find the exciting work at the University of Chicago that he had hoped for. He had therefore accepted a position at the Illinois Eastern Hospital for the Insane at Kankakee, where, for several years, he tried to carry out anatomical research.

The experience had been a nightmare. As he complained in an 1895 letter to a colleague: "The worst and fatal defect was that I was expected to examine brains of people who never had been submitted to an examination; the notes which were available would be full of reports of queer and 'interesting delusions.'" More than thirty years later, Meyer again recalled this miserable experience, with some feeling: "I had to make autopsies at random on cases without any decent clinical observation, and examinations of urine and sputum of patients whom I did not know, and for physicians who merely filed the reports. . . . Whenever I tried to collect my results, I saw no safe clinical and general medical foundation to put my findings on."[28]

His goal became to develop a method that would generate those missing clinical foundations. In 1895 he gratefully left Kankakee and accepted a new position as director of pathology at the Worcester Lunatic Hospital. In that capacity, he began to develop and teach, not the neuroanatomical methods in which he had been trained, but a new quasi-Kraepelinian approach to clinical case recording. The intemperate search for brain lesions in the absence of clinical data had been a dead-end project. In contrast, the disciplined recording of clinical facts—without prejudice as to the greater importance of some over others—could never mislead. As Meyer wrote in 1908, "I started out from the realization that in some diseases we are continually promising ourselves lesions, and over that we neglect facts which are even now at hand and ready to be sized up and the very things we must learn to handle."[29] He was thus one of the first to promote Kraepelin's vision of longitudinal clinical observation in the English-speaking world and to teach it to Americans.[30]

The facts he was interested in observing and recording, however, were far more expansive and eclectic than even Kraepelin had pursued. A patient's clinical file, Meyer began to insist, should include detailed and ongoing records of his or her family history and key life events prior to hospitalization; a description of his or her changing clinical presentations over time; notes on his or her behavior on the ward and interactions with staff; results from blood and urine tests; and yes, results of autopsy work when possible. Basically, the records should include *all* plausibly relevant mental, physical, and developmental facts about the patient.

Even as Meyer taught a generation of American psychiatrists to follow the facts—all the facts—he also encouraged them to think of the mentally ill patient less as someone suffering from a discrete disease than an individual who was "reacting" in psychotic or neurotic ways to the world—who had failed, in one way or another, to "adjust" to its demands. Every patient was a biological organism with inherited strengths and weaknesses, but every patient was also an individual with a unique life history.[31] Inheritance and life history might well both shape his or her ability to react effectively and adjust successfully.

In conceiving mental illness this way, Meyer believed he was laying the foundations for American psychiatry to be medical and biological— without being reductionistic. To do justice to mental illness, he taught, psychiatrists needed to act more like naturalists in the field than like scientists in the laboratory. They needed to make room for the facts of both mind and body—for data from brain tissue and heredity studies, and for the developmental, social and mental facts that could only be gathered from a patient's life story. Meyer called this vision *psychobiology* but also sometimes "common sense" psychiatry, because it eschewed dogmatism and arcane theory and focused on gathering facts in plain view, without prejudice.

In 1901 Meyer took over the directorship at the New York Pathological Institute, abandoned its previous singular focus on neuroanatomical and physiological research, and refocused it on training New York hospital staff in his new methods of clinical observation and record keeping.[32] Then in 1908 he left New York to take up a professorship at Johns Hopkins University, and in 1914 he accepted a position as director of its newly established Henry Phipps Psychiatric Clinic, where he stayed until his retirement in 1941.[33] Over the course of his tenure at Johns Hopkins, it is estimated that he personally trained as many as 10 percent of the country's psychiatrists. Diagnostics had a place, Meyer conceded, but it should never be used to limit the clinician's focus on sifting and resifting through all the available facts—developmental, environmental, and biological—to find out what might have gone amiss. By the middle of the twentieth century, such sifting and resifting would brand "the well-trained Meyerian psychiatrist," in the words of J. Raymond DePaulo (a more recent director of the Henry Phipps Psychiatric Clinic) as "someone who could argue for and against any diagnosis in the same patient."[34]

BLEULER INVENTS SCHIZOPHRENIA

Meanwhile back in Europe, the Swiss psychiatrist Eugen Bleuler was disrupting both anatomical and classical Kraepelinian diagnostic approaches to mental illness in a different way. In 1898, Bleuler had been appointed director of the Burghölzli psychiatric hospital near Zurich. Since the 1870s, the Burghölzli had been headed by German and Swiss alienists who cultivated its reputation as a center for biological (especially neuroanatomical) research on mental illness. (Auguste-Henri Forel, Bleuler's immediate predecessor, had also tackled the hospital's previous reputation for corruption and poor living standards.)[35] Bleuler was not hostile to biological research, but he began his tenure with a different agenda: cultivating relationships with his patients.

This happened partly because he was a native of the same canton of Switzerland from which most of the patients came, and hence shared both their culture and their dialect, a fact that had considerable emotional meaning for him. In 1874, when he was seventeen, his sister had developed a catatonic psychosis and been hospitalized at the Burghölzli. At that time, the hospital was headed by the German neurologist Eduard Hitzig, famous for animal laboratory work that had led to the identification of motor centers in the cortex. During her hospitalization, the family was outraged by Hitzig's aloof attitude toward the girl, and especially by the fact that he could not understand a word she said. Her Swiss-German dialect was quite different from the "high German" Hitzig spoke. Bleuler's sister wasn't the only patient Hitzig couldn't understand—he couldn't understand *any* of his Swiss-German-speaking patients. Both his family and his biographers later said that this experience was so traumatic for Bleuler that he determined to pursue a career as a psychiatrist who would literally be able to speak his patients' language.[36]

And so when Bleuler did become a psychiatrist, he adopted an unusually pastoral attitude toward his patients, spending a great deal of time on the wards talking with them and becoming familiar with their delusions and idiosyncrasies. And this practice unexpectedly led him to some important observations. During an earlier stint as the director of a backwater hospital in Rheinau, Germany (designed for the incurably mentally ill), he had found that his patients' symptoms were not constant but varied in intensity, depending on what was going on in their lives. A visit from a beloved relative could improve them; a visit from a detested one could set them back. If a pretty woman was present, normally disorderly patients might pull themselves together.[37] In other words, patients with mental disorders—even incurable ones—were not just collections of symptoms; they were human beings who responded to other human beings. As Carl Gustav Jung—Bleuler's junior colleague—later put it:

> Hitherto we thought that the insane patient revealed nothing to us by his symptoms save the senseless products of his disordered cerebral cells; but that was academic wisdom reeking of the study. When we penetrate into the human secrets of our patients, we recognize mental disease to be an unusual reaction to emotional problems which are in no way foreign to ourselves, and the delusion discloses the psychological system upon which it is based.[38]

Jung's reference to the "human secrets" of these patients alerts us to something else going on: the growing influence of Sigmund Freud's ideas at the Burghölzli. In 1898, when Bleuler was appointed director of the Burghölzli, he was already an admirer of Freud's work. He called Freud's 1895 study on hysteria "one of the most important additions of recent years in the field of normal and pathological psychology."[39] In a review of Freud's 1900 *Traumdeutung* or *Interpretation of Dreams*, he gushed that the Viennese neurologist "has shown us part of a new world."[40]

Freud, for his part, could hardly believe his luck. For the first time, a university professor in mainstream psychiatry—who ran a prestigious mental hospital to boot—had given him an enthusiastic endorsement. As he marveled to his close friend Wilhelm Fliess, it was "an absolutely stunning recognition of my point of view . . . by an official psychiatrist, Bleuler, in Zurich. Just imagine, a full professor of psychiatry [supporting] . . . my . . . studies of hysteria and the dream, which so far have been labeled disgusting!"[41]

It was Bleuler who introduced Jung to Freud's work. For a while, the two men were an inspired double act at the Burghölzli, working out ways to integrate psychoanalytic ideas into their study of psychosis. Jung invented a well-regarded word association test, designed to reveal repressed material buried in the unconscious minds of psychotic patients. Subjects would be told a word and asked to say what other word immediately came to mind. Any hesitation was supposed to indicate unconscious struggles. Bleuler and Jung claimed to have found that even the most psychotic and delusional patients responded in ways that suggested a range of Freudian-style desires and instincts at work.[42]

Ultimately Bleuler's pastorally oriented, Freudian-minded approach to his patients led him to propose a significant reframing of psychotic disorders, but especially Kraepelin's dementia praecox. To begin, he denied that all patients with that disorder inevitably became demented, and that the disorder always began in early life. As a first order of business, therefore, psychiatry needed a new word for the disorder, and in his major 1911 founding text, he proposed the term *schizophrenia*. The word itself means "split mind," but Bleuler did not intend to suggest that patients with schizophrenia have "split personalities," another disorder that interested people in those years. Rather he meant the word to refer to a primary fraying or breakdown in the mind's ability to make stable associations among thoughts, feelings, and perceptions. Bleuler assumed these breakdowns were rooted in some metabolic imbalance or toxic internal process and were ultimately the result of genetic defects. For this reason, he would later advocate legislation making it impossible for people with schizophrenia—sympathetic as he was with their plight—to "propagate themselves."[43]

At the same time, Bleuler believed that the biological perspective on schizophrenia went only so far. Beyond the primary symptoms caused by defective biology, patients with schizophrenia also suffered from a wide range of secondary symptoms. They heard disembodied voices, experienced thoughts echoing in their head, practiced strange rituals, hewed to delusions, suffered catatonic spells, and more. There was no point, Bleuler said, in trying to find a biological cause for those symptoms, because they were not caused by brains gone wrong. They were instead caused by patients' use of psychological mechanisms (especially the kinds identified by Freud) to defend themselves against a world that they experienced through brains that didn't work right. Biochemistry and psychoanalysis were *both* needed to make sense of this disorder, said Bleuler. It was possible to walk a middle path.[44]

But in those days, Freud had no patience with middle paths: he pushed Bleuler to toe the line. Bleuler resisted. The tension between the two men grew to such a point that Bleuler finally decided that he could no longer associate himself with a movement that did not tolerate dissent. At the end of 1911, he submitted a letter of resignation to the International Psychoanalytic Association, which read in part: "In my opinion, saying 'he who is not with us is against us' or 'all or nothing' is necessary for religious communities and useful for political parties. Thus, I can indeed understand the principle, all the same I find that it is harmful for science."[45]

With Bleuler's withdrawal from the movement, Freud lost his main champion in European academic psychiatry. The consequences, certainly for the movement in Europe, were great. Lacking a foothold in the academy, psychoanalysis now largely went its own way: establishing its own societies, its own training methods, and its own vision of research and clinical practice.

Meanwhile Bleuler's new term for dementia praecox, *schizophrenia*, spread, its appeal heightened because it seemed to convey a less desperate, fatalistic course than *dementia praecox* had done. By the 1910s, American alienists were beginning to use the new word, and by the 1920s, the term *dementia praecox* was on its way to becoming archaic.[46]

What largely failed to travel to the United States, though, was Bleuler's insistence that schizophrenia was best understood through a double lens: both neurobiologically *and* psychoanalytically. Instead, views on the disorder fractured. On the one side were those who assumed that schizophrenia was best understood in strictly biological terms, even as they disagreed over what those terms should be. On the other side were clinicians who were more interested in the degree to which the disorder resulted from bad experiences, bad habits, and bad upbringing. As early as 1914, the Harvard pathologist Elmer Southard referred to these two camps as the "brain spot men" and the "mind twist men."[47]

BRAIN POISONING

The American "brain spot men" are of greatest interest to us here. Unlike the aloof neuroanatomists of the previous generation, who cared only about their specimens and showed little interest in treating patients, the men of 1914 were expected to try to do something about mental illness. Therapeutic nihilism was going out of fashion. And for many, schizophrenia—the purest embodiment of "being crazy"—was the great nut to be cracked. But how would they crack it—that is, how would they treat schizophrenia in patients?

Convinced that the nineteenth-century hunt for anatomical evidence of localized brain damage had been the wrong strategy, some of the brain spot men looked to the exciting new fields of bacteriology, toxicology, and serology (the study of blood serum) for answers. The early twentieth-century discoveries linking the syphilis spirochete to GPI were an important reference point for them. By this time, understandings of infectious diseases had become more refined than they had been in the days when the spirochete was first found in the solid brain tissue of dead GPI patients. It had become clear that people often fell ill from infections not simply because microorganisms were present in a particular organ but because once such organisms were inside the body, they produced toxic (waste) chemicals that could cause systemic poisoning. And this meant that mental afflictions with an infectious origin did not necessarily need to be caused by microbes directly infiltrating the brain. A microbial infection in the gut, the teeth, or the sinuses might end up producing waste products that had intoxicating effects on the brain and thereby mental functioning. Maybe, some suggested, this insight opened up the door to a new explanation—and treatment—for schizophrenia. If one could identify and remove all sources of infection from the bodies of schizophrenic patients, perhaps one could cure them.[48]

By the 1920s, at least two therapeutic efforts thus emerged that involved surgically removing allegedly infected organs from the bodies of schizophrenic patients: teeth, appendixes, ovaries, testes, colons, and more. The most prominent advocate for this therapy was Henry Cotton, the medical director at the New Jersey State Lunatic Asylum, in Trenton. At Cotton's instruction, starting in 1916, more than two thousand patients at the asylum were subjected to systematic colonic irrigations and successive extractions of presumed infected organs. Cotton claimed astonishingly high cure rates—exceeding 80 percent.[49] Newspaper reports trumpeted the exciting news of a treatment for a disease previously believed to be hopeless. Families implored Cotton to operate on their devastated relatives.

Throughout this work, Cotton was encouraged by his mentor, Adolf Meyer. More than encouraged: in fact, as historians Andrew Scull and Jay Schulkin have shown, Meyer later actively worked to suppress the emerging evidence that Cotton's surgeries, far from curing patients, were making virtually all of them worse than before—if they survived at all. Postsurgical fatalities were estimated to be as high as 30 percent.[50]

Meanwhile in Chicago, the American bacteriologist and surgeon Bayard Holmes also fervently advocated treating schizophrenia by "cutting out" infections that might be poisoning patients' brains. Holmes's efforts seem to have been carried out completely independently of Cotton's. There is no evidence that the two men ever met or corresponded, though—perhaps tellingly—both were close to Adolf Meyer.[51]

Although Holmes was not a psychiatrist, he had thrown himself into the quest to find a cure for schizophrenia after witnessing the devastating effects of the disease on his teenage son Ralph. He came to believe that in patients with schizophrenia, fecal stasis (immobile or blocked fecal matter in the colon or small intestine) led to bacterial growth that produced toxic alkaloids. And those alkaloids, he thought, were similar to those implicated in ergotism, a form of poisoning often associated with psychotic symptoms. Surgical extraction seemed the obvious solution.[52]

In May 1916 Holmes performed his first surgery—on his son. Four days later Ralph Holmes died. Adolf Meyer was one of the very few, outside the family, to whom Holmes spoke about this tragedy. Possibly on Meyer's advice, Holmes expunged the record of this failed effort from the public medical reports. He continued to carry out additional operations on patients and even successfully lobbied for the establishment of an experimental ward and laboratory dedicated to this work: the short-lived Psychiatric Research Laboratory of the Psychopathic Hospital at Cook County Hospital in Chicago.[53]

STERILIZING

Meanwhile the nineteenth-century degenerationist biological approach to mental illness was not dead. A widespread consensus still held that some mental defects were inherited and incurable no matter what one did. Those who thought this way understood schizophrenia (dementia praecox) to be one of these incurable and inherited disorders, alongside epilepsy and intellectual disabilities, in people known variously (depending on the degree of defect) as morons, idiots, imbeciles, and the feebleminded.

The final category—feeblemindedness—was particularly widely used by early twentieth-century degenerationists because it was so flexible. A developmentally disabled child unable to speak might be called feebleminded, but so might a chronic shoplifter or a pregnant teenage girl who ran wild with the boys. What supposedly distinguished all these people was the incorrigibility of their defects, their presumed imperviousness to therapy, training, or discipline. In the 1910s Henry H. Goddard, director of the New Jersey Vineland Training School for Feeble-minded Girls and Boys,[54] did family genealogies and provided photographic evidence purporting to show how feeblemindedness passed from one generation to the next. (Much later the photographs he offered as evidence were shown to have been doctored.)[55] Moreover, in his 1912 book *The Kallikak Family: A Study in the Heredity of Feeble-Mindedness*, he suggested—alarmingly—that "feeble-mindedness" was most likely caused by a single recessive

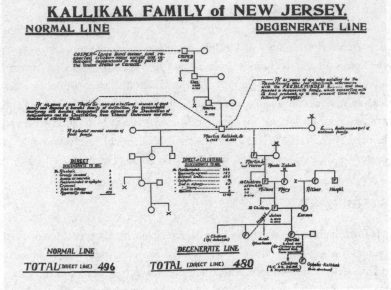

Heredity chart demonstrating inheritance of "feeble-mindedness" in the Kallikak family of New Jersey. Eugenics Record Office Records. Courtesy of the American Philosophical Society.

gene—meaning that citizens could carry the trait without showing symptoms themselves but pass it on to their offspring.[56]

What should be done with all of these incorrigibly defective people? For decades, there had been only one answer: warehouse them in custodial institutions. But now the will to do more was growing. Medicine might not be able to salvage them, some physicians said, but it could at least ensure that they did not reproduce. Such people—especially those institutionalized at taxpayers' expense—should therefore be required to undergo a simple operation of the reproductive organs that rendered them sterile. And in cases where medical judgment agreed on a person's incorrigibility, such an operation should be done regardless of whether the person agreed to it or was even capable of agreeing.

The Committee on Eugenics, an organization of scientists originally under the auspices of the American Breeders Association, took the lead in providing the scientific justification for these calls to sterilize. The biologist

Charles Benedict Davenport, who headed the committee, set up a Eugenics Record Office at Cold Spring Harbor, New York, that eventually housed an archive with hundreds of thousands of family records, pedigrees, and medical reports.[57] He and his allies worked hard to persuade legislators to act. In due course, they did. In 1907 Indiana passed the first state law permitting mandatory sterilization. Over the ensuing years, other states had followed Indiana's lead, with California and Virginia emerging as especially zealous.

One of the allies on whom Davenport depended was the psychiatrist Adolf Meyer. In 1910 Meyer agreed to head a subcommittee on insanity on behalf of Davenport's committee.[58] In 1916 he allowed himself to be elected the third president of the Eugenics Research Association. He served on the advisory council of the American Eugenics Society from 1923 to 1935. With his growing influence in psychiatry, all these actions left their mark.

Ironically, Meyer seems to have done all these things less because he was a hard-nosed advocate of eugenics than because his "allegiance to the rich harvest of fact" (his words) meant that he was reluctant to rule out any potentially important avenue of research.[59] In 1917 Meyer did gently criticize the zealots within the eugenics movement, saying in his presidential address that eugenics research had done more to stir up "*fear* of tainted families" than to provide "wider and clearer knowledge" about their actual existence.[60] Nevertheless, in 1921 he was still welcoming Davenport to Johns Hopkins, hoping he would give medical students there "a correct and real conception" of the work of the eugenics movement.[61] And while he seems to have privately written to colleagues about his distaste for legislation allowing the involuntary sterilization of the insane, it was not until the mid-1930s that he finally denounced it publicly.[62]

What was life like for psychiatric patients living in states where sterilization laws were being aggressively implemented? We can get a sense from a 1932 anonymous memoir, penned by a patient at the Eastern State Hospital in Vinita, Oklahoma:

> The spectre of sex sterilization has been thrust over us. The legislature has passed and the governor has signed a measure permitting the desexualization under certain circumstances of any male or female inmate who is not too aged to procreate. And the patients

are frightened, wrought up, angry and muttering. They know little about the law, therefore they are the more frightened. . . . They gather in knots and discuss the fate which may be hanging over them.

But they do not do it where the attendants can hear. They are afraid to do that. And so the fears, the loneliness, and the near hopelessness of the Locked-ins have an added terror.[63]

By 1924 an estimated three thousand institutionalized persons in the United States had been involuntarily sterilized. But critics of the laws argued that they violated rights guaranteed in the U.S. Constitution. In 1924 eugenicists decided to force the issue and bring a case to the courts, hoping it would settle the matter in their favor once and for all. To this end, they chose a young woman in Virginia, Carrie Buck.

Carrie was an eighteen-year-old unmarried teenager with a baby daughter, Vivian, who had been sent by her foster parents to the Virginia Colony for the Epileptic and the Feebleminded, near Lynchburg, Virginia. Carrie's birth mother, Emma Buck, was already an inmate in this asylum; some said she had been a prostitute. The foster parents said Carrie was mentally subnormal and morally depraved, pointing to her out-of-wedlock pregnancy. We now know that the foster parents lied: Carrie had been raped by her foster mother's nephew and was sent to the asylum to avoid shame being cast on the foster family.

By chance, on March 20, 1924, shortly before Carrie's incarceration, the Virginia General Assembly had passed a law allowing for the involuntary sterilization of institutionalized patients deemed to be suffering from mental or moral defects that were likely to be hereditary in nature: "An Act to Provide for the Sexual Sterilization of Inmates of State Institutions in Certain Cases" (more generally known as the Sterilization Act). In case the eugenicist agenda motivating the legislators should be in any doubt, that same day they passed the Racial Integrity Act, which criminalized all interracial marriages. To ensure compliance, that second law required that the "race" of every person be recorded at birth, with only two options: "white" and "colored."[64]

Albert Priddy, superintendent of the Virginia Colony, the institution where teenage Carrie was sent, decided to sterilize her under the terms of the new sterilization law. First, though, he and his eugenicist colleagues arranged for an "appeal" in her name. The prosecution argued that her case involved clearly inherited defects. Carrie was the daughter of an allegedly depraved mother, she was herself "feebleminded," and she had now given birth to a daughter whom a nurse judged to be "not quite normal."[65] Technically, her defense was that the state was denying her due process and equal protection under the law, as required by the Fourteenth Amendment. In fact, as legal historian Paul Lombardo has shown, the whole appeal was a setup: she had no true voice in the process as it made its way through various courts. The lawyer who was supposed to defend her had been hired by the eugenicists, was in constant communication with them, never cross-examined any of their witnesses, and at times seemed to testify himself in support of their cause. In Lombardo's words, "A bystander might reasonably have reached the conclusion that there were two lawyers working for Dr. Priddy and none for Carrie Buck.[66]

By the time Carrie Buck's case reached the Supreme Court in the spring of 1927, Priddy had died. The new superintendent of the Virginia Colony was his former assistant, John H. Bell, so the case that went to the Supreme Court was called *Buck v. Bell*. The justices heard no witnesses of their own: instead, they chose 8–1 to uphold the legality of Carrie's sterilization based on their reading of (largely trumped-up) records from the original trial and the appeal. The majority opinion was written by Associate Justice Oliver Wendell Holmes, Jr. In words that have echoed down over the decades, he summed up his support for Carrie's sterilization:

> It is better for all the world, if instead of waiting to execute degenerate offspring for crime or to let them starve for their imbecility, society can prevent those who are manifestly unfit from continuing their kind.

He went on to link the Court's decision to the era's larger public health and hygiene imperatives: "The principle that sustains compulsory vaccination is broad enough to cover the cutting of the fallopian tubes." He then famously concluded: "Three generations of imbeciles are enough."[67]

The Supreme Court's 1927 ruling transformed the debate over sterilization in the United States. Over the ten years, new laws were passed, and some 28,000 Americans were sterilized. In 1933 Germany's Nazi government would cite the 1927 *Buck v. Bell* decision in defending its own "Law for the Prevention of Hereditarily Diseased Offspring." The Nazi law mandated the sterilization of intellectually disabled people (the "feeble-minded"), people with inherited neurological disorders like Huntington's chorea, and people diagnosed with schizophrenia and epilepsy.

Germany's sterilization program, in turn, paved the way in 1939—after Germany went to war—for an originally secret decision not to steril-ize but to murder thousands of mentally ill and disabled institutionalized persons. The justification was that such people had no life "worth living," and as they were "useless eaters," the rest of society was better off with them dead as well. Between 1939 and 1945, some 200,000 to 275,000 peo-ple (estimates vary), including some 8,000 children, are estimated to have been killed under this program, by lethal injection, by deliberate starva-tion, or (later) in gas chambers.[68] The methods of extermination developed for this program—especially the gas chambers—were later utilized for the so-called "Final Solution," the genocide of more than six million Jews.

In 1942, while these atrocities were unfolding, the *American Journal of Psychiatry* published two short articles, side by side, on the question of whether killing "feebleminded" children was ever permissible. The first, by Dr. Foster Kennedy, argued in favor of such killing, but only when the cases in question were "hopelessly defective," "nature's mistake," "something we hustle out of sight, which should never have been seen at all." In such cases, he said, "we may most kindly kill, and have no fear of error."[69]

The second paper, by Dr. Leo Kanner (later better known for his work on autism), disagreed, pointing out that we should not judge people's value based on their IQ. He spoke of a "mentally deficient" man who had worked in his neighborhood for many years as a "garbage collector's assistant." This "sober, conscientious, and industrious fellow" made an indubitable contribution to society, and there were many like him. In fact, without all the menial labor such people performed, he suggested that it was doubtful that society could function:

> For all practical purposes, the garbage collector is as much of a pub-
> lic hygienist as is the laboratory bacteriologist. All performances
> referred to snobbishly as "dirty work" are indeed real and necessary

contributions to our culture, without which it would collapse within less than a month.[70]

But what about those who were so impaired that they could not contribute on any level to the common good? Here the growing shadow of Nazism seems to have influenced Kanner. He spoke of recent reports coming out of Germany that the Gestapo was "systematically bumping off the mentally deficient people of the Reich." (He made no mention of doctors' roles in such killings.) He then asked rhetorically, "Shall we psychiatrists take our cue from the Nazi Gestapo?" While he was prepared to defend the sterilization of "persons intellectually or emotionally unfit to rear children," he could not see any situation in which "we are justified in passing the black bottle" to accomplish murderous goals that some "dignify with the term 'euthanasia.'"[71]

With these apparently contrasting perspectives before them, the editors of the *American Journal of Psychiatry* weighed in. In an unsigned editorial, they came down decisively in favor of legislation permitting euthanasia in cases where the severity of the mental disability clearly (in their eyes) warranted it. They were aware, though, that public sentiment in the United States was largely opposed to such legislation, largely because many parents of such children generally claimed to be fond of them and wanted them to live. This fact, the editors noted, was frustrating because clearly no sane parent could feel "normal affection . . . for a creature incapable of the slightest response." Any apparent feelings of affection must therefore actually be a morbid state rooted in "obligation or guilt." "If euthanasia is to become at some distant day an available procedure," the editors concluded, then one needed to find ways to modify such feelings of parental pseudo-affection "by exposure to mental hygiene principles." Herein lay an important practical task for psychiatry: help such parents realize that they did not truly love their severely disabled children after all.[72]

WATER AND WALKING

Of course, most rank-and-file hospital psychiatrists were not involved in debates like these but soldiered on in their hospitals with pessimistic stoicism. Some practiced sterilization, but most did not see that it made much difference to their everyday work. Tellingly, a few hospitals insisted that sterilization was actually a kind of therapy in its own right, reducing patients' aggression, and even making some of them more lucid.[73] Tellingly, too, they put the best face on other longstanding managerial practices, especially painful needle showers, soaks in hot baths, and ice-cold wet sheet wraps. A 1927 article in the *American Journal of Nursing* insisted, without irony, that baths and showers represented a cutting-edge treatment approach, "designed to give the patient the benefit of water applied externally by a number of scientific methods."[74] Sedative drugs such as potassium bromide, chloral hydrate, and chloroform were also widely used. No one thought that they actually touched the underlying disease, but they did often make everyday care easier. Long, exhausting exercise routines and work sessions were other preferred methods used to tire patients out and make them easier to handle.

In 1972 a former employee of Jacksonville State Hospital in Illinois was interviewed about his memories of being a ward attendant in the 1920s. He recalled the daily routines as follows:

> Now we used to do what we called walking the loop. Well, we got this loop here on the ground. . . . We'd go out around nine o'clock in the morning and we'd walk until about eleven o'clock or eleven-fifteen. Then we'd go in for dinner. . . . Then as quick as they got through their lunch, we'd take them in on the ward for a while. We had polishers, that were made out of six by sixes and they were about three feet wide. They had rugs nailed on them, and you line these patients up with those polishers and they'd go around and around in the halls. You walk a patient a little while and then take him off and let him rest and give it to another one.
>
> Q. I don't think I understand yet, why did they walk?
>
> A. . . . Now I'm no doctor, but the doctors told me that was supposed to be good treatment for them. But I think they just got so doggone tired that when they come in they was ready to go to bed, see, and they naturally was pretty quiet, you know.[75]

It was a discouraging state of affairs, to be sure. But then during the late 1920s and especially the 1930s, the mood within the state hospitals began to perk up because, in quick succession, five new treatments found their way into these institutions. These treatments all promised not just to manage patients but to fix their minds. And taken together, they sent a clear signal that mental hospitals were no longer just in the business of providing custodial care or palliative therapies: they now also offered real treatments— medical treatments. Foster Kennedy—who would defend euthanasia in 1942—spoke out in strong support of these treatments in 1938 in a comment that also served as a clear dig at the Freudians: "The scholasticism of our time is being blown away by a new wind, and . . . we shall not again be content to minister to a mind diseased merely by philosophy and words."[76]

Of the five treatments in question, only one—electroconvulsive therapy (ECT)—is still used today. Three others—malaria fever treatment, insulin coma treatment, and metrazol shock treatment—have largely faded from memory. The fifth one—psychosurgery, or lobotomy—has not been forgotten, but only because it has become associated with the most barbaric and arrogant face of psychiatry's ignorance. But how were they all understood at the time? Let us briefly look at each in turn.

MALARIA FEVER TREATMENT

Malaria fever treatment was focused on GPI, still an incurable disease in the 1910s, although exciting advances in treating early-stage syphilis (using the arsenic compound Salvarsan) had made some clinicians less fatalistic than they had previously been about the prospects of treating it. Salvarsan was the original "magic bullet" drug for malaria but had proved disappointingly ineffective against GPI.

A chance observation by the Austrian psychiatrist Julius Wagner-Jauregg would inspire the development of a different treatment approach for GPI. In 1887, while he was working at an asylum in Vienna, a mentally ill patient under his care contracted the infectious skin disease erysipelas and succumbed to high fever, chills, and shaking. When she recovered, she seemed far more lucid than she had been before falling ill.

This intriguing fact prompted Wagner-Jauregg to undertake some studies in which he deliberately induced fever in psychotic patients using an experimental vaccine that had been developed by Robert Koch against tuberculosis (tuberculin). He felt the results were particularly promising for GPI patients. Unfortunately, though, the vaccine proved more toxic than expected and some of the patients died.

Wagner-Jauregg then considered inducing fever in GPI patients using blood contaminated with malaria. His reasoning was simple: unlike other infections, the high fever of malaria could be controlled with quinine. In 1917 he had a chance to test this new approach when a shell-shocked soldier sent to his clinic turned out to be suffering from malaria (a major problem in the Great War for soldiers stationed in Africa). Before treating the soldier, Wagner-Jauregg drew blood from him and injected it into nine GPI patients.

Within a week, these patients all showed the typical symptoms of malarial infection: chills, shaking, temperatures as high as 106, and profuse sweating. Wagner-Jauregg let the disease run its course for several weeks, then terminated it with quinine. Six out of the nine patients, he reported, experienced mental improvement after their ordeal. Four years later, he wrote, three of those six were "actively and efficiently at work." Given that they had suffered from a disease that typically killed its victims within two years of its first symptoms, these results were remarkable. Encouraged, Wagner-Jauregg pressed on and eventually tested the treatment on more than two hundred patients. In 1922 he reported that fifty of these GPI patients were in complete remission.[77]

While this 25 percent success rate may not seem all that impressive today, back then it was vastly better than anyone else had done for GPI. In 1927 Wagner-Jauregg received a Nobel Prize for Physiology or Medicine in recognition of his work. On the occasion of his award, *Scientific Monthly* summed up the consensus: "the whole . . . world should join his patients and students in their congratulations."[78]

Malaria fever treatment spread into hospitals around the world, and as it did, something unexpected happened: many patients with GPI underwent, in the eyes of their clinicians, a kind of moral rehabilitation. For decades, hospital staff had dismissed these patients as degenerate, repugnant, and unsalvageable. The historian Joel Braslow discovered a case note from a doctor's

file in an American mental hospital, written a few years prior to the introduction of malaria fever therapy: "An extremely vulgar paretic who has led
an immoral life. Had been treated for syphilis.... This is the place for her."[79]

But now, with a treatment available that might help them, patients like
these seemed deserving of compassion—all the more so, perhaps, because
their path to redemption involved an almost literal trial by fire. In 1933 a
Reader's Digest article, "The Pale Horror," captured the new understanding. "Give your paretics the right kind of malaria," its author, Paul de Kruif,
explained, "and, though it burned them, the whole bodies of these paralyt-
ics seemed cleansed by the malaria fire. Thin, washed out by the terrible
fever, they ... began to turn into new people."[80]

The rehabilitation of one set of patients, however, was sometimes
achieved at the cost of objectifying another. Maintaining adequate stocks
of malaria-tainted blood for the purposes of treatment was difficult (outside tropical settings where malaria was endemic). Some research centers
maintained colonies of mosquitoes, but hospitals were not set up for such
an undertaking. Many coped by adopting a kind of recycling system: they
inoculated one GPI patient with malaria, then used the resulting infected
blood to inoculate the next paretic patient. At St. Elizabeths, however,
William Alanson White insisted (overriding the reluctance of his staff)
that only blood known to be unaffected by syphilis be used for treatment
(to avoid the risk of accidentally infecting patients who had been wrongly
diagnosed).

Clinicians therefore identified a small number of psychiatric patients
deemed clean of syphilis and arranged for them to serve as "malaria reservoirs." These patients—among the most socially marginalized in the
hospital— were repeatedly infected with malaria (and then cured with quinine) so the clinicians could use their contaminated blood. Both black and
white paretic patients were offered this treatment, apparently without prejudice. In these years, it had become accepted, at least among clinicians, that
blood did not carry any kind of racial marker, so there would be no need to
worry (as the general public still so often did) about "mixing." Still, it may
be significant that one of the hospital's most reliable malaria reservoirs was
a man named Hussein, whose swarthy complexion made him, in the eyes of
the staff, a racially ambiguous figure.[81]

The full details of the practice of turning some patients into "malaria reservoirs" are still coming to light, but evidence is growing that the practice was used in other hospitals besides St. Elizabeths. In 2014 a commission was set up in Austria to investigate claims that hundreds of Viennese patients, including unknown numbers of orphaned children, were also used as malaria reservoirs in the same way that patients at St. Elizabeths were.[82]

The death knell for malaria fever treatment was the discovery of penicillin (rather than any ethical qualms about the trade-offs required to practice this treatment). Penicillin, the first antibiotic, was mass-produced during World War II, where it was used initially to save the lives of wounded soldiers, who would previously have died of infection. In 1945 the U.S. government released the drug for unrestricted civilian use. By the early 1950s, GPI patients were routinely given a course of antibiotics instead of a shot of tainted blood. And by the end of the decade, with penicillin treatment for early-stage syphilis also readily available, the number of GPI cases plummeted.

Today malaria fever therapy plays almost no role in psychiatric practice. Wagner-Jauregg's personal reputation has plummeted, certainly in Austria, as facts have come to light about his later advocacy of racist Nazi policies.[83] Nevertheless, at the time, Wagner-Jauregg's Nobel Prize–winning treatment marked a turning point for biological psychiatry. It raised hopes that at least some patients who had previously been deemed incurable and, on some level, expendable might be salvageable after all. The recognition given to Wagner-Jauregg's achievement also persuaded some clinicians that if they were bold enough, they could win status and professional recognition in ways that had previously been unthinkable in psychiatry.

INSULIN-INDUCED COMAS

In the 1920s Frederick Banting and Charles Best isolated insulin and used it to save the lives of diabetic children. The fanfare that followed (including another Nobel Prize) inspired other clinicians to experiment with this new drug. Today we think of insulin as a specific treatment for diabetes, but at the time some hoped it might alleviate symptoms of other disorders as well. In some hospitals, clinicians gave insulin to malnourished patients to encourage appetite. Others used it to treat the symptoms of delirium tremens in alcoholics.[84]

In the late 1920s, a number of attempts were also made to use insulin to calm agitated psychotic patients. In Switzerland, several clinicians experimented with injecting such patients with doses of insulin large enough to produce light hypoglycemic comas. They claimed to achieve good sedative results.[85] In Vienna a young and intensely ambitious clinician, Manfred Sakel, also tried his hand at using insulin for psychosis, but in one case in 1934, he took a bolder route. When lower doses of insulin failed to produce much of an effect on the patient in question, he increased the dose to such a high level that the patient began to convulse and sweat profusely, then fell into a deep coma. Apparently, Sakel had not intended to cause convulsions in this patient, though he later claimed he had (especially after other convulsive therapies became popular).[86] Whatever the case may be, Sakel's aggressive insulin treatment produced a gratifying result, in his eyes: after he reversed the patient's coma artificially with a glucose infusion, the patient was so lucid that, after a couple of weeks of top-up treatment, he could be released from the hospital and resume work.

This result suggested that insulin-induced coma might be more than a palliative treatment for calming schizophrenic patients: it might be working directly on the underlying disease. Filled with excitement, Sakel was now convinced that he was "on the road to great discoveries"[87]—maybe even a Nobel Prize. (He did not receive one.) He worked hard to both refine and promote his new treatment, publishing between November 1934 and February 1935 no fewer than thirteen reports that claimed improvement rates of over 80 percent.

Sakel's method caught the eye of the young American psychiatrist Joseph Wortis, who by chance was in Vienna in 1935 to undergo a training analysis with an aging Sigmund Freud.[88] After watching Sakel demonstrate insulin coma therapy, he was sold. In 1936 he helped Sakel relocate to New York and arranged for him to demonstrate the method at various venues in the United States. Interest grew rapidly, not least because the demonstrations were accompanied by a frenzy of sensationalistic newspaper reports: "New Hope for Mental Patients: Insulin 'Shock Treatment' "

(1938); "Insane Now Get Chance to Live Life Over Again" (1937); "Thousands of 'Living Dead' May Live Again Through 'Insulin Shock'" (1937); "Dementia Praecox Curbed by Insulin:... Treatment Is Hailed as by Far the Most Effective Discovered to Date" (1937); "Insulin Rocks the Foundations of Reason and Yet Seems to Restore Sanity in Many Cases. Science Today Is Engaged in No More Exciting Adventure" (1940).[89]

In 1938 Wortis expressed regret about "unfortunate and premature press releases" like these, but he spoke optimistically about the "solid and sympathetic support" Sakel had received from American psychiatric leaders like Adolf Meyer. That same year, Wortis noted, at a meeting of the American Psychiatric Congress in Pittsburgh, clinicians "from over a score of hospitals throughout the country" reported on the results of their own experiments with the treatment. In Wortis's words: "The degrees of enthusiasm varied, but no one rose to intrude a single dissenting note."[90] Indeed, a review of the outcome of one thousand cases, published in 1938, suggested that, while Sakel's near-miraculous claims to 80 percent recovery were not replicated, he did seem to be on to something. Eleven percent of schizophrenic patients treated with insulin were said to have completely recovered, 26.5 percent were declared greatly improved, and another 26 percent were said to show evidence of some improvement.[91]

And so more and more hospitals set up special insulin coma therapy (ICT) wards to pursue this new treatment—at least, the better-endowed ones. The fact is, ICT was expensive. It required dedicated space, special equipment, and intensive nursing care. A hospital that might house thousands of patients could accommodate only 20 or 30 ICT patients. But in hospitals that could afford such wards, they seem to have been often experienced as strangely wonderful. Staffers later recalled that the wards felt like a world apart from the tedium and pessimism that prevailed in the rest of the hospital. The twenty or so patients under their care—hand-selected for their presumed ability to benefit from the treatment—were nursed and even indulged in ways that would have been inconceivable anywhere else in the hospital. One 1947 British handbook went so far as to suggest that a good "insulin nurse" would "keep the patients occupied and interested during the exercise by organizing games or competitions, picking flowers, gathering sticks, visiting various parts of the hospital estate, map-reading,

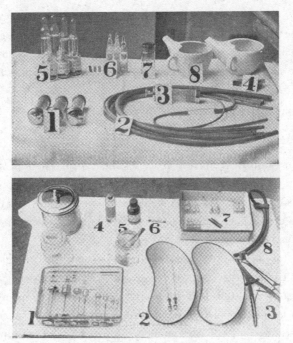

Insulin coma therapy trolley. Eric Cunningham Dax, *Modern Mental Treatment: A Handbook for Nurses* (London: Faber & Faber, 1947), 75.

etc."[92] Physicians, meanwhile, carried out the exacting routines required by the treatment using an impressive arsenal of medical equipment. All these workers felt as if—finally—they were real clinicians, looking after real patients.[93]

In 1958, reflecting back on all this, the British psychiatrist Harold Bourne would suggest that insulin coma therapy was—and always had been—an ineffective biological treatment but, ironically, a rather effective psychological one. That is to say, the insulin injections were not effective in reducing psychosis, but the special attention given to patients undergoing the treatment likely did them considerable good. After all, the patients selected for ICT were first identified as promising candidates for improvement, and then were brought into a special, quiet ward, where they received good food and lots of attention. Finally, they were subjected to an apparently cutting-edge, dramatic medical treatment that their clinicians were excited to give them. As Bourne put it: "Insulin coma treatment may come to be remembered as the first application of psychological healing for schizophrenics in the mass, and its achievement as an inadvertent one—the supply to persons hitherto considered impervious to it, of daily, devoted, personal care."[94]

METRAZOL SHOCK TREATMENT

By the time Bourne published this assessment, ICT was in decline: confidence in its efficacy was waning, it was expensive—and another treatment was becoming available. Like insulin coma therapy, this treatment produced convulsions and unconsciousness, but much more quickly and cheaply than ICT had done.

The story of metrazol shock treatment begins with a Hungarian psychiatrist, Ladislav Meduna, who proposed a theory (no longer accepted) that schizophrenia and epilepsy are antagonistic diseases; the presence of one disease inhibits the expression of the other. There had indeed been a report published in 1929 that some epileptic patients who developed symptoms of schizophrenia showed a marked reduction in the frequency of their epileptic attacks.[95] The authors, Nyirö and Jablonszky, had been sufficiently inspired by this finding to inject some epileptic patients with the blood of schizophrenic patients, to see if it reduced their incidence of convulsions. It didn't, and they had abandoned the effort.

Meduna, though, was interested in the opposite possibility: that epileptic convulsions could have a beneficial effect on schizophrenia, much as high malarial fever had a beneficial effect on GPI.[96] Schizophrenic patients might not need to develop a true epilepsy in order to experience improvement, he thought—experiencing seizures might be enough. If so, an enterprising clinician might be able to induce them pharmaceutically. Quite a few drugs were known to have convulsant properties, if given in large enough doses.

It was an exciting thought, and Meduna began to pursue it. He moved to a psychiatric hospital outside Budapest that was willing to allow him to experiment on patients. After briefly using camphor as a convulsant agent, he settled on the circulatory and respiratory stimulant pentylenetetrazol (also known as metrazol and cardiazol). It could be administered intravenously and, unlike camphor, produced convulsions almost immediately. Meduna's 1937 text, *Convulsion Therapy for Schizophrenia*, described results of the treatment for 110 patients. He was bullish, judging that a good half of the treated schizophrenic patients fully recovered, and many others—especially ones who had been ill less than a year—had considerably improved.[97]

Within three years, this treatment too was being used in hospitals worldwide, and it clearly had effects. Clinicians reported that patients became more subdued, in ways that the ward staff quite appreciated. As one American psychiatrist reflected in 1938:

It was found generally ... that ... the necessity for sedation dropped to the vanishing point; and about half the patients became capable of productive work. Open masturbation, obscenity, ready irritability, incoherency of speech and escape attempts were much diminished. Apart from the psychiatric implications of these data, the observations appear to have significance for the administrative problems involved in the custodial care of chronically disturbed patients.[98]

Yet from the outset a sense of unease hovered over this treatment. Some clinicians spoke of patients being held down on the table in "panicky states of fright."[99] Others worried about the fact that convulsions produced by metrazol could not be easily controlled and often became so extreme that patients broke bones, lost teeth, and suffered other injuries. In 1939 the New York State Psychiatric Institute reported that no fewer than 43 percent of its patients treated with metrazol had suffered spinal fractures.[100]

ELECTROCONVULSIVE TREATMENT (ECT)

Such concerns led the Italian neurologist Ugo Cerletti, working in the 1930s, to suggest that, rather than using drugs to produce convulsions in patients, clinicians should use a controlled electrical current. He envisioned an approach modeled on the technologies used in slaughterhouses to stun (but not kill) pigs just before they were killed.[101] Of course, as he later recalled, he knew it would not be easy to get past immediate reactions that such an idea was "barbaric and dangerous." He knew that "in every-one's mind was the spectre of the 'electric chair.' "[102]

Nevertheless, he instructed his assistant, Lucio Bini, to build a proto-type device. It was duly tested, first mostly on stray dogs (brought to the hospital every day by the dog catcher). By 1938 Cerletti and his students finally felt ready to run a test on a human patient. An opportunity to do so presented itself in April 1938, when a thirty-nine-year old engineer from Milan, known today only by his initials S.E., was arrested at the railway station in Rome. Because the man did not seem to be in full possession of his mental faculties, the city police commissioner arranged to have him sent to Cerletti's hospital for observation.

S.E. was clearly quite deranged: he spoke in a strange jargon and believed himself to be telepathically influenced. Equally important, he was far from his hometown, and the chances seemed low that a family mem-ber would show up and make inquiries, if something went terribly wrong with the experiment. Just to be on the safe side, Cerletti instructed his staff to see whether anyone was looking for S.E., and as one of his students recalled years later, they "could not find anyone who was searching for him or seemed to care about him."[103]

And so the decision was made to proceed. Reports of the first test, many of which were recorded years after it happened, are filled with high drama. S.E.'s head was shaved, and he was strapped to a table. Electrodes were affixed to his temples with rubber bands. Ferdinando Accornero, Cer-letti's assistant, later recalled that a total of three sets of shocks were given, each at a progressively higher voltage. After the second set resulted in sud-den, involuntary muscle spasms, the patient "relaxed with a deep breath. . . . After about a minute, he opened his eyes, shook his head, sat up, and started to sing a popular, dirty song, out of tune." This surreal development broke the tension in the room, but the task at hand had yet to be achieved. Accord-ing to Accornero, Cerletti then said: "Well, another time at a higher voltage and with a longer duration, then no more." At that time, the patient himself protested—calmly—for the first time: "Be careful: the first one was a nui-sance, the second one was deadly." Everyone was startled. Maybe it was a warning. But Cerletti, the "Maestro," pressed on: "Let's proceed."

The device was set to "maximum current." The button was pushed, and this time it worked: the patient began to convulse. For some forty-eight seconds, he stopped breathing. Sweat broke out on the brows of all the witnesses. Finally, the patient recommenced breathing. People exhaled in relief.

According to Accornero, Cerletti then broke the silence by speaking in a "calm and decisive voice": "I can therefore assume that an electric current can induce a seizure in man without risks."[104] Cerletti himself would later tell a slightly different version of the conclusion of this experiment, saying the patient sat up "calm and smiling." Unable to recall what had just happened to him, he suggested that he must have been "asleep."[105]

All accounts agree, though, that S.E. continued to improve. The clinicians reported that he voluntarily underwent a further course of treatments. And after several weeks, he was released from the hospital in much better health.

Of all the somatic treatments introduced in the 1930s, none became more widely used than Cerletti and Bini's shock treatment, which in the

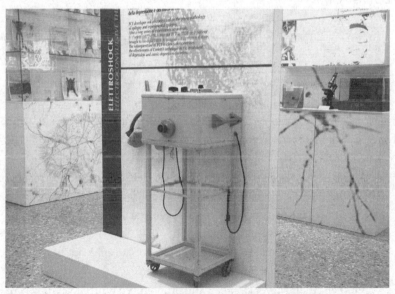

Prototype of the electroshock machine used by Ugo Cerletti. A. Aruta / Courtesy of Museum of History of Medicine, Department of Molecular Medicine, Sapienza University of Rome.

United States came to be called electroconvulsive therapy (ECT). It could be controlled; it was cheap; it was easy; and it seemed to bring real therapeutic benefits. Ironically, as ECT's use spread, it became clear that it was not particularly effective for the disorder for which it had been invented: schizophrenia.[106] But for unknown reasons, it did seem to be quite effective in alleviating symptoms of otherwise intractable forms of depression (for which it is still used today). In that sense, ECT raised more questions than it answered about the specific biology of different mental disorders. From the beginning, the reputation of the treatment also suffered from credible claims that it could cause memory loss, either temporary or long-lasting (see Chapter 6).

Still, the overall feeling among clinicians was that ECT gave them reason to be more optimistic about their mission than they had been in a long time: the mental hospital might not have made much progress in understanding the biology of mental illness, but at least it now had something concrete to offer many patients.

LOBOTOMY

The last treatment to emerge out of 1930s-era somatic therapeutic experimentation involved the deliberate surgical destruction of brain tissue in the frontal lobe. Called variously lobotomy (the term I will use), psychosurgery, or in England, leucotomy, it was pioneered in Portugal by the ambitious neurologist Egas Moniz. It was originally described as a treatment of "last resort" for people crippled with debilitating levels of anxiety and obsessive thoughts. And it was seen, even at the outset, as a treatment that pushed the boundaries of permissible therapies.

We know this because, in late November 1936, the American psychiatrist Walter Freeman and his neurosurgeon colleague James Watts spoke about their first experiments with the procedure at a meeting of the Southern Medical Association in Baltimore. After they finished, the neurologist Bernard Wortis expressed horror at the specter of "an epidemic of progressive eviscerating experiments." Others agreed.[107]

But then Adolf Meyer stood up and pronounced himself cautiously in support of the work. He admitted that, like Wortis, he had some "hesitation at the thought of a great many of us having our distractability or our worries removed" with a knife. Still, he said, "I am inclined to think there are more possibilities in this operation than he does." The key to proceeding was prudence:

> The work should be in the hands only of those who are willing and ready to follow up the experiments with each case, such as Dr. Freeman and Dr. Watts are doing. Their procedure in the hands of responsible persons seems permissible as an experimental attempt, but it is important that the public should not be drawn into an expectation of this and that being done to their brains. In the hands of Dr. Freeman and Dr. Watts I know that the work will not take that turn.[108]

The historian Jack Pressman has suggested that Meyer's intervention in the conversation at that moment was a decisive turning point in lobotomy's history: it gave license for Freeman and Watts to carry on.[109] Two months after their presentation in Baltimore, they published their results in the *Southern Medical Journal*, describing six cases. One was a middle-aged woman wracked with anxiety about illness and fears of aging. She then underwent the procedure with striking consequences:

> When seen recently she stated that her anxiety and apprehension were no longer present, that she could sit down and plan out a course of procedure better than she could before because of freedom from distraction; that she was content to grow old gracefully.... She noticed some loss of spontaneity which she described as being subdued. Her husband said that she was more normal than she had ever been.[110]

Soon others felt encouraged to try the procedure. Some were pleasantly surprised, like the English neurosurgeon Jason Brice. One patient on whom he performed the operation had an overwhelming fear of fire. "Funnily enough," he told a journalist in 2011, "she finished up after I had done the operation very much better, but she went and bought herself a fish and chip shop with grossly hot oil in it."[111]

At the same time, Meyer's rather pious hopes that the public would not be given unrealistic expectations about the procedure were quickly dashed.

An uncritical media saw to that.[112] In the late 1930s and early '40s, newspaper headlines in the United States and elsewhere touted its benefits: "Sever 'Worry Nerves' of Brain, Restore Insane to Normal"; "Brain Surgery Urged as Aid in Mental Illness"; and "Using Soul Surgery to Combat Worry, Fear."[113] A critical moment in the American media firestorm came in 1941, when the prominent science journalist Waldemar Kaempffert collaborated with Walter Freeman in crafting a fawning long-form article for the popular mainstream *Saturday Evening Post*. Lobotomies, he explained, were bringing light and hope into the lives of those who had previously only known misery:

> From problems to their families and nuisances to themselves, from
> ineffectives and unemployables, many... have been transformed
> into useful members of society. A world that once seemed an abode
> of misery, cruelty and hate is now radiant with sunshine and kind-
> ness to them.[114]

Kaempffert did acknowledge there were risks associated with the procedure. Of a group of patients discussed in the article, three had died (with Kaempffert noting, "Curiously enough, all three were tormented with the desire to die"), and some became "careless happy drones." Yet in the end, he concluded, "Doctor Freeman thinks it is better so than to go through life in an agony of hate and fear of persecution."[115]

In 1949 (thanks in part to Freeman's intense lobbying), Egas Moniz was awarded the Nobel Prize in Physiology or Medicine for pioneering the use of lobotomy in relieving certain kinds of mental illness. No one was particularly outraged; those reactions were still decades away. On the contrary, the press largely heralded this outcome.[116]

As word of the procedure spread, more families reached out to Freeman and Watts. One was Joseph P. Kennedy, recently (until 1940) ambassador to the Court of St. James's of the United Kingdom and father to John, who in 1960 became president of the United States. One of Joseph's other children, Rosemary, had been a pretty and vivacious child but always struggled to learn, possibly because of an oxygen deficit she experienced at birth. Over the years, she had been painstakingly trained

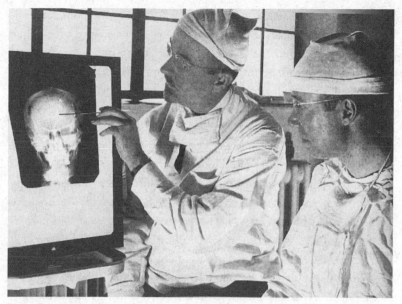

Walter Freeman and James Watts, as pictured in "Turning the Mind Inside Out" by Waldemar Kaempffert, *Saturday Evening Post*, May 24, 1941.

to "pass" in the social circles that the large Kennedy family frequented. As she matured, however, she chafed against the restraints imposed on her, to the point of running away. The family feared that her headstrong nature and impetuousness might lead to a pregnancy, with potentially costly and embarrassing consequences for the family.

Joseph Kennedy was desperate enough to take drastic action. In November 1941, while his wife, Rose, was out of the country, he arranged for Freeman to lobotomize Rosemary at George Washington University. The operation was a disaster. It erased all of Rosemary's intellectual gains. It would take months of therapy before she could walk or talk again. The devastated family then arranged for her to be secretly institutionalized in a hospital in Wisconsin, where she remained until her death at eighty-six in 2005. "All along I had continued to believe that she could have lived her life as a Kennedy girl, just a little slower," Rose Kennedy sadly told a biographer many years later. "But then it was all gone in a matter of minutes."[117]

As the Kennedy family worked through the fallout from this terrible experience, Freeman was seeking to make lobotomy a more accessible and widely available procedure. To this end, he developed a technique that changed it from a major surgical intervention into a practice that virtually anyone could perform swiftly. Transorbital lobotomy (as it came to be called) did not involve opening the patient's skull; it made use of a special pick (Freeman originally used an ice pick) to penetrate a patient's brain via the eye socket. The pick, once in place, was then quickly twisted to sever connections between the brain's prefrontal area and the areas directly below. When Freeman's longtime collaborator Watts expressed outrage and refused to support this new procedure, Freeman struck out on his own. He performed the first transorbital lobotomy in his Washington, D.C., office on January 17, 1946. The test patient was a twenty-nine-year-old depressed and suicidal housewife, Sallie Ellen Ionesco.[118] Freeman felt she responded well.[119] More operations followed in quick succession.

With the simple new technique in hand, Freeman saw an opportunity to vastly expand the scope of its use. Originally, he and Watts had emphasized that it was not appropriate for schizophrenic patients or others deemed "truly insane." But the new transorbital technique changed the equation for him. He did not believe the procedure would remove the hallucinations and delusions from which schizophrenic patients suffer, but he did think it might make them less preoccupied with themselves, less agitated, less tormented by their delusions, more docile, and ultimately easier to care for. Some might even be able to leave the hospital, return to their families, and get jobs.[120] Yes, many might experience a dulling of their personality or lose their capacity for creativity and initiative, but that seemed to Freeman to be a fair price to pay, all things considered. As he put it bluntly in 1945: "Even if a patient is no longer able to paint pictures, write poetry, or compose music, he is, on the other hand, no longer ashamed to fetch and carry, to wait on tables or make beds or empty cans."[121]

In the early 1950s, he undertook a cross-country road trip (which he puckishly referred to as "Operation Icepick") to demonstrate the transorbital procedure in as many state mental hospitals as possible. In one twelve-day period, he supervised or performed 228 such operations.[122] The road show paid off handsomely. Ever more hospitals began to use the procedure, including many VA hospitals that were desperate to do something about the large number of war-shocked soldiers in their care.[123]

Then in 1954, the Food and Drug Administration (FDA) approved the use of the first pharmaceutical treatment for schizophrenia: chlorpromazine (discussed in detail in Chapter 3). It accomplished many of the therapeutic and managerial goals of the lobotomy, but in apparently far less destructive ways. Tellingly, in the early years, many clinicians described this new drug as a "chemical lobotomy." By the early 1960s, the incidence of actual lobotomies was in sharp decline.

For some years afterward, the media and the medical profession maintained an uncomfortable silence about this whole chapter in psychiatric therapeutics. Not until the late 1970s—against a backdrop of mounting vocal criticism of psychiatry more generally—did more and more clinicians begin to say that actually they had never liked this procedure and had always considered it unwarranted and even barbaric. In October 1980 Dr. Thomas Knapp—who had been director of Spencer State Psychiatric Hospital in West Virginia when Freeman came to demonstrate his procedure— told the *Charleston Gazette* that Freeman had just "dropped in. . . . He was a big name in neurology and he had all the proper papers and signatures—all I could do was watch. It was a real grisly thing." He went on with emphasis: "I was never convinced that the operation was helpful, and it appeared to me we were dealing with a sadistic bastard."[124]

CHAPTER 3

A Fragile Freudian Triumph

FIGHTING MALADJUSTMENT

Adolf Meyer never accepted that different approaches to mental illness were in conflict. All "facts," from whatever source, were welcome and would, in due course, contribute to understanding and combating mental illness. Thus, as we have seen, Meyer was an encouraging presence in the rise of virtually all the new biological treatments of the 1920s and '30s. Prior to that, as we have also seen, he left his mark on the American eugenics movement.

But Meyer also played a decisive role in the rise of an important new American movement to combat mental illness that was not biological. Called mental hygiene, it was animated by the belief that many mental illnesses had their roots not in bad brains but in bad habits picked up from living in bad neighborhoods or being raised by bad parents. It was Meyer who named the movement and provided many of its original framing ideas. After World War II, when a new generation of American Freudians inherited mental hygiene's mantle, Meyer's stamp on their thinking was visible everywhere.

The story of mental hygiene begins in 1909, when Meyer co-founded the National Committee on Mental Hygiene, with a mission to research the social and environmental causes of mental illness and to develop strategies for ameliorating them.

In setting up this committee, Meyer worked (not always very harmoniously) with former asylum patient and wealthy citizen activist Clifford Beers. In 1908 Beers had published a widely noted memoir, *A Mind That Found Itself*, in which he described his appalling experiences in a mental hospital. He himself had originally envisioned a movement focused on reforming the often abusive and underfunded state hospital system, and had reached out to Meyer for help.[1] Meyer persuaded Beers to focus instead on reducing the number of people who ended up in such institutions in the first place. And as mentioned, Meyer coined the term *mental hygiene* for this initiative, thereby aligning it with other public hygiene movement of this time: *social hygiene* (which aimed to combat promiscuity and reduce the spread of sexually transmitted diseases), *physical hygiene* (which aimed to teach habits of cleanliness, good nutrition, and fitness), and what was sometimes called *race hygiene* (eugenics, in which Meyer of course was also active).[2] All of these movements in turn came of age during a period in the early twentieth century known as the Progressive Era, when the United States was first coming to terms with the effects of rapid industrialization, urbanization, and immigration. The Progressive Era was marked by great moral contradictions. It was a time when so-called robber barons— late nineteenth-century American businessmen like the Carnegies and the Rockefellers—made huge wealth by exploiting workers and using cutthroat business methods, but it also saw the establishment of the first worker unions and efforts to improve child labor laws. The National Association for the Advancement of Colored People was established in 1909, even as Jim Crow segregation laws structured virtually all aspects of American life. White suffragettes fought to extend the vote to women, but did so in ways that often explicitly contributed to black disenfranchisement. Finally, it was the age of the expert, when lots of things were supposedly going to be fixed by the people who knew best.[3]

With the help of other prominent figures in the field, Meyer and Beers's movement of experts aimed to broaden psychiatry's remit along preventive lines. Psychiatrists should no longer sit in their cavernous hospitals, waiting for mentally ill patients to come to them. They should instead seek to combat incipient mental illness before institutionalization was needed. In setting this goal, the mental hygienists created a new kind of patient for psychiatry: the so-called *maladjusted* person, also a term coined by Meyer. Maladjusted people, he explained, were not truly mentally ill but were at risk of becoming so. One saw such people everywhere: they were the socially awkward ones, the introverts, the evasive ones, the shy ones, the excessively "good" ones, or conversely, the troublemakers or rebels. What all these people shared (different as they might have superficially seemed) was a deficiency in the ability to effectively "react" or "adapt" to the demands of life. As one of Meyer's colleagues, C. Macfie Campbell, put it in 1917, "Mental disorders are disorders of human adjustment, maladaptations, unhygienic compromises, immature or distorted methods of meeting the complex situations of life."[4]

In their effort to prevent or at least reduce incidences of maladjustment, the hygienists initially focused on education. They mounted traveling exhibitions, produced and distributed pamphlets, hired and promoted public speakers, and pitched local newspapers stories. They taught ordinary people how to identify the early signs of disorder, urging parents in particular to bring their maladjusted children to a doctor at once. They offered tips for practicing good mental hygiene at home: avoid alcohol abuse, become aware of the fatal risks of syphilis, avoid overwork, reduce strain, don't suppress feelings but also don't brood, avoid taking refuge in fantasy, and partake in normal social activities. These tips may strike us today as homilies that equated mental health with Progressive-Era understandings of productive citizenship, but the mental hygiene movement wrapped them in a patina of medical authority, and at the time they were taken seriously.[5]

After World War I, the mental hygienists became both more ambitious and more focused. Efforts by Thomas Salmon and others to manage the new disorder of shell shock gave their movement new visibility and status, and now they sought to leverage that goodwill. Having concluded that childhood was the "golden period" for teaching good mental hygiene habits, they reached out to schools and (to a lesser extent) universities, to recruit them as allies in the cause.[6] And they enjoyed considerable success.[7] By the 1920s, teachers in public schools across the country had accepted

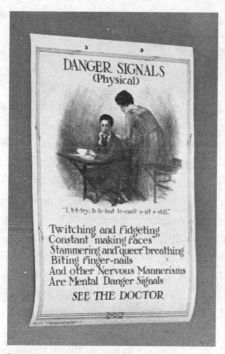

Poster from a public exhibition on mental hygiene, Washington, D.C., 1924. Detail from "Exhibit: Mental Hygiene," National Photo Company Collection (Library of Congress).

that part of their work was to create classroom environments designed to cultivate "well-adjusted" youth, even as they kept a watchful eye out for signs of maladjustment. Books with titles like *Educating for Adjustment* and *Mental Hygiene for the Classroom Teacher* provided guidance for novices.[8] In 1927 the National Congress of Parents and Teachers (with 1.5 million members) went so far as to elect a member of the National Committee on Mental Hygiene as its chairman.

By the early 1930s, some institutions of higher education had joined the cause. The University of Missouri required all college freshmen to take a course on mental hygiene. The 1932 course materials included advice such as "Face reality and all painful situations. . . . Be objective; lose your sensitiveness. . . . Be cool, calm and collected at all times; practice this attitude.... Turn attention from unhealthy ideas but do not repress them.... Regard *Balance* and *Adaptability* as the key-words to mental health and strive for this condition."[9]

When education failed, mental hygienists favored a range of early interventions—and the creation of new kinds of clinics to treat the less seriously mentally disordered. Here too they saw significant success, not least because they were able to attract funding from wealthy, public-minded foundations like the Rockefeller and the Commonwealth. The new clinics went by various names: psychopathic clinics, mental hygiene clinics, psychiatric dispensaries, and child guidance clinics. Some of them offered strictly outpatient services. Others maintained a small number of beds for short-term residential treatment.

One of the first—and certainly one of the most impactful—of such clinics was the Henry Phipps Psychiatric Clinic, set up in 1913 at the Johns Hopkins University School of Medicine. It offered both short-term residential services and an outpatient "psychiatric dispensary."[10] It was the brainchild of William H. Welch, the first dean of the medical school, who had been involved in the mental hygiene movement since its founding. Welch persuaded the philanthropist Henry Phipps to fund such a clinic and then promptly recruited Adolf Meyer to become its founding director.

About this same time, the State of Massachusetts established the Boston Psychopathic Hospital for patients thought to require short-term care only. Imbued with a mental hygienist sensibility, it became an important platform for the development of psychiatric social work (even as its founding director, Elmer Southard, retained classical interests in neuropathology).[11] A few years later, in 1916, the Rockefeller Foundation gave $10,000 for the creation of a Psychopathic Clinic at Sing Sing Prison, near Ossining, New York. The foundation suggested that such a place might be able to "improve greatly the mental and physical standard among prisoners, at the same time supplying the other prisons with a stream of sane, sound men in excellent condition, or with their specific defects accurately known."[12] By the early 1920s, Bellevue Hospital in New York City was running a thriving Mental Hygiene Outpatient Clinic, modeled on Phipps.[13]

The clinics that ultimately had the broadest influence on everyday psychiatric practice, however, were those that targeted children.[14] Known first as juvenile psychopathic institutes and later as child guidance clinics, in the 1920s they focused mostly on the special problems of children born to poor, immigrant families who were presumed to be unfamiliar with modern scientific understandings of parenting. By the 1930s they concentrated more on mostly white, middle-class children with emotional problems ranging from bedwetting to truancy to stuttering.[15]

Each center was staffed by a team: a clinical psychologist ran tests on the apparently troubled child; a psychiatric social worker met with the parents (usually just the mother) to understand the problems at home that might be causing the child's difficulties; and a psychiatrist devised and executed a treatment plan, usually with a broadly didactic, psychotherapeutic focus. By the 1930s, such clinics were fixtures in American cities big and small. Many worked closely with schools, which were glad to refer their most difficult charges to these experts.

During the period that some scholars now call "the long civil rights era" (stretching from the late 1930s through the late 1960s),[16] a small number of African-American activists and clinicians and white liberal allies worked to extend child guidance services to African-American children, at a time when such children were routinely denied care. The pioneering Northside Center for Child Development, founded in 1946, was headed by the African-American husband-and-wife team, Kenneth and Mamie Clark. Later, this couple, but especially Kenneth Clark, offered testimony to the Supreme Court on the degree to which black children living in an oppressive society suffered from self-hate. This testimony played a seminal role in the outcome of the landmark 1954 case outlawing school segregation, *Brown v. Board of Education of Topeka*.[17]

The year 1946 also saw the opening of the Lafargue Mental Hygiene Clinic (named after the Cuban Marxist reformer and physician Paul Lafargue). This clinic was a joint initiative of the white Jewish psychiatrist Fredric Wertham (formerly director of Bellevue's Mental Hygiene Clinic), the African-American novelist Richard Wright, and Earl Brown, the first African-American staff writer for *Life*. Run by an interracial staff, the then-radical position of the clinic was that their patients were no different from white children in their inherent capacities, but their potential was being thwarted by the endemic racist structures of Jim Crow society. As Wright

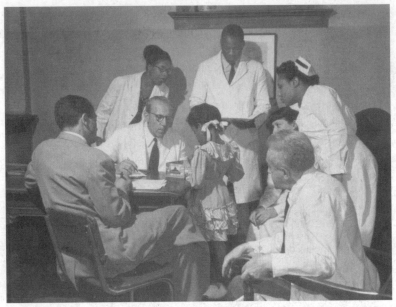

Evaluating a child at the Lafargue Mental Hygiene Clinic, date unknown. Container 215, Fredric Wertham Papers, Manuscript Division, Library of Congress, Washington, D.C.

explained to a journalist from the *Chicago Defender* (an important activist newspaper largely serving African-American readers), "The Clinic has found that the most consistent therapeutic aid that it can render Harlem's mentally ill is instilling in them what Wertham calls 'the will to live in a hostile world.'"[18] For eleven years, the Lafargue Clinic worked out of a basement in a parish house attached to an Episcopal church in Harlem, New York.[19]

By the 1930s, the mental hygiene movement had helped changed American psychiatry's mission. It consolidated an understanding that psychiatry should not focus solely on the mentally ill but should also regard people who were distressed, troubled, dis-ordered, or struggling to "adjust" even if they were not (or not yet) victims of a disease. As this message spread, so did another one: namely, that there was not just "mental illness" but also "mental health," and mental health was something no one could afford to take for granted.

By the late 1930s this "new psychiatry" (as people called it) was becoming increasingly "Freudianized." Concerns about "adjustment" and "maladjustment" blended more and more with concerns about unconscious aggression, anxiety, and repressed feelings. Clinicians in child guidance clinics increasingly looked at troubled children in their offices, and asked, not what bad habits might have brought them there, but what unconscious attitudes their mothers might hold toward them.[20] In these ways and others, rank-and-file Freudianized mental hygienists helped lay the groundwork for the ascendency, after World War II, of a new generation of Freudian psychiatric leaders.

THE "NEW PSYCHIATRY" GOES TO WAR

In the 1930s the groundwork for the postwar Freudian surge was also laid by a shift in the intellectual center of gravity for psychoanalysis from Europe (especially Vienna and Berlin) to the United States (especially New York and Chicago).

In May 1930 Washington, D.C., hosted the First International Congress on Mental Hygiene, with President Herbert Hoover acting as the congress's honorary president.[21] Between May 5 and 10, some four thousand participants from around the world showed up in the nation's sweltering capital. Virtually every American organization with an interest in the prevention and treatment of mental illness organized parallel events: the American Psychiatric Association, the American Psychoanalytic Association, the American Association for the Study of the Feebleminded, the American Occupational Therapy Association, and the American Association of Psychiatric Social Workers. There was even a Conference on Nursing and Nursing Education designed to prepare nurses for work in psychiatric settings. "Never in the world's history has there been such a large gathering of people actively interested in psychiatry and allied subjects," exclaimed J. R. Lord, the British psychiatrist and co-editor of the *Journal of Mental Science*.[22]

He may well have been right; in any event, the congress was a tremendous symbolic triumph for its American hosts and especially for American psychoanalysts, who turned out in force. They gave their European colleagues a royal welcome, warmer than many had ever experienced back home. Some of these Europeans began looking to relocate, and by the mid-

1930s, with the rise of Nazism, the exodus of European psychoanalysts to the United States was in full force. Collectively, these refugee analysts helped infuse American psychoanalysis with new gravitas and intellectual energy. Some also brought in new resources, winning grants from American philanthropic organizations like the Rockefeller, Rosenfeld, and Macy foundations.

The European psychoanalysts did not, however, speak with one voice. On the one side, were the orthodox Freudians who were concerned to safeguard Freud's legacy. On the other side were the analysts who sought to reform the orthodox tradition in a range of ways. In the end, many American-born psychoanalytic psychiatrists allied themselves with this second, apparently more progressive contingent. These American neo-Freudians (as they were sometimes called) tended to be less interested in the sexual secrets of the unconscious than in how to live an authentic life of love and work. Most saw anxiety (rather than sex) as the great problem fueling mental disorders. Many emphasized the central role played by real experiences of safety and love in early childhood (rather than fantasies involving breastfeeding, castration and so on). And virtually all were attracted to the idea that psychotherapy could and should be emotionally nurturing rather than aloof.[23]

Most significantly, adherents of the neo-Freudian tradition emerging in the United States saw it as a *medical* tradition—indeed, as the most progressive and cutting-edge medical path available to psychiatry at the time. Freudian psychoanalysis offered something that neuroanatomy and even serology had failed to offer: a coherent causal explanation for disease that led logically to a strategy for treatment. The psychoanalyst-historian Gregory Zilboorg's 1941 *History of Medical Psychology* helps us recapture this virtually lost understanding. With the arrival of psychoanalysis, he wrote, "the symptoms generated by the cause, and the therapeutic agent revealing and removing the cause were combined in one succession of factors. . . . It was this combination," Zilboorg concluded, "that made clinical psychopathology *a true medical discipline for the first time.*"[24]

When the United States went to war in 1941, many of the new psychoanalytically-oriented psychiatrists went to war as well. As early as December 1940, the psychiatrist Harry Stack Sullivan joined the Selective

Service System as a consultant to develop a screening program designed to identify recruits who were unfit to serve. Sullivan believed the program should exclude not just individuals suffering from mental illness but also those on the border, those deemed to be neurotic or maladjusted. The military officials Sullivan worked with were particularly interested in detecting evidence of homosexuality in potential recruits, since they believed the presence of homosexuals in the military destroyed combat effectiveness and morale.[25] Sullivan (who is generally believed today to have been a closeted gay man) quietly tried, and failed, to have homosexuality removed as a disqualification for military service. Between 1941 and 1944, his screening methods excluded 12 percent (almost two million) of some fifteen million men examined—six times the rate of rejection in the previous war.

Nonetheless, once drafted, huge numbers of men who had passed the screening test succumbed to what was then called "war neurosis" (the word *shell shock* had been abandoned)—double the rate of breakdown during World War I. In 1943 the military therefore shifted resources from screening and into attempts at early intervention.[26] The psychoanalytic psychiatrist William Menninger was appointed director of psychiatry for the U.S. Army and was given generous leeway to develop educational programs to help soldiers cope with emotions that could lead to breakdown: fear, loneliness, hopelessness. He personally drafted a guide, *Neuropsychiatry for the General Medical Officer*, that was sent to army physicians everywhere.[27] Its urgent message was that "every man has his breaking point." Given sufficiently stressful circumstances and inadequate coping strategies, any man could break. The challenge was to understand the conditions that might push one man to that point sooner than another, while implementing sensible policies for rest and recovery to avoid pushing all men beyond their capacities.

What should be done, though, when men did break? Starting in 1943, the psychoanalytic psychiatrists Roy Grinker and John P. Spiegel developed a strategy to treat "broken" air force pilots. The pilots were given the opportunity to rest and enjoy good food, engage in brief, supportive talk therapy, and participate in low-strain occupational therapy. At the same time, they were put through a rapid-fire approach to psychoanalysis called "narcosynthesis." They were injected with sodium pentothal, a newly synthesized short-acting barbiturate that put them in a disinhibited trancelike state that was believed to open up a road to the unconscious mind. The idea was that, in their drugged state, the pilots would be able to identify and work through the repressed memories and feelings that were responsible for their symptoms.

The psychiatrists were, to put it mildly, hugely encouraged by the results: "the stuporous become alert, the mute can talk, the deaf can hear, the paralyzed can move, and the terror-stricken psychotics become well-organized individuals."[28] In 1945 they published a manual on their method, entitled *War Neuroses*. Some 43,000 copies were distributed to officers across various theaters and battlefields.

At the end of the war, as the soldiers all prepared to return to civilian life, the army commissioned the prominent film director John Huston (who had written and directed the 1941 Hollywood film *The Maltese Falcon*) to make a documentary about the therapeutic efforts undertaken during the war to help soldiers recover from war neurosis. Huston, then serving as a captain in the Army Signal Corps, had already made two documentaries on commission for the military, one of which, *Report from the Aleutians* (1943), had won an Oscar for best documentary. This was to be his final commissioned film. It went into production with the working title *The Returning Psychoneurotics*.

To make the film, Huston and his film crew spent three months in 1946 at Mason Hospital on Long Island, focusing on the progress of a small group of young soldiers who were undergoing an intensive eight-week therapeutic program. The film shows them first in extreme distress: shaking, weeping, vacant, mute, stricken with hysterical paralysis, and so on. In ways very much like what Grinker and Spiegel recommended, the men then undergo a mix of group support therapy, occupational therapy, hypnosis, and narcosynthesis, using sodium amytal (a barbiturate similar to sodium pentothal). In the final minutes of the film, the results of all this effort are made clear. They are shown playing that all-American pastime, baseball: the previously paralyzed lad hits a home run; the previously mute soldier is the fast-talking umpire. The final shots show the soldiers departing from the hospital in buses, presumably heading home, while pretty nurses wave them off.

Huston completed the film, now called *Let There Be Light*, in late 1946. But literally minutes before its scheduled premiere at the Museum of Modern Art in New York, two military policemen showed up and demanded

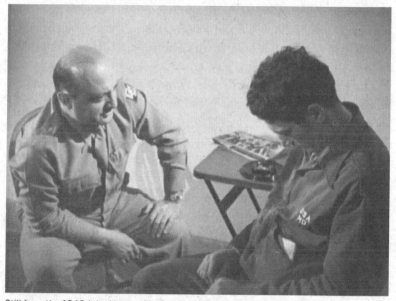

Still from the 1946 John Huston film *Let there Be Light*, showing the military psychiatrist Benjamin Simon inducing hypnosis in a soldier under treatment.

that the print be handed over to them. The War Department then banned all public showings of *Let There Be Light*. For the next thirty-five years, no one other than designated members of the "medical profession and allied scientific groups" was allowed to see this film.

The department's official reason for the ban was concern to protect the identity of the soldiers. Indeed, when Huston looked for the signed releases he had obtained from the participants, they had disappeared. It was obvious to all that the military just did not want the film to be seen: someone in the system had judged it a piece of failed propaganda. Huston himself felt the film was confiscated because it challenged (in his words) "the 'warrior myth' which said that our American soldiers went to war and came back all the stronger for the experience, standing tall and proud for having served their country well."[29] Right or not, the military's decision to ban a film originally supposed to showcase psychoanalytic psychiatry's wartime successes was a disconcerting way to ring down the curtain on this unprecedented collaboration.[30]

After the war, psychiatrists themselves privately agreed that their wartime efforts had been a mixed success at best. They repeatedly noted that, despite the screening program that rejected close to two million men, almost one million additional men broke down in the line of duty—this was two to three times more than in World War I. There was a consensus that too much time and money had been spent on screening and not enough in intervention.

In public, though, William Menninger and other leaders of the wartime effort struck a more upbeat tone. They acknowledged, to be sure, that some returning vets would need help for their psychological problems; for that reason, these years saw the expansion of mental health services within the Veterans Administration (VA) hospitals.[31] But the overall message to the public was that neo-Freudian psychiatry had been critically important to victory in ways (for example) that biological psychiatry, with its shock and surgical methods, had not.[32] The historian Ben Shephard has drily remarked, "It might seem paradoxical that American [Freudian] psychiatry should have emerged from the war with its reputation enhanced when its wartime record was so poor," but it did.[33]

The consequences of that public relations victory would be profound. The Freudian clinicians who had led the effort within the military now felt emboldened to turn their attention to a new project: caring for the mental health of the nation's civilians. "Every man has his breaking point," the wartime mantra went, but not just on the battlefield. How would Americans cope in a troubled, dangerous world that had just witnessed the birth of the atomic age, that was reeling under the recent revelations of Nazi atrocities, and that feared the brutality and anti-Americanism of the Soviet Communist regime? It was time for psychiatry as a whole to commit to tackling this question—and all the arrows to solutions, these postwar psychiatrists said, pointed broadly down the psychoanalytic road.

POSTWAR VICTORIES

In May 1948 William Menninger asked President Harry Truman if he would be willing to send "a message of greeting" to the upcoming annual meeting of the American Psychiatric Association. Truman approved the following statement, which was probably drafted by Menninger himself:

> Never have we had a more pressing need for experts in human engineering. The greatest prerequisite for peace, which is uppermost in the minds and hearts of all of us, must be sanity—sanity in its broadest sense, which permits clear thinking on the part of all citizens. We must continue to look to the experts in the field of psychiatry and other mental sciences for guidance in the evaluation of our mental health resources.[34]

"The greatest prerequisite for peace . . . must be sanity": these words make clear the audacious scope of the proposed postwar agenda for American psychoanalytic psychiatry. The great social problems facing the United States (it was now believed) had their origins not in institutional, political, or policy decisions but in individual psychological deficits. Psychiatry in the postwar era was therefore crucial for any and all efforts to address the great social and political scourges of the age. These included the psychological traits that led populations to succumb to dictators, the persistence of anti-Semitism, the shame of racism, the persistence of chronic poverty, and the problems of social deviance and crime.

And the country, for a while, paid attention. In 1946 Congress passed the American Mental Health Act, which President Truman signed into law on July 3. For the first time, federal support was available to the states for research and professional training in psychiatry and clinical psychology. A key focus was to develop a new generation of clinicians ready to deal with urgent postwar needs—that is, trained in psychodynamic theory and psychotherapeutic methods. William Menninger and his equally active older brother Karl—now running a training center in Topeka, Kansas—were critical in developing the prototype programs.

That this legislation was enacted in support of "mental health," rather than against "mental illness," is telling. "Mental health" was the fashionable new way of talking about issues that had previously been discussed under the rubric of "mental hygiene."[35] True, the public-minded psychoanalysts now calling the shots (Adolf Meyer had retired in 1941) insisted they were a new generation with a new agenda,[36] but most of them had come of age during the heyday of Meyerian psychiatry—and it showed. Though they now mostly spoke of "mental health" instead of "mental hygiene," they were still keen to help people understand the importance of being "well-adjusted," they still worried about the dangers of being "maladjusted," they still spoke of most mental illness as a pathological "reaction" to life's challenges rather than a disease, and they still encouraged schools to teach students principles of good mental health and appropriate social comportment.

The postwar world of mental health, however, differed from the prewar world of mental hygiene in one important respect: it was far less tolerant of biology. The revelation of German Nazi atrocities had tanked the reputation of eugenics, whose agenda had once been seen as complementary to that of mental hygiene. Postwar psychoanalysts also regarded the varied shock treatments being conducted in mental hospitals as palliative at best and destructive at worst, in contrast to their own methods, which they believed went to the heart of mental disorder in humane and effective ways.

In May 1946, impatient with the seemingly hidebound agenda of the American Psychiatric Association (still dominated by clinicians from mental hospitals), fifteen progressive-minded psychiatrists—all influenced by various wartime experiences—met with William Menninger in a "crowded, smoke-filled room" at Palmer House in Chicago to plot a way forward. Should they break with the APA or try to reform it? In the end, they opted for reform, creating the Group for the Advancement of Psychiatry (GAP) to pressure the APA to take action on the critical problems of the time.[37] The psychiatrists responsible for GAP—who often fondly referred to themselves as "Young Turks"—agreed that they would advance their agenda through a range of working committees that would focus on particular pressing issues and release public reports.

Tellingly, the very first report that some of these Freudian "Young Turks" produced was on electroshock therapy—a clear shot across the bow at the APA's biological faction. The report harshly condemned the "indiscriminate use of the technique," the frequency with which it was "abused," and the "complications and hazards" associated with it. In an implicit contrast to the Freudian methods, the authors pointed out that ECT was not grounded in any "adequate theory" and did not get to the heart of disease. Nevertheless, too many hospitals now resorted to electroshock in lieu of "adequate psychotherapeutic attempts," in ways that led "to the neglect of a complete psychiatric program."[38]

A year later, in 1948, another GAP committee produced a report slamming lobotomy — one of the earliest to do so. Lobotomy, the authors said, represented a retrograde "mechanistic attitude" toward mental illness that was "a throwback to our pre-psychodynamic days." It was less a therapy than a "man-made self-destructive procedure that specifically destroys" parts of the brain essential to being human. The report quoted the clinician Gösta Rylander, who had pointed out that after undergoing an operation, patients generally "are shallow and show no depth of feeling." Relatives complained that their family member, postsurgery, seemed to have "lost his soul."[39]

Chafing at attacks like these, some biologically oriented psychiatrists within the APA tried to fight back. Charlton Farrer, editor of the *American Journal of Psychiatry*, declared that he was establishing a rival group to GAP, that he, tongue in cheek, called GUP, or the "Group of Unknowns in Psychiatry." Believing that the GAP leaders had abandoned real medicine for airy psychoanalytic and political agendas, Farrer proposed that GUP's slogan should be "Back to Hippocrates." Again, mocking the alleged absurdities of the Freudian agenda, he concluded by saying that to join GUP, one had first to write a thesis on a topic such as "Group Psychotherapy During Passage in the Ark Which Permitted all Passengers to Land with Sound Minds" or "The Malign Influence of Grandpopism."[40]

But the times were not favoring the biological psychiatrists. They were losing control of training. A 1954 study of psychiatric resident training centers reported that in 1951 (when the information was collected) "the orientation of most centers is described as Freudian or neo-Freudian; however, the resident's own orientation is apt to be in this direction regardless of his center's orientation."[41] By the 1950s psychoanalysts also chaired most academic departments of psychiatry and wrote most of the textbooks.[42]

Biological psychiatrists were also losing control of their field's research agenda. The year 1949 had seen the founding of the National Institute of

Mental Health (NIMH), the first federal center for research into mental illness and mental health. Its founding director was Robert Felix, a psychiatrist who had previously been chief of the mental hygiene division of the government's Public Health Service. Felix's vision for the NIMH's research agenda emphasized both the social roots and the social consequences of mental health challenges. He had been deeply influenced in his youth both by Freudian ideas and by a slew of studies that linked mental illness to urbanization, poverty, social isolation, overcrowding, poor education, and violence.[43] He saw not just psychoanalysis but also social science research as a critical partner in psychiatry's work. For years thereafter, the NIMH's funding patterns would reflect the strategic priorities established by Felix and his cohort. As late as 1963, 35 percent of external grants awarded by the NIMH were for "studies on the psychological, social and cultural bases of behavior." Only 24 percent of grants were awarded to research that had a biological or more conventional medical focus.[44]

A CRISIS OF BAD MOTHERS

The postwar psychoanalytic psychiatrists disagreed on many issues, but they were unanimous on one thing: when it came to mental health, the social environment that mattered most was the family. And the person in the family who mattered most was the mother.[45]

There was nothing inevitable about the fact that they had come to this view. Classical Freudian theory had not taken mothers very seriously. Indeed, Freud himself had sometimes seemed to believe that the only reason a woman might want to be a mother was to compensate for her feelings of inferiority that resulted from not having a penis. And he had sometimes implied that the mother-child relationship was just the prelude to the great Oedipal drama focused on the father.

It took a new generation of Freudian theorists—including strong female therapists like Helene Deutsch, Anna Freud, and Karen Horney—to insist that these classical understandings were nonsense. The experience of motherhood, they argued, was a fundamental and—for the most part—emphatically positive dimension of female psychology, one that should be understood on its own terms. "Its chief characteristic," Deutsch insisted, "is *tenderness*."[46] This was not to say that motherhood was always easy or without pain, as Deutsch also underscored: "There is hardly a woman in whom the normal psychic conflicts do not result in a pathological distortion, at some point, of the biologic process of motherhood."[47] But that was all the more reason, these women analysts insisted, for psychoanalysis, as both science and clinical practice, to take it seriously.[48]

What about the children cared for by these mothers? For most of his career, Freud had portrayed mothers rather instrumentally, as simply a means for satisfying infants' physiological needs for food, warmth, and safety. Only at the very end of his career did Freud consider that the mother-infant relationship might be psychologically critical in itself (perhaps especially for girls). But even as he tried out this (to him) new idea, he confessed himself personally unable to follow through on all its implications: "Our insight into this early, pre-Oedipus phase in girls comes to us as a surprise, like the discovery, in another field, of the Minoan-Mycenaean civilization behind the civilization of Greece."[49]

It fell to others, therefore, to clarify how the maternal relationship mattered—and actually mattered most—for the emotional development of both girls and boys. The initiative was undertaken by a new generation of analysts who came of age in the 1930s and helped spearhead a series of major revisions of psychoanalytic theory in Europe and the United States (ego psychology, object relations theory). While the rise of both ego psychology and object relations theory was a complicated affair, for our purposes the most important thing to know about them is that in contrast to classical psychoanalysis, they gave great weight to the emotional effects of experiences that happened in the first years and even months of life. In so doing, they turned attention away from imaginary castrating fathers and toward real experiences of early maternal care. When it came to infant and child development, mothers mattered, and usually mattered most.

Many of those who insisted on this point had had first-hand encounters with neglect that told them just how true it was. During World War II, many young English children had been separated from their families to avoid the bombings of the big cities or because both parents were working. Some were boarded out to foster families in the countryside, while others were housed in purpose-designed children's residences, such as the famous "war nursery" in Hampstead. There they received generally good physical care, but it soon became clear that something was amiss. Anna Freud, who had by now fled to England with her aging father, observed that many of the children at Hampstead, when they first arrived, first showed signs of severe distress, then descended into apparent listlessness. Many regressed developmentally, stopped speaking, and ceased to be toilet trained. She pronounced them victims of "maternal deprivation" and called for changes in their care. Only when the staff created small family-style units consisting of children and dedicated caretakers did the situation improve.[50]

This work was reinforced by the equally influential work of the child researcher and psychoanalyst René Spitz in the United States. During the 1940s, Spitz studied children who were raised in orphanages or forced to spend prolonged periods in hospitals. His reports documented that they didn't simply regress and become emotionally stunted; sometimes they wasted away physically and died. He called this condition "marasmus" or "hospitalism."[51]

By the early 1950s, the studies of children institutionalized or displaced during World War II had helped create a consensus: children needed an emotional attachment to a caregiver, especially a loving mother, to grow and thrive. Such an attachment was as essential to good health as milk, fresh fruit, and vegetables. The British psychiatrist John Bowlby, who helped formulate the consensus on behalf of the World Health Organization, put it this way: "Prolonged deprivation of a young child of maternal care may have grave and far-reaching effects on his character . . . similar in form . . . to deprivation of vitamins in infancy."[52]

GENDER TROUBLE

All children needed a mother's care, but all mothers were not equal, as the staff working in child guidance clinics since the early 1930s knew well. What kinds of inadequate mothers did these guidance clinics see? A few neglected their children or seemed hostile toward them, but they were deemed rare. The most common problematic mother erred in the opposite direction: she was too involved with her children, in ways that stifled their development and their capacity for long-term independence. David

Levy, a child psychiatrist in New York City, coined a term for this kind of woman: the *overprotective mother*.[53] White middle-class families seemed to have an enormous number of these women, but up through the 1930s there was no real sense that this fact added up to a crisis. Clinics encouraged these mothers to seek therapy (and some of the social workers staffing these clinics even offered it). Some psychoanalysts suggested that overprotective parenting put a child at risk for asthma.[54] Some clinicians posited a relationship between maternal overprotectiveness and marital discontent.[55] Newspapers and magazines warned mildly about the problems of overprotective parenting: "Mother's Perplexing Problems: How Does One Stop Being Over-Protective?"[56] But all in all, not too much seemed at stake.

World War II dramatically changed the stakes, making all questions to do with mental health much more fraught and political. And mothers, because of their assumed critical role in raising mentally healthy offspring, were suddenly a key part of the new conversations. Some of these conversations were catalyzed by struggles within the military to come to terms with the failure of the recruit screening process, which had rejected close to two million young men for "neuropsychiatric" (neurotic) reasons. As we know, a million additional men who passed the screening process nevertheless became emotionally incapacitated during the war, sometimes under circumstances that did not strike their supervising officers as excessively adverse. So what was wrong with America's young men? Why were they so weak, immature, and unstable?

In 1946 Dr. Edward Strecker, a psychiatrist who had advised the surgeon general during the war, proposed that the fault lay with a certain kind of overprotective and domineering mother that he called a "mom." For Strecker, moms were mothers who tied their sons to their apron strings for their own gratification and in this way failed to fulfill the most fundamental responsibility of parenting: to help their boys become mature men. Their coddling had almost lost the country the war, Strecker said, and it was now threatening America's capacity to defend itself against Communism. These women, he said, were "our gravest menace," a "threat to our survival" as a democratic civilization.[57]

Such comments were taken seriously, repeated and discussed by military analysts, by *Ladies' Home Journal* magazine writers, and by *New York*

Times journalists. Some expressed skepticism, but many did not. "His central thesis—that Mom is bad for the son and therefore bad for the country— more than justifies the writing and publication of the book. . . . I want to see her hide pegged out to dry on a tepee," John L. Zimmerman wrote in *Military Affairs* in 1947.[58] Amram Scheinfeld, writing in the *Ladies' Home Journal* in 1945 (and reporting on a lecture by Strecker), did not mince words: "Are American Moms a Menace?"[59]

Strecker's analysis was taken so seriously in part because it resonated with a general postwar fear that the United States was in the throes of a crisis of masculinity. Women had become too dominant, people complained; they were resisting their traditional roles, while men were having difficulty asserting their traditional authority.[60] This perception that traditional gender roles were in crisis had some historical basis. During the war, women had been vigorously recruited to work in factories and other industries that supported the war effort because so many men were overseas. These employment arrangements were supposed to be temporary, as the men would need the jobs when they returned, but at war's end many women resisted leaving the workforce. Consequently, in the 1950s new efforts were undertaken, just as vigorous as the earlier ones, to reconcile women with a strictly domestic role.

By and large, American women did go back into the home, but for many, things were not the same. Discontented and restless, some tried to have careers alongside marriage or demanded more from their marriages. And while some mental health professionals worried about the effects of such discontent on the husbands, most were more concerned about the effect these discontented women were having on their children's (especially their sons') emotional well-being and mental health.

As the consensus took hold that men (and boys) were in trouble because motherhood was in a state of crisis, clinicians gradually broadened their focus beyond the needy, narcissistic mom who had so worried Strecker. There were many ways to fail as a mother, and over time a typology developed. There was the type of bad mother who was seductive and smothering with her sons—she put them at risk of becoming homosexuals. There was the type who was cold and distant—she created an emotionally withdrawn child (who would come to be called autistic). There was still another type who was excessively permissive to the point of being neglectful—she put her children at risk of delinquency. One bad mother type had a specific ethnic identity: the African-American mother, generally supposed to be raising her children on her own, who was said to dominate the household in ways that emasculated her sons. In this way, she failed to help them develop the masculine confidence they needed to survive in a world where the odds were stacked against them.[61]

Of all the types of bad mothers, however, arguably none was more terrifying than the schizophrenogenic mother, who literally drove her children into a state of psychosis. The schizophrenogenic mother was not overprotective; she was also not neglectful. The original view of her instead was that she was a bad-faith mother, a woman with a superficially loving veneer that covered a tyrannical and bullying nature. Refugees from Nazi Germany were among the first to describe this type of bad mother—the term *schizophrenogenic mother* was actually coined by a German refugee psychoanalyst, Frieda Fromm-Reichmann. It did not take long for some of them to suggest connections between her personality type and those of the fascists who flourished under Nazism. A research team based at a VA hospital went so far as to test a cohort of mothers of schizophrenic patients for fascist traits, using a so-called F-scale test (in which F stood for "fascism"). It found that, when mothers tested high for F traits, her schizophrenic children tested high on other personality traits that were supposed to make a person submissive to fascist dictators.[62]

The schizophrenogenic mother in this sense represented the extreme edge of the psychoanalytic discussions about the effects of inadequate or perverse mother love on children. In addition, ideas about her role in creating schizophrenia directly challenged older biological understandings of this disorder. This is significant. Postwar clinicians and social scientists who claimed that juvenile delinquency, racism, military unpreparedness, and even homosexuality had maternal roots were met with occasional skepticism, but they did not encounter an entrenched alternative set of biological perspectives. With schizophrenia, they did.

Why didn't the neo-Freudians just leave schizophrenia to the biological psychiatrists, who had been treating psychotic patients with shock and surgery since the 1930s? The answer, in part, was: exactly *for this reason.*

As we saw in GAP's incendiary report, many neo-Freudians believed the biological treatments for schizophrenia of their day were misguided at best and harmful at worst, and that only psychotherapy could get to where the wounds really were. Only psychotherapy could really cure—and do so in ways that were both effective *and* humane. Understanding this helps us make sense of a comment that Frieda Fromm-Reichmann made in the early 1940s, when staff were considering the use of insulin, barbiturates, or Benzedrine on an unruly psychotic patient: "Do you want to knock him out completely or give him enough to relax and then be able to talk to you as he comes out of it? . . . It seems to me you should give [the medicine] but not deprive him of his doctor."[63]

In the eyes of analysts like Fromm-Reichmann, the "real medicine" for patients with psychosis was their relationship with the doctor, not the drug, because only a healthy relationship could heal them. Something had gone wrong, terribly wrong, for them in early childhood. The mothers who should have loved them and kept them safe had failed to do so. The cure they needed therefore had to be relational as well.[64] By the 1940s, a small number of psychiatrists in Europe and the United States—Marguerite Sechehaye, Lilly Hajdu-Gimes, Sandor Ferenczi, Gertrude Schwing, Frieda Fromm-Reichmann, and John Rosen—began to adapt psychoanalytic psychotherapy into forms that might be suitable as a treatment for schizophrenia. Strikingly, a significant number of these therapists were women, who implicitly saw themselves as the "good mother" their patients had never had.

In a few cases, the assumption was more implicit. The Swiss therapist Marguerite Sechehaye, working in the 1940s, actively encouraged her young adolescent patient to call her "Mama," physically cradled her as if she were a baby, and talked to her as if she were a tiny child. At one point in the therapy, when the patient's desperate pleas for apples appeared to be a cry for a loving maternal breast, Sechehaye symbolically breastfed the girl. In Sechehaye's words:

> To the remark that I gave her as many apples as she wanted, Renee cries: "Yes, but those are store apples, apples for big people, but I want apples from Mummy, like that," pointing to my breasts. "Those

apples there, Mummy gives them only when one is hungry." I understand at last what is to be done! Since the apples represent maternal milk, I must give them to her like a mother feeding her baby: I must give her the symbol myself, directly and without intermediary.[65]

Insight having dawned, Sechehaye sliced an apple and invited her patient to lay her head on her breast and "drink the good milk." The girl did so, while slowly eating the apple, finally at peace.

In the United States, Frieda Fromm-Reichmann for her part became renowned for her willingness to do whatever it took to make an emotional connection with her severely disturbed patients. She would sit in their urine to show them she was no better than they were. She would accept a gift of feces from them to show that she was not rejecting them. In the admiring words of one of her colleagues, Edith Weigert:

> Sooner or later the schizophrenic patient experienced that he was no longer alone, that here was a human being who understood, who did not turn away in estrangement or disgust. This rare moment of discovery—unpredictable and unforeseen like a gift of grace— sometimes became a turning point in the patient's life. The gates of human fellowship were opened, and thereby the slow way to recovery was opened also.[66]

How could shock therapy or insulin injections compete with that?

DRUGS IN A FREUDIAN WORLD

And then drugs arrived.

Until the early 1950s, drugs in institutional psychiatry were notable not only by their absence but also by the extent to which they weren't even being pursued as an option. The psychiatrist Heinz Lehmann recalled the scene in the late 1940s: "No one in his right mind in psychiatry was working with drugs. You used shock or various psychotherapies."[67]

Psychiatrists did not pursue drugs as therapeutic tools before the 1950s in part because they *already used* drugs—as managerial tools, to sedate and calm unruly patients. Since the 1920s, most drugs used in this way were barbiturates. Sold under such brand names as Veronal and Luminal, they were not cures but the "quieting hand" (as one ad put it) to soothe agitated patients and/or help them sleep. The patients who took them may have found temporary relief or been easier to handle, but everyone was clear that their underlying illness was not affected. These drugs did not help patients think more clearly or act more rationally.

Elsewhere in medicine, however, new kinds of drugs were coming onto the market that *did* seem to cure and correct. Insulin, synthetic hormones, synthetic vitamins, and penicillin all became available in the 1950s and received wide public exposure.

Hand in glove with these developments was another, equally important one: the rise of the modern pharmaceutical industry. This industry was the product of a marriage between traditional pharmacy (which for centuries had made medicines from compounds of botanical and naturally found elements) and industrial chemistry (which had emerged out of the businesses that developed the first synthetic dyes for fabrics). By the early twentieth century, industrial chemical companies had discovered that some dyes had physiological effects and might therefore be of interest to pharmacists. The sensible and lucrative result was a series of mergers between various pharmacies and industrial chemistry companies. Ciba-Geigy in Switzerland (now owned by Novartis) and Rhône-Poulenc in France were early and powerful examples of such partnerships. Before the 1950s, however, none of the modern pharmaceutical companies were focused on mental illness, and no one expected any breakthroughs on that front.

And then a substance called chlorpromazine appeared on the scene. It looked a little like sedative of some sort, but it also seemed a completely different kind of fish from the old barbiturates. Quietly, slowly, and inexorably, it began to change almost everything.

The story of chlorpromazine as a breakthrough drug for psychiatry began in France during World War II, when the French Navy surgeon Henri Laborit tried to develop a pharmacological means of reducing or eliminating postsurgical shock. Surgical shock is a life-threatening condition in which the blood vessels constrict, the heart may stop pumping properly, and the body's tissues become unable to properly absorb oxygen and nutrients. No one knew for sure what caused it, but one theory held that it might involve the body overreleasing histamines, a chemical involved in immune and inflammatory responses. That theory was based on the observation that the symptoms of postsurgical shock resembled the severe allergic reactions suffered by some people when they were stung by bees or exposed to pollen. Such reactions were known to be mediated by histamine release. A class of synthetic drugs known as antihistamines had been around since the 1920s, and they were used to alleviate allergic reactions. Laborit now wondered if any of these drugs might be helpful in preventing surgical shock. He turned to Rhône-Poulenc, one of France's major pharmaceutical manufacturers, because he knew they were developing new antihistamines. They sent him samples of a class of antihistamines known as phenothiazines. Like many early pharmaceuticals, these had been originally developed by the dye industry; they made a wonderful blue color when dissolved in water but now were being tested for their medicinal properties.

Laborit, working with the anesthetist Pierre Huguenard, experimented with several of these phenothiazines. The one that gave the most promising results was 4560 RP, which a company chemist, Paul Charpentier, later named chlorpromazine (a simple description of its chemical structure). Mixed with other drugs into a "cocktail" and taken before surgery, chlorpromazine seemed to reduce patients' susceptibility to postsurgical shock by lowering blood pressure and body temperature. But Laborit and Huguenard noticed that patients who received the cocktail also became distinctly "indifferent" about their upcoming surgery, even if they had been very anxious about it before. After surgery, they needed less morphine to manage their pain and anxiety than those who didn't take it.[68] Intrigued, Laborit wondered if the mixture he and Huguenard had devised might have psychiatric uses.

He persuaded some colleagues to investigate this possibility by giving the cocktail to a psychiatric patient. They chose a middle-aged laborer who had been admitted to the hospital because he liked to walk down the street with a flowerpot and occasionally berate strangers; he also liked to stand up and make impassioned political speeches in cafés. In the hospital, this patient had been given a succession of insulin and ECT shock treatments, to little effect. Within one day of receiving the cocktail, though, he was noticeably calmer and less inclined to outbursts. The staff thought his new behavior resembled nothing so much as that of a successfully lobotomized patient.[69]

If mere drugs could accomplish the managerial and therapeutic goals of lobotomies (but presumably without the risks), that would be a real advance. Laborit's efforts to encourage further investigation paid off when a fellow surgeon agreed to ask his brother-in-law, the psychiatrist Pierre Deniker, whether he would do more systematic testing of the drug. Deniker agreed. It was also agreed that these tests would involve only chlorpromazine, without any other sedating drugs in the mix.

In March 1952 Deniker collaborated with his colleague Jean Delay on an open trial. They gave the drug to thirty-eight of the most agitated, uncontrollable patients at the Centre hospitalier Sainte-Anne in Paris. No one was expecting anything remarkable, but the effects of the drug, now used on its own, seem to have startled everyone. The hospital staff said mute and frozen catatonic patients suddenly looked up and connected with them, and violent patients became rational and calm. They spoke of how, within a matter of weeks, Sainte-Anne had become a new kind of place, a quiet place, *un endroit tranquille*.[70]

Several decades later, many would declare that moment a turning point in the history of psychiatry. An early (1978) history of psychopharmacology, published as part of a medical textbook, offered the following, rather breathless account:

> By May 1953, the atmosphere in the disturbed wards of mental hospitals in Paris was transformed; straitjackets, psychohydraulic packs and noise were a thing of the past! Once more, Paris psychiatrists who long ago unchained the chained, became pioneers in liberating their patients, this time from their inner torments, and with a drug: chlorpromazine. It accomplished the pharmacologic revolution of psychiatry.[71]

The revolutionary significance of this new pharmaceutical was visible more in hindsight, however, than it was at the time. Even though Rhône-Poulenc came to believe that the drug had potential for psychiatry, it also continued to investigate its other possible therapeutic uses.[72] And it seemed to have many, from aiding sleep, to reducing nausea and gastric distress, to diminishing the inflammatory response to wounds. Thus, when the company introduced chlorpromazine to the market in France in 1953, it did so under the brand name Largactil—"large action"—to underscore its perceived versatility.

Meanwhile, the American pharmaceutical company Smith, Kline & French bought the rights to chlorpromazine from Rhône-Poulenc. They gave it a different brand name—Thorazine—and marketed it initially as a pediatric antiemetic, mixing it with a sweet-tasting syrup to make it more palatable to children.

With interest spreading in Europe about the possible psychiatric uses of chlorpromazine, though, Rhône-Poulenc decided to market the drug as a new kind of sedative in North America as well. Smith, Kline & French had exclusive rights to market it in the United States, but Canada was fair game. The French company thus sent one of its salesmen to francophone Canada to test the waters. Years later the Canadian psychiatrist Heinz Lehmann, who earlier had said that "No one in his right mind in psychiatry was working with drugs," described a visit that this salesman paid to him and hinted at the enormous consequences that resulted. "It all happened because of a drug salesman." Lehmann was irritated by the salesman's cocky attitude (as described by his secretary—he never actually met the man), and partly for that reason he read the reprints (written in French) that the man had left behind. "It was very strange, they made statements such as this is a sedative that produces something like a 'chemical lobotomy.' Somehow it was different from other sedatives."[73]

Lehmann decided to try the substance on a small number of agitated patients, and in early 1954 he and a resident published their findings in the American journal *Archives of Neurology and Psychiatry*. They suggested that chlorpromazine was actually not just a special kind of sedative and not just a chemical lobotomy but a substance that had a *specific and selective* tranquilizing effect on what they called the "affective drive."[74]

It was a big moment, but it was also still partly a psychoanalytic one. Psychoanalysts knew all about "affective drives"—they talked about them all the time. Logically, if chlorpromazine acted to reduce such drives, psychoanalysts should welcome it. Others soon echoed Lehmann's Freud-friendly way of talking about the drug. The psychopharmacologist Nathan Kline suggested early on that chlorpromazine worked by reducing the amount of "psychic energy" (a Freudian term) in the brain and "thereby lessened the necessity for defense against unacceptable urges and impulses."[75] Later both Kline and Lehmann would talk rather differently about the drug, but at the time the strategy was clear: make it possible for this useful new drug to find a comfortable place for itself in a Freudian world.[76]

In late 1954 the FDA approved chlorpromazine (under the brand name Thorazine) for psychiatric use. It was the first drug ever approved as a specific treatment for mental disorder. Practically every psychiatric hospital in the United States stocked up. Powerful and seductive advertisements placed in psychiatric and mental hospital journals helped create demand. "Disturbed wards have virtually disappeared," trumpeted a 1956 ad in *Mental Hospitals*. Thorazine "reduces or eliminates the need for restraint and seclusion; improves ward morale; speeds release of hospitalized patients; reduces destruction of personal and hospital property; reduces need for shock therapy and lobotomy; increases capacity of hospitals to serve more patients than ever before."[77]

Within a year of FDA approval, Thorazine had singlehandedly boosted the sales of Smith, Kline & French by a third. Within ten years of approval, some fifty million prescriptions had been filled. The revenues of Smith, Kline & French doubled three times over a period of fifteen years.[78]

As remarkable as chlorpromazine was, its coming was only half the quiet revolution effected by the 1950s introduction of drugs into psychiatry. The other half was catalyzed by a different class of drugs, the so-called "minor tranquilizers." They were marketed quite explicitly to the bread-and-butter patients of the psychotherapists: patients deemed anxious, neurotic, not quite well, or "worried well." Manufacturers stressed that they were quite different from chlorpromazine (sometimes now called a "major tranquilizer") given to psychotic patients in hospitals. The minor tranquilizers existed merely to take the edge off things for everyone else.

As with chlorpromazine, no one had been actively looking for a

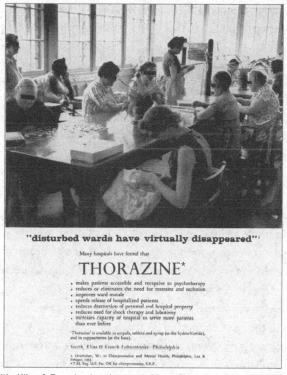

"disturbed wards have virtually disappeared"

Many hospitals have found that

THORAZINE*

- makes patients accessible and receptive to psychotherapy
- reduces or eliminates the need for restraint and seclusion
- improves ward morale
- speeds release of hospitalized patients
- reduces destruction of personal and hospital property
- reduces need for shock therapy and lobotomy
- increases capacity of hospital to serve more patients than ever before

'Thorazine' is available in ampuls, tablets and syrup (as the hydrochloride), and in suppositories (as the base).

Smith, Kline & French Laboratories Philadelphia

1. Overholser, W.: in Chlorpromazine and Mental Health, Philadelphia, Lea & Febiger, 1955.
*T.M. Reg. U.S. Pat. Off. for chlorpromazine, S.K.F.

Smith, Kline & French advertisement. *Mental Hospitals* 7, no. 8 (1956), 2.

minor tranquilizer. Carter-Wallace, the company that created the first one, meprobamate, had previously actually been best known for personal care products, such as Arrid deodorant and Trojan condoms, as well as pet products.

It had, however, once been famous for its patented treatment for neurasthenia, Carter's Little Liver Pills, whose active ingredient was basically a laxative. In the 1940s, it had decided to try to reestablish a profile in pharmaceuticals, hiring several chemists to explore new avenues. One of them was Frank Berger, who in 1950 (working with a colleague, Henry Hoyt) had synthesized a new molecule called meprobamate. Berger had reason to believe that meprobamate would have a muscle-relaxing effect because it was chemically related to myanesin, an existing compound whose muscle-relaxing effects on rodents he had previously observed with interest. (He had been especially intrigued that these effects happened without affecting respiration.)[79]

When Berger tested meprobamate on animals, however, he found to his surprise that it seemed to work less on the muscles than on behavior. It was calming but not sedating, which led him to wonder if the drug might be useful in psychiatry. However, when he broached the possibility of developing it for that market, his Carter-Wallace bosses told him they were not interested. Their own market research had suggested that psychiatrists were unlikely to prescribe such a drug.

After chlorpromazine received FDA approval in 1954, however, the market situation looked completely different. In 1955 Berger therefore masterminded a kind of wake-up call for Carter-Wallace executives. He and a few colleagues produced a short film demonstrating the drug's effects on rhesus monkeys and screened it at a psychiatric meeting in San Francisco. Against the backdrop of excitement over the "tranquilizing" effects of chlorpromazine, no one was indifferent now. Berger's film in fact inspired the head of another pharmaceutical company, Wyeth Laboratories, to ask Carter-Wallace's chief executive if Carter-Wallace would license meprobamate to Wyeth. The executive, hearing this, decided that Carter-Wallace would produce the drug commercially itself, but so as not to miss an opportunity, he also arranged to sell Wyeth *non*exclusive licensing rights to meprobamate. Wyeth came out promptly with a branded version of meprobamate it called Equanil, which is still on the market today.

Carter-Wallace, for its part, rushed out its own branded version of meprobamate that it called Miltown (after the small hamlet in New Jersey, where the company was based). Its ad campaign insisted that Miltown was the "original" brand of meprobamate. According to Berger, there was some concern that clinicians might favor the chemically identical drug Equanil because they liked the name better.[80]

Within a year, meprobamate (and indeed Miltown) had become the best-selling drug ever marketed in the United States, far outstripping even Thorazine. Pharmacies could not keep it on their shelves. Signs reading "Out of Miltown" and "Miltown Available Tomorrow" became familiar sights on drugstore windows. By the end of the 1950s, one in every three prescriptions written in the United States was for meprobamate. In 1957 *Scientific American* marveled that "more than a billion tablets have been sold, and the monthly total of 50 tons falls far short of the demand."[81]

Why did this happen? There are several likely reasons. For one, meprobamate seemed like the perfect Cold War drug. The 1950s was widely viewed (and even ambivalently celebrated) as an "age of anxiety." It was also a time of wonder drugs in medicine. Meprobamate was an apparent wonder drug that combated anxiety. What more could one want?

At the same time, and somewhat in tension with this, the drug was also consumed so freely because there was a common perception that it was hardly a serious medicine at all—no more problematic than a cup of coffee. The popular press did much to frame it this way, calling Miltown and Equanil "peace pills," "peace of mind pills," "wonder pills," "emotional aspirins." Fashionable ladies and hard-driving male executives alike kept their supplies close at hand. In these early days of television, the comedian Milton Berle said frequently that he depended on Miltown, jocularly observing that he had even thought about renaming himself Miltown Berle. Greeting card companies created cute Valentine's Day designs that incorporated the drug, and bars introduced the Miltini—a martini with a Miltown tablet in place of the traditional olive.[82]

Inevitably, some began to worry. Was Miltown contributing to the "softening" of American men? Was it making them complacent and uncompetitive? Was it likely to "make millions of people significantly indifferent to politics—or to their responsibilities as automobile drivers?" asked *Time* magazine in 1957.[83] That same year a nervously humorous *New Yorker* cartoon captured the unease in a different way: "Now remember," the wife admonishes her husband as he departs for the office. "You skip your tranquilizer. Watch for him to take his. Then hit him for a raise."[84]

Unease notwithstanding, the market for minor tranquilizers only got hotter after 1960, when the pharmaceutical company Hoffmann–La Roche came out with an alternative to Miltown that it called Valium. Its chemical structure differed from meprobamate's (it is a benzodiazepine), and Hoffmann–La Roche claimed it acted faster and worked longer. Within a year of its introduction, sales of Valium outstripped those of Miltown, and it became the new most commonly prescribed drug in the United States, a position it maintained until 1982. At the peak of its popularity in 1978, some 2.3 billion pills were sold.

As Valium overtook Miltown in popularity, a shift occurred in the gendering of these drugs. In the 1950s minor tranquilizers were often touted as aids for the pressured and overworked male; they were the "executive's Excedrin." By the 1960s, however, women were almost twice as likely as men to receive a prescription for an antianxiety drug. The profile of the typical patient in the 1960s was the mother unable to cope with her responsibilities, the wife who wanted to work but didn't want to have sex with her husband, the career girl who failed to get married, then feared it was all too late.

The "feminization" of minor tranquilizer consumption has attracted a lot of historical attention. One of the most provocative analyses, put forward by the historian Jonathan Metzl, is that it was one way for clinicians to manage the problem of the inadequate mother and restless wife and thereby mitigate the damage that these women were supposed to be causing their families. If women were less neurotic, dissatisfied, and restless, everyone would benefit, but especially husbands and children. Put another way, the neurotic mother and wife who in the 1950s had been blamed for causing mental illness in her children had, by the 1960s, herself become the patient. If right, this could be seen as yet another way in which the new drugs not only failed to specifically challenge the era's Freudian hegemony but also actively worked to advance a broadly Freudian social agenda.[85]

CHAPTER 4

Crisis and Revolt

WHILE REAL, THE TRIUMPH OF THE NEO-FREUDIAN PERSPECTIVE IN postwar American psychiatry was fragile. Less than two generations on, there was growing talk of its "decline." But drugs, as we have already seen, did not directly cause this decline, certainly not right away. Nor, as we will see in later chapters, did the emergence of new biological theories of mental disorder. American psychoanalysis rather faltered first under the weight of a series of largely self-inflicted wounds. On a number of fronts, its leadership overreached. There were unintended consequences, and as they became clear, more and more critics sharpened their knives, and more and more proponents of alternative biological perspectives saw an opportunity to assert their authority.

DEINSTITUTIONALIZATION

The first front on which the American Freudian leadership overreached and miscalculated had started out, in many ways, with the best of intentions. When, during World War II, psychiatrists worked with soldiers suffering breakdowns, they had found themselves again learning the old mental hygiene lessons about the importance of keeping care within the community. They had repeatedly observed that soldiers who were starting to break down could be turned around more quickly if they were treated near their platoons—the army communities to which they would eventually return. The standard treatment that thus developed was to offer brisk, matter-of-fact, but sympathetic treatment to soldiers on site, while telling them they were suffering from "exhaustion." (Stigmatizing psychiatric language was eschewed.) Standard practice during the First World War had been to ship disturbed soldiers to special hospitals for treatment, but that had generally led to delays in recovery, and some patients had gotten worse. By contrast, the "community-based" approach seemed to really work.[1]

After the war, when psychiatrists turned their attention to the mental health problems of civilian populations, they remained convinced of the importance of basing treatment, as much as possible, in the community. As one former military psychiatrist put it as late as 1971: "From the experiences of military psychiatry have come . . . repeated demonstration that locally based facilities furnish optimum conditions for the prevention, intervention and treatment of mental disorders."[2] The new consensus was clear: admission to a state mental hospital, often far from the patient's home, should always be a last resort.

One of the most passionate advocates of the community-based approach was Robert Felix, a former military psychiatrist, a former chief of the mental hygiene division of the Public Health Service and now the director of NIMH. In the late 1950s, he wondered whether some version of the model of care developed during the war could be adapted to be a model for U.S. mental health care in general.[3]

In considering his options, Felix was particularly inspired by the work of two Boston-based psychiatrists, Erich Lindemann and Gerald Caplan, who had developed a community-based therapeutic approach for survivors of the infamous Cocoanut Grove fire that occurred in Boston on November 28, 1942. Some 492 persons had perished, making this the deadliest nightclub fire in history. Lindemann and Caplan had been summoned to find a way to ease the overwhelming grief, anger, despair, and guilt experienced by survivors. In the end, they mobilized the whole community—hospital staff, schools, youth centers, churches—to help survivors recover. In 1964, Caplan's *Principles of Preventive Psychiatry* described the "community mental health" method they had developed; Felix wrote the foreword, gushing, "This book is not only a primer for the community mental health worker—it is a bible. It should be read by every psychiatric resident and mental health worker in training."[4]

Even as "community" was increasingly touted as the touchstone of progressive mental health care, the mental hospital was denounced more and more as a failed institution. While it had long been criticized, some exposés published right after World War II helped put its problems on the front burner. Spearheading these exposés were a group of young conscientious objectors who had refused to serve in the military on religious grounds and had instead been drafted into the so-called Civilian Public Service Camps. Some 3,000 (out of a total of 13,000) of these young men were assigned duties in mental hospitals. (The other 10,000 were pressed into other kinds of work.) Most of them were appalled by what they saw.[5]

To be fair, they probably could not have come into the system at a worse time: during the Depression, the budgets of mental hospitals had been severely cut, and most of their trained staff were now off fighting in the war. Be that as it may, some of these conscientious objectors felt called to action by what they had seen. They secretly took photographs of the conditions, and after the war, they contacted journalists with their shocking stories.

One of the most famous of the resulting articles was written in purple prose by the journalist Albert Maisel. Published in *Life* magazine in 1946, it was called simply "Bedlam 1946":

> Thousands spend their days . . . locked in devices euphemistically called "restraints"; . . . Hundreds are confined in "lodges"—bare, bedless rooms reeking with filth and feces—by day lit only through half-inch holes . . . by night merely black tombs in which the cries of the insane echo unheard from the peeling plaster of the walls.[6]

Maisel's article was extensively illustrated with photographs smuggled out by the conscientious objectors. These photos, as much as anything else, galvanized public outrage: the patients in those images looked like nothing less than the emaciated and abused prisoners in Nazi concentration camps. The United States had just fought a war to rid the world of the evil of Nazism. Did similar institutions from hell exist in this country?

Maisel's exposé was condensed later that year in *Reader's Digest* under the title "The Shame of Our Mental Hospitals." Editors from the *Cleveland Press* then took up the cause, and the State of Ohio subsequently became the scene of energetic reform efforts.[7] In 1948 the journalist Albert Deutsch came out with one of the most comprehensive exposés to date: *The Shame of the States* documented on a state-by-state basis the appalling conditions of the mental hospitals and called for deep reform.[8]

Some people, though, wondered if calls for reform of any sort might be misplaced. By the 1950s, a growing body of social science research was suggesting that, even under the best conditions, life in a mental institution did not encourage recovery. Instead, it tended to facilitate dependency, cognitive sluggishness, and lack of initiative that made mentally ill patients worse than they would have been otherwise. The British psychiatrist John Wing and the sociologist George Brown, who spearheaded much of the relevant work, christened this syndrome "institutionalism."[9]

At this point some began to suggest, quietly at first, that the existence of the new drugs, especially chlorpromazine, might just possibly open a door through which some patients could escape from institutions like these. In 1956 the journal *Mental Hospital* published a transcript of a discussion led by the psychiatrist Addison Duval, who practiced at St. Elizabeths Hospital in Washington. Duval described how most of the patients under his care who had left the hospital on convalescent leave (a break from treatment), and were on a regime of chlorpromazine, had not returned. In contrast, patients who had been released on leave without drug therapy had returned. Did this not suggest, Duval asked, that under drug treatment, overburdened hospitals might be able to release at least some of their patients?

His question sparked further questions from participants in the discussion. What if patients were stable only on the drugs but not otherwise? Should they still be released? Yes, said one doctor. We should think about the use of the drugs in mentally ill patients the way we think about the use of insulin with diabetes; as a treatment the patient should expect to have to take for the rest of his life. But what if the patients stopped taking the drugs? some asked with concern. Who would monitor them to ensure compliance? Although the discussion raised such questions, it did not answer them.[10]

That said, the existence of the new drugs did not directly drive a decision to begin to empty the mental hospitals.[11] The truth is that since at least the 1930s, American mental hospitals had already been discharging more and more of their patients, not to spare them the indignities of institutionalization but to save money. (A recent examination of census records over this period, however, shows that readmission rates also increased, suggesting that discharged patients may not have done very well.) Nothing much changed in the first years after the drugs were introduced.[12]

The turning point in the historical event we call deinstitutionalization was not the availability of the drugs but the development of a new federal policy conceived not by psychopharmacologists but by the neo-Freudian leadership. The policy was designed to move large numbers of patients out of hospitals and into community-based forms of treatment. And it was in the course of developing and arguing for this policy that the drugs came to matter—as *rhetorical* reference points. The neo-Freudian leadership promised that the policy would work because the drugs would reliably stabilize severely mentally ill patients while they lived and continued to receive care in the community.[13]

The path to this conclusion had been a long one. It was in the mid-1950s that the postwar neo-Freudian psychiatric leadership first persuaded the Eisenhower administration to review the American mental health care system. In 1955 the Joint Commission of Mental Illness and Mental Health was established under the directorship of NIMH director Robert Felix and charged to investigate and make recommendations. The committee took its time. In 1961 it finally produced its report, a ten-volume analysis that boiled down to two unsurprising recommendations: (1) shift most mental health treatment from an institutional to a community-based model, and (2) invest federal funds to reform the state hospital system in ways that would allow it to work in an integrated fashion with this proposed community mental health system.

In the words of the final report:

The objective of modern treatment of persons with major mental illness is to enable the patient to maintain himself in the community in a normal manner. To do so, it is necessary

1) to save the patient from the debilitating effects of institutionalization as much as possible,
2) if the patient requires hospitalization, to return him to home and community life as soon as possible, and
3) thereafter to maintain him in the community as long as possible.[14]

By the time this report came out, Eisenhower was no longer president. The charismatic young John Kennedy, now in the Oval Office, was determined to take broad and bold action on this front. Partly because his sister Rosemary was intellectually disabled, however, he was also keen to ensure that, whatever legislation was passed would improve care not only for the mentally ill but also for persons with intellectual disabilities (who at the time were called "mentally retarded"). His advisers, however, told him that the cost of fully reforming both systems of care would be prohibitive; Congress would never approve it. Still, it was suggested, he could preserve some funds to support new programs for the care of the intellectually disabled if he pushed for just one of the committee's two recommendations: the creation of community mental health centers. Let the federal government invest in those, and let the states then be responsible for reforming the mental hospitals.

And so on February 5, 1963, Kennedy sent a message to Congress urging action. Entitled "Remarks on Proposed Measures to Combat Mental Illness and Mental Retardation," it painted a picture of a world in which "reliance on the cold mercy of custodial isolation will be supplanted by the open warmth of community concern and capability." He provided context: "The new knowledge and new drugs acquired and developed in recent years . . . make it possible for most of the mentally ill to be successfully and quickly treated in their own communities and returned to a useful place in society." Such "breakthroughs," he concluded, "have rendered obsolete . . . a prolonged or permanent confinement in huge, unhappy mental hospitals."[15]

In 1963 Congress passed the Mental Retardation Facilities and Community Mental Health Centers Construction Act.[16] It gave the NIMH responsibility for distributing block grants to the states for the building of new community mental health centers. The states were of course happy to accept the new federal funds, but they proved less willing to invest large amounts of their own funds into improving their own mental hospital systems. Instead, they saw the block grants as an opportunity to downsize and economize. The state hospital system had always cost too much anyway.

Thus began the long exodus of patients from state mental hospital systems, some of whom had been living there for many years, and many of whom left with no clear plan regarding what would happen to them next. Fewer than half of the envisioned 1,500 community mental health centers were ever built—about 650. In addition, federal funds were provided only for their construction, not for maintaining their staff, and the states were generally not prepared to provide funds to run the centers at the levels needed.[17] For these reasons, they were increasingly staffed not by psychiatrists but by social workers and psychologists. These professionals were often good at looking after a troubled child, or a divorcing family in crisis, but were not permitted to prescribe drugs and did not necessarily know how to deal with the severe mental health needs of a psychotic patient.

Meanwhile most state hospitals were never reformed in the ways necessary for them to become part of the overall care of such patients. They were never integrated into the new community mental health system. Instead, as they released more of their patients, their budgets were slashed by fiscally conservative governors and legislators. The final straw came when an extended recession hit the economy in the 1970s. At that point, many of them closed permanently.

The Mental Retardation Facilities and Community Mental Health Centers Construction Act was not the only legislation that drove deinstitutionalization. After Kennedy's tragic assassination and Lyndon Johnson's assumption of the presidency, Congress passed two new federal health insurance programs as part of Johnson's Great Society initiative: Medicare (which funds health care for all persons over the age of sixty-five) and Medicaid (which funds health care for persons living in poverty).

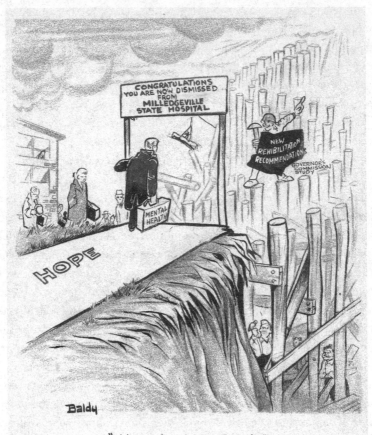

"...You're free to Go Folks!..."

This Clifford "Baldy" Baldowski cartoon depicts people leaving the Milledgeville State Hospital in Georgia. From the *Atlanta Constitution* (c. 1978). Clifford H. "Baldy" Baldowski Editorial Cartoons. Courtesy of the Richard B. Russell Library for Political Research and Studies, the University of Georgia Libraries.

Because Medicare covered the cost of caring for the elderly in nursing homes, patients with dementia who might previously have been sent to a state hospital suddenly qualified for federally funded care in nursing homes. The conclusion seemed obvious: adapt the nursing home structure to allow it to service people with dementia, then move such patients out of the state hospitals and into nursing homes. The rationale was that Medicare and Medicaid between them would then generally cover their costs. But what started off looking like welcome relief for hospitals turned into a growing burden on nursing homes. By the 1990s, that system was in danger of sinking under the strain, partly because payouts for Medicare were significantly cut in the late 1970s.

Medicaid, for its part, had transformed the treatment of the poorest mentally ill, not necessarily for the better. This program covered costs that low-income people incurred when they received care in general hospitals, but it did not cover the costs for transfer to a state mental hospital. For this reason, a system evolved in which many of the poorest mentally ill would receive care for acute conditions in a general hospital setting, and then be discharged, possibly with a prescription in hand, but with no long-term follow-up. Many would repeatedly return, creating what some began to call a "revolving door" of care.[18]

Litigation in the 1970s accelerated the process of deinstitutionalization further, for reasons that, in many cases, were rife with ironies. In 1970, in the case of *Wyatt v. Stickney*, the Bryce psychiatric hospital in Alabama was sued on the grounds that many of its patients had been committed there against their will and lived there without receiving appropriate and adequate treatment. This state of affairs, the prosecution argued, turned such patients into prisoners who had committed no crime and amounted to a gross violation of their civil rights. The court agreed and declared that patients had a right to adequate treatment, which was defined by the court as a humane environment with the least restrictions, guarantees of exercise, religious worship, therapeutic occupation, individualized treatment plans, and qualified staff in numbers sufficient to administer such treatment. Hospitals would have to comply or face huge fines. Unfortunately, virtually all hospitals lacked sufficient funds to comply, so what they did instead was release more patients. Bryce Hospital, for example, was forced by the ruling to discharge half its patient population by 1975.

In 1972 a federal court further ruled that patients in mental health facilities could no longer work at state mental hospitals without appropriate compensation.[19] For over a century, hospitals had sustained themselves by requiring patients to labor on their farms, in their kitchens, and in their laundries. The hospitals called such work occupational therapy, but it was also an economic necessity. Now they had to stop because they didn't have enough money to pay the patients. They also didn't have enough staff to do the work that the patients no longer performed. The result was that most hospital farms and laundries had to close down, the costs of feeding and clothing patients increased dramatically, patients had to spend their days in rooms with largely inadequate programming, and the pressure to move increasing numbers of them out of the system increased further.

Some numbers tell the story. In 1955 the United States had 350 state hospitals with a resident population of about 560,000. By 1977 there were only 160,000 patients in public mental hospitals, a reduction of 71 percent. By 1994 only about 70,000 patients were being treated in mental hospitals around the country. During those years—1955 to 1994—the U.S. population more than doubled, from 150 million to about 260 million. If we assume that the proportion of people with serious mental illness stayed stable over this time, this means that 92 percent of the people who would have been living in public psychiatric hospitals in 1955 were no longer doing so in 1994.[20]

The drugs, as explained, were supposed to stabilize these patients. By the 1960s, however, the initial high hopes for what these drugs would accomplish had been significantly dampened. Clinicians realized that while chlorpromazine (and later alternatives like haloperidol, brand name Haldol) was often effective in reducing delusional thinking and hallucinations—the so-called positive symptoms of schizophrenia—it had little effect on the so-called negative symptoms: lack of motivation and problems in interpersonal relations. This meant that even medicated patients often failed to keep appointments and had continuing trouble caring for themselves. Instead, they might spend all day staring at a TV in a cheap apartment or in one of the many for-profit boarding houses established in the wake of deinstitutionalization. The lucky ones moved back in with their families, who then struggled with their ongoing care (see also Chapter 4). True, the availability of federal entitlement programs (Supplemental Security Income) helped some of these patients scrape by, and many did say that they had no desire to return to the institutions that had released them.[21] Still, even for those who adjusted reasonably well and stayed on their medication, life was usually by no means filled with the "warmth of community concern" that the architects of the community mental health system had promised.

Many, though, did not stay on their medication. With no one forcing them to comply, they stopped taking the drugs that were supposed to allow them to live in the community because they hated how these substances made them feel. Side effects ranged from chronic nausea to a sense of restlessness that some described as wanting to crawl out of one's skin. Many also gained a lot of weight, and a significant number also developed tardive dyskinesia, a neurological disorder that causes abnormal limb movements, disabling facial twitches, and tongue protrusions, usually permanently (today it is believed to be caused by drug-induced supersensitivity of a specific group of subcortical dopamine receptors). Even more developed a (usually reversible) Parkinson's-like side effect of the drugs: a strange shuffling way of walking that was so common that it became known among patients as the "Thorazine shuffle." By 1961, one American survey estimated that as many as 40 percent of schizophrenia patients on a regime of long-term drug treatment suffered from some combination of these symptoms.[22]

One patient, interviewed many years later, painted a fuller picture of what they felt like:

I remember these drugs having a number of unpleasant effects. They wanted me to do ward work . . . and my muscles were so shot from the medication that I couldn't even mop the floor. . . . I also had a dystonic reaction where I couldn't control my tongue and it would contract wildly. Another reaction that would happen was called akathisia. I would get very restless and I would shuffle forward and back.[23]

In the 1990s the short-lived music comedy group Bongos, Bass and Bob summarized the side effects this way:

Well now you take your right arm and you shake it all around,
and then you open up your mouth and you drool on the ground,
and then you try to speak but you just mumble a lot,
so you hold onto your head, cuz it's the only one ya got,
and then you're doing the shuffle, the Thorazine shuffle.[24]

Off medication, many of these patients experienced relief, but they also generally became more psychotic and detached themselves from all support systems. Some ended up homeless, sleeping rough on the street and some even dying of exposure to the elements or a treatable medical illness. Others wound up in prison, after being picked up by the police for anything from disorderly conduct to loitering. Once there, many were put back on medication and given basic care. This happened partly because there were not enough hospital facilities, and partly because the array of court cases and new legislation in the early 1970s had made involuntary hospitalization of the mentally ill vastly more difficult. In this way, prisons slowly became the de facto institutional alternative to the American state mental hospital system, especially for African-American mentally ill persons.[25] Today the three largest mental health providers in the United States are jails: Illinois's Cook County Jail, the Los Angeles County Jail, and New York's Rikers Island.

And even though fiscally conservative politics had largely driven the pace of deinstitutionalization, and drugs had been used to justify the policies, the failure to create any kind of robust alternative system of care for these patients had happened on the neo-Freudians' watch. In due course, their failure to deliver would come to haunt them (see Chapter 5).

WHO'S CRAZY? SOCIAL THEORIES OF MADNESS COME HOME TO ROOST

Meanwhile other trouble was brewing for this group, also largely of their own making. For decades, the neo-Freudians had focused relentlessly on the mental health consequences of bad families, bad neighborhoods, and bad cultural conditions. Over and over again they had insisted that mental disorder was less a medical condition as such than a "problem in living" (to use the language of Harry Stack Sullivan) or a failure to "adjust." Over and over they had turned to social scientists to help them better understand the social origins and enabling conditions for mental illness. By the 1960s, they would start to pay a steep political price for all these choices and approaches, as critics found ways to use these understandings of mental disorder against them. If psychiatry was not in the business of medicine, then what was its business?

One early answer was proposed by the sociologist Thomas Scheff, who received funding in the early 1960s from the Advisory Mental Health Committee of Midwestern States to support hospital-based fieldwork. After watching psychiatrists screen potential patients for involuntary commitment purposes, he concluded that the profession was interested less in disease than in deviance.[26] What did that mean? In his groundbreaking 1963 book *Outsiders*, the sociologist Howard Becker had defined *deviance* as "*not a quality of the act the person commits, but rather a consequence of the application by others of rules and sanctions to an 'offender.'* The deviant is one to whom the label has successfully been applied; deviant behavior is behavior that people so label." Scheff was persuaded that this approach, far more than any medical understanding, could illuminate the psychiatric diagnostic practices he had witnessed: "we can characterize most psychiatric symptoms as instances of . . . rule breaking or . . . deviance."[27]

While Scheff was doing his work in the Midwest, another young sociologist, Erving Goffman, was doing observational research (funded by the NIMH) at St. Elizabeths Hospital in Washington (where he also worked as a physical therapist's assistant). The result was a stunningly critical—and widely hailed—book, published in 1961, called *Asylums: Essays on the Condition of the Social Situation of Mental Patients and Other Inmates*. Goffman's argument was that mental hospitals were less like medical facilities than like prisons and concentration camps. All these institutions worked by taking all personal autonomy from their "inmates" and rigidly defining their social roles. The mental hospital, Goffman suggested, was one of the most insidious of all, because it did not even offer any opportunity to resist—all acts of resistance by the so-called mentally ill (who, after all, had committed no crime) became just further evidence, in the eyes of the staff, of their mental incompetence and illness.[28]

The idea that the mentally ill were an oppressed group who had no ability to resist or assert themselves was taken considerably further in the early 1960s by the philosopher Michel Foucault, whose 1961 history of psychiatry, *Folie et déraison*, made waves almost as soon as it was translated and published in English under the title *Madness and Civilization*. Foucault's argument was that the history of psychiatry was not a story about a medical encounter with the suffering of the mentally ill, but a story of morality and politics pretending to be medical but actually working to discipline and silence the authentic truths of people labeled mad.[29]

Meanwhile the Scottish psychiatrist R. D. Laing was explaining to increasingly enthralled audiences how such bad-faith attitudes still operated in clinics and hospitals. Over the course of the 1960s, he moved in his writings from an existentialist analysis of schizophrenia as a disorder with roots in profound "ontological insecurity" caused by dysfunctional families ("I have never known a schizophrenic who could say he was loved"),[30] to an attack on his own profession for colluding with these families by officially turning these children into patients,[31] then finally to a radical political analysis of the schizophrenic as a kind of thwarted mystic struggling to tell the truth about the ugly state of the world.[32] By the time he published his final major work in 1967, *The Politics of Experience*, he had concluded that the truly dangerous family was not the so-called psychotic family but the so-called normal family who successfully brainwashed its sons and daughters into supporting the era's mad political and social policies:

> The ["normal"] family's function is to repress Eros; to induce a false consciousness of security; to deny death by avoiding life; to cut off transcendence; to believe in God, not to experience the Void; to create, in short, one-dimensional man; to promote respect, conformity, obedience; to con children out of play; to induce a fear of failure; to promote respect for work; to promote respect for "respectability."[33]

At the same time, Laing had decided that the so-called mentally ill—and especially those labeled "schizophrenic"—were not just victims of a dishonest collusion between bad families and bad-faith doctors but were actually heroes: people who, having lost their moorings in the inauthentic world we call normal life, were now on a perilous journey to discover what the world might be like without the masks of false consciousness that the rest of us habitually wear. In Laing's words, "Future men will see ... that what we call 'schizophrenia' was one of the forms in which, often through quite ordinary people, the light began to break through the cracks of our closed minds."[34]

The young Hungarian émigré psychiatrist Thomas Szasz was also emerging in these years, alongside Laing, as a voice of radical dissent within his own profession—and one potentially even more dangerous to his colleagues than Laing. More than any of the other critics of the 1960s, Szasz exposed just how risky it had been for the neo-Freudians to claim that psychiatry was a medical field that nevertheless was concerned not so much with disease as with social and psychological "disorders" that it explained using constructs like "unconscious anxiety," "neurotic reactions," "maladjustment," "inauthenticity," and "problems of living." All real medicine, Szasz insisted, dealt with diseases, and all real medicine was clear that before something could be specified as a disease, there had to be some evidence of organic malfunctioning. There had to be some biology in play.

Psychiatry, however, did not seem to either know or accept this understanding. There was no blood test for schizophrenia, and no X-ray could reveal the presence of a disease called depression or mania. What psychiatry did instead, Szasz said, was to identify persons who behaved in strange, distraught, or unacceptable ways and decide they were sick and therefore in need of its special treatment. It imposed these treatments even if the person in question insisted that he or she didn't want them (something that did not happen in other areas of medicine). Mental illness was thus a "myth" in the sense that it was a false, or at least unproven, belief that gave license to a group of self-identified professionals to infringe on the civil liberties of others. Significantly, it also gave license to psychiatry's so-called patients to play the role of victim and abdicate responsibility for their actions. The 1961 book in which Szasz first articulated these arguments was called *The Myth of Mental Illness*.[35]

The larger real-world stakes of Szasz's argument quickly became clear. In 1962, a year after Szasz came out with *The Myth of Mental Illness*, the University of Mississippi admitted its first African-American student, James Meredith, in accordance with new federal requirements but in defiance of Mississippi's still-extant Jim Crow laws. In response, the white Southern segregationist and former army general officer Edwin Walker successfully orchestrated a night of rioting on campus. The so-called "Ole Miss riot of 1962" led to over three hundred injuries, two deaths, and one-third of the entire corps of U.S. marshals (some 166 men) being deployed to restore order.

Walker was arrested for "inciting, assisting, and engaging in an insurrection against the authority of the United States." Before he could post bond, however, Attorney General Robert F. Kennedy ordered him committed to a mental asylum for a ninety-day evaluation, on the grounds that psychiatrists might judge Walker's violent racism to be a kind of mental illness—a way of thinking that some neo-Freudians had been promoting for decades. If found medically unfit to stand trial, he could then avoid prosecution.

Thomas Szasz at this point intervened and eventually persuaded the hospital staff (who were under no real doubts as to Walker's sanity) to release Walker so he could face justice. In the end, to its shame, a federal grand jury refused to indict Walker, and the charges against him were dropped. Nevertheless, Szasz wrote up the incident in a blistering chapter of his 1965 book *Psychiatric Justice*, which explicitly aimed to expose the willingness of at least some psychiatrists to reframe unacceptable or abhorrent political and ethical behaviors as signs of mental illness, in ways that did not serve justice but actually undermined principles of legal accountability and due process.[36]

In the end, Szasz's colleagues were less alarmed by his critique of neo-Freudian psychiatry's drift toward sociological and nonbiological understandings of mental illness than by his impulse to use that critique to challenge psychiatry's right to operate in the legal arena. By 1963, his position was clear and uncompromising: "My objections to many current practices . . . rest on a fundamental proposition: We should value liberty more highly than mental health, no matter how defined."[37] In 1964 some of his colleagues decided to stage a collective intervention. They invited him to speak at the APA's annual gathering, not so much to engage him as to try to humiliate and (in the frank words of one discussant) "corral" him. One of the speakers, the forensic specialist Henry Davidson, made the stakes clear: "People think that we psychiatrists are a menace to our patients. It is as if, out of all American psychiatrists, only Dr. Szasz has been given the mission of protecting people from the plotting of the other twelve thousand."[38] After this episode, Szasz increasingly sought and found allies and audiences outside his own profession, often with left-leaning political views quite different from his own libertarian commitments.[39]

Among them were various leaders of new patient activist groups, who came of age in the early 1970s and modeled their rhetoric and agendas partly on the civil rights and feminist movements of the 1960s. They were more of a loose consortium than a single, coherent movement, and they went by many different names—the Insane Liberation Front, the Mental Patients' Liberation Project, the Mental Patients Liberation Front, the Ex-Patients' Movement, and the Network Against Psychiatric Assault. All agreed, though, that psychiatry regularly labeled innocent people "crazy" in order to deprive them of their liberties; that its treatments often caused more harm than good; and that the so-called mentally ill were generally an oppressed group who had finally begun to assert their right to live unfettered lives. (The group differed over whether they thought mental illness actually existed.) The world was being educated to recognize the evils of racism and of sexism, these groups said; it was time now to recognize equally the evil of "mentalism"—that is, prejudice against people whom psychiatry has labeled mentally ill. In the words of one of its leaders, Judi Chamberlin, "We must work to eliminate the racism, sexism, and *mentalism* which makes lesser people of us all."[40]

These groups kept in touch with one another—and with the latest radical critiques from academia—through the journal *Madness Network News*, first published in August 1972. Browsing through the issues, one finds repeated excerpts, pithy quotes, and references to Goffman, Laing, but especially Szasz, interspersed with first-person testimonies of abuse. "The history of psychiatry," read one 1974 approving quote from Szasz, "is largely the account of changing fashions in the theory and practice of psychiatric violence, cast in the self-approbating idiom of medical diagnosis and treatment."[41]

Meanwhile the lawyer Bruce Ennis, who came of age during the 1960s civil rights movements, was inspired by Szasz's claim that psychiatry was a profession that engaged in systematic violation of the civil rights of the mentally ill. Ennis had worked for the New York Civil Liberties Union and was particularly struck by Szasz's arguments against involuntary psychiatric confinement. While Ennis was inclined to think that there was such a thing as mental illness—that it was not just a "myth"—he concluded that this hardly mattered. What mattered was the more basic point that innocent people who had committed no crime—even mentally ill ones—should not be hospitalized or given treatment against their will. As Ennis told a journalist for the *New York Times* in 1971, "What Szasz has done is make it respectable for lawyers to challenge the myriad psychiatric assumptions that are the foundations of our current mental hygiene laws."[42]

In 1972 Ennis laid out the legal argument as he saw it against involuntary commitment and forced treatment in his widely read *Prisoners of Psychiatry*—to which Szasz wrote a warm introduction.[43] That same year, 1972, Ennis established, with three other attorneys, the Mental Health Law Project, dedicated to taking the argument to the courts. Within two years, they had about a thousand lawyers on their mailing list. Defendants were identified, and suits were filed. And out of this work came a number of landmark cases—*Wyatt v. Stickney* (1971), *Lessard v. Schmidt* (1974), *Rennie v. Klein* (1978), *Addington v. Texas* (1979)—that would slowly have the effect of shrinking the legal landscape within which psychiatrists could enforce their authority over patients.[44]

In the end, Szasz's most notorious (and, in the eyes of even many sympathizers, unfortunate) alliance was with the science fiction writer and founder of the Church of Scientology, L. Ron Hubbard. Scientology had emerged out of a system of quasi-spiritual mind "cleansing" called Dianetics (originally promoted as a "mental health" practice). In the late 1950s Hubbard had hoped Dianetics would find a prominent place within psychiatry. When that failed to happen, Hubbard's church committed itself to destroying psychiatry using any means at its disposal (as laid out in a once-secret 1966 memo Hubbard issued entitled "Project Psychiatry"). While no Scientologist, Szasz found strategic value in joining forces with Hubbard on his anti-psychiatric crusade. In 1969 he and Hubbard co-founded the Citizens Commission for Human Rights, with close financial and ideological ties to Scientology. Its ostensible mission was a civil rights one: to fight psychiatric abuse and expose corruption; its deeper mission was to destroy psychiatry's authority outright. The organization persists to this day, with Szasz (who died in 2012) remaining its most important in-house intellectual. If one searches the internet, one can still find photos from the early 2000s of Scientology's most famous Hollywood convert, the actor Tom Cruise, cheerfully posing with an elderly Thomas Szasz.[45]

For a period, many psychiatrists working in the trenches did their best to dismiss these various disconcerting challenges to their authority as so much irresponsible noise on the margins. In 1973, however, something happened that was harder to ignore. *Science* published a provocative article written by the psychologist (with an expertise in law) David L. Rosenhan, "On Being Sane in Insane Places." The importance of the article lay not just in what it said, but also in where it was published. *Science* is the flagship journal of the American Association for the Advancement of Science and one of the world's most influential scientific journals.

Rosenhan opened his paper with the provocative question: "If sanity and insanity exist, how shall we know them?" Alluding to the labeling theories of the sociologists, he suggested that mental illness might not actually exist. Diagnoses of mental illness might just be stigmatizing labels that psychiatrists imposed on patients for various disciplinary ends. "The view has grown," Rosenhan observed, "that psychological categorization of mental illness is useless at best and downright harmful, misleading, and pejorative at worst. Psychiatric diagnoses, in this view, are in the minds of observers and are not valid summaries of characteristics displayed by the observed."

This view had "grown" in influence, but was it true? Rosenhan explained how he had tested the matter empirically. Eight sane persons, including himself—people with no previous history of mental illness— went to twelve psychiatric hospitals and pretended they were mentally ill. They told the admitting clinicians that they were hearing voices that said such things as "hollow" and "thud." They reported no other symptoms. The specific symptom they reported was chosen because it had never been reported in the clinical literature before, implying a kind of "existential psychosis." All eight were given diagnoses of either manic-depressive psychosis or schizophrenia and admitted. The minute they entered the wards, they started behaving normally, but now that they had been diagnosed as mentally ill, all their behaviors were interpreted as symptoms of their presumed disease. These behaviors included taking field notes for the study (documented in their charts as "excessive writing behavior").

All the sane pseudopatients were released within 9 to 52 days, all with a diagnosis of "schizophrenia in remission." In no instance did any psychiatrist realize that these people were not mentally ill and never had been, even as other patients on the wards appreciated that fact. Rosenhan recorded how fellow patients would say such things as: "You're not crazy. You're a journalist or a professor. You're checking up on the hospital."[46]

Rosenhan concluded his article by discussing the results of a second, more informal study that involved an unnamed "research and teaching hospital" whose staff had heard about his original study and been told the results but "doubted that such an error could occur in their hospital." They had challenged him to send pseudopatients to their hospital, and Rosenhan accepted. Over a period of several weeks, the hospital staff felt they had identified 41 "stooges" who had illicitly gained entry onto their wards. In fact, Rosenhan had not recruited any pseudopatients for this part of his study: all the people identified by the staff as pseudopatients were genuinely seeking help. Rosenhan concluded, "It is clear that we cannot distinguish the sane from the insane in psychiatric hospitals."[47]

A PALACE REVOLT

Against the growing sense that the Freudian leadership of the past three decades had presided over a slow train wreck, a small but increasingly animated group of psychiatrists began to plot a different course forward. Many of the key instigators were based in the department of psychiatry at Washington University in St. Louis, one of the only major American psychiatry departments that was not chaired by a Freudian (the University of Iowa became another, after George Winokur left Washington University to become chair of psychiatry there in the early 1970s). Not surprisingly, Washington University was dominated by people who didn't have much time or patience for Freudian ideas. As Samuel Guze, one of this cohort, later recalled, "Residents who were looking for something other than psychoanalytic training were always told to go out to St. Louis. We got a lot of interesting residents that way."[48] Another psychiatrist at Washington University during those years, Richard Hudgens, fondly recalled the atmosphere as follows: "What are your data? That became the question. Freud would say something, and it became like Moses saying it. There was a whole concept of orthodoxy in psychoanalysis. Well, here they didn't have anything to do with that kind of, 'because I said so it's so,' thinking."[49] Guze recalled that many of his colleagues began to feel a sense a growing destiny around their approach: "One of the things we began to realize is that there were people around the country who felt that they wanted something different and were looking for some place to take the lead."[50]

Guze and two fellow psychiatrists latched onto *diagnostics* as the starting point for their efforts. To understand why, we need to back up several decades, to 1952 when, with very little fanfare, the APA released the first edition of the *Diagnostic and Statistical Manual* (*DSM*). This manual was designed to replace the *Statistical Manual for the Use of Institutions for the Insane*, first published in 1918 and used by hospitals (in various revised versions) for government census purposes and record keeping. That older book had recognized twenty-two diagnoses, including dementia praecox, manic-depression, general paralysis of the insane, senility, chronic mental retardation, and alcoholic psychoses.

World War II, however, had unmasked lots of new forms of mental distress, and it had become clear that both VA hospitals and the average psychiatrist needed a guide to the new terrain.[51] Written by psychiatry's new psychoanalytic leadership, the *DSM* thus recognized two main classes of disorders: disorders "associated with impairment of brain tissue," and disorders of a "psychogenic" nature "or without clearly defined physical cause." In this second category, the authors included "psychotic reactions," "psychoneurotic reactions," and "personality disorders."[52]

It was an important but not exactly world-shaking moment. Much of the leadership within postwar American psychiatry appreciated the practical need for a system of diagnostics, especially for administrative purposes. They did not, however, believe diagnostics was very important for treatment purposes because what really mattered, most Freudian-leaning psychiatrists thought, was (as Karl Menninger had said) finding out what lay "behind" the symptoms. The psychiatrist Robert Spitzer remembered how, at APA meetings in the 1960s, "the academic psychiatrists interested in presenting their work on descriptive diagnostics would be scheduled for the final day in the late afternoon. No one would attend. Psychiatrists were not interested in the issue of diagnosis."[53]

Knowing this also helps explain the field's rather low-key response to research showing that, when American psychiatrists were asked to independently diagnose the same patient, they tended to agree on the diagnosis only about 30 percent of the time. That is to say, two typical psychiatrists examining the same patient failed to provide the same diagnosis *about 70 percent of the time*.[54] In any other branch of medicine, that would have been scandalous. In psychiatry, it barely registered as a problem.

The St. Louis group was determined to change this state of affairs. In 1978 one of their admirers, Gerald Klerman—then head of the Alcohol, Drug Abuse and Mental Health Administration—described their situation as rather like that of Emil Kraepelin in the late nineteenth century, when he decided it was time to revise psychiatry's approach to diagnostics and bring the profession back into the fold of medicine. Klerman christened the Washington University group "neo-Kraepelinians" and penned a manifesto that summed up what they stood for—one that at the same time implicitly offered a devastating critique of psychiatry's current wayward state:

1) Psychiatry is a branch of medicine.
2) Psychiatry should utilize modern scientific methodologies and base its practice on scientific knowledge.
3) Psychiatry treats people who are sick and who require treatment for mental illness.
4) There is a boundary between the normal and the sick.
5) There are discrete mental illnesses. Mental illnesses are not myths. There is not one, but many mental illnesses. It is the task of scientific psychiatry, as of other medical specialties, to investigate the causes, diagnosis, and treatment of these mental illnesses.
6) The focus of psychiatric physicians should be particularly on the biological aspects of mental illness.
7) There should be an explicit and intentional concern with diagnosis and classification.
8) Diagnostic criteria should be codified, and a legitimate and valued area of research should be to validate such criteria by various techniques. Further, departments of psychiatry in medical schools should teach these criteria and not depreciate them, as has been the case for many years.
9) In research efforts directed at improving the reliability and validity of diagnosis and classification, statistical techniques should be utilized.[55]

On a mission to reform the field, the St. Louis group's first concern was to review all the major diagnostic categories used in psychiatry and better understand how they were being applied in clinical practice. A resident, John Feighner, was assigned to review much of the literature, and in 1972 the group published one of the most influential papers since Freud's *Interpretation of Dreams*: "Diagnostic Criteria for Use in Psychiatric Research" (with over six thousand citations since publication and still counting).[56] Its basic argument was that clinicians could make diagnoses much more consistent across different research sites by operationalizing the criteria, through a method that involved applying standardized checklists consistently. Feighner, the most junior member of the team, became the paper's first author, and the approaches outlined in this paper came to be known as the Feighner criteria.[57]

The psychiatrist Robert Spitzer was heavily influenced by the paper. He had recently finished revising a second (1968) edition of the *DSM* and was now working on a project for the NIMH to develop a diagnostic protocol for assessing depression that would be used for a major epidemiological study. He visited the group at Washington University and eventually collaborated with them. Like them, he became thoroughly convinced that the profession's casual approach to diagnostics was a scandal and a major impediment to its ability to justify its standing as a legitimate branch of medicine.

As Spitzer was contemplating these issues, he found himself unexpectedly recruited by his colleagues to help manage a brewing crisis, one with direct relevance for the diagnostics question. It concerned the status of homosexuality as a mental disorder. For some decades, psychiatry had assumed that homosexuality was a form of mental illness. The first *DSM*, published in 1952, had called it a "sociopathic personality disorder." The 1968 *DSM-II* had defined it more narrowly as a form of sexual deviance, listing it alongside disorders like pedophilia and fetishism. Most psychiatrists felt that the disease model of homosexuality was progressive, certainly preferable to the previous understanding of homosexual behavior as a crime of "gross indecency."[58]

To be sure, as early as the 1950s, a minority perspective had held that homosexuality might be best conceived neither as a crime nor as a disease but simply as an alternative sexual identity. In the early 1950s, during the height of the McCarthy era (when gay baiting was also at a peak), the psychologist Evelyn Hooker had received NIMH funding to study what she called "normal homosexuals."[59] Working with a former student who had first introduced her to the underground gay culture in Los Angeles, she recruited thirty gay male subjects and used standard projective tests to compare their mental health to that of thirty matched heterosexual male subjects. She found that the two groups were effectively indistinguishable.[60]

This would have come as no surprise to many members of the gay community, who had long been forced to hide their sexual identity while living otherwise unexceptional lives. Through the 1960s, momentum quietly grew within this community to find ways to insist on their own mental health and on the right to love whom they chose.

Then in late June 1969, a riot broke out in front of the Stonewall Inn, a gay bar in New York City's Greenwich Village. For years, police had regularly raided and closed the bar down on a range of pretexts. However, on June 28, the crowd decided not to go quietly. Instead, they fought back, first by throwing coins at the police, then by resisting with beer bottles and sticks, as a sympathetic crowd gathered.

The Stonewall Inn riot is generally seen as a key catalyst for the gay liberation movement. Radicalized, energized, and angry, its leaders rapidly developed a political agenda and a list of demands. One of the most important was the right not to be pathologized for their sexual choices. Their fight, the radicals now said, was against not only the police but also the psychiatrists.

Just months after the Stonewall riot, activists attended the annual convention of the APA and demanded a hearing. In one of the most notorious moments from the 1970 meeting, gay activists hurled profanities and accusations at the psychiatrists participating in a session on the use of so-called aversion therapy (electrical shocks) to "cure" people of any tendency to have sexual responses to homoerotic material. The psychiatrists were frightened and enraged; in the heat of the moment, one demanded that the police shoot the protesters.[61]

Fortunately, a more conciliatory mood prevailed. The protesters said, "Stop talking about us and start talking with us," and the APA leadership agreed. At the following year's meeting, the APA organized a panel on "Lifestyles of Non-Patient Homosexuals," in which people talked about their lives as homosexuals and made clear that being homosexual was compatible with perfectly normal and successful functioning. They reminded the psychiatric community of studies conducted by Alfred Kinsey which showed that homosexual behavior—male and female—was a remarkably durable and widespread feature of American society, and that most of the people who engaged in such practices never came to the attention of psychiatrists. Maybe, they said, this was because these people weren't mentally ill. They proposed that the APA eliminate homosexuality as a category from the *DSM*.

This primed the pump, but not until 1972 did matters begin to really change. At that year's meeting, a panel was organized under the title "Psychiatry: Friend or Foe to Homosexuals?" The moderator agreed to add a gay psychiatrist if one could be found. Only one came forward, and only on condition that he could wear a wig and mask and use a voice-distorting microphone. He called himself Dr. H. Anonymous.

Before the assembled company, he explained why he was there and dressed the way he was.

> I am a homosexual. I am a psychiatrist. I, like most of you in this room, am a member of the APA and am proud to be a member. However, tonight I attempt to speak for many of my fellow gay members of the APA as well as for myself. When we gather at these conventions, we have a group, which we have glibly come to call the Gay-PA. And several of us feel that it is time that real flesh and blood stand up before you and ask to be listened to and understood. . . . I am disguised tonight in order that I might speak freely. . . . I can assure you that I could be any one of more than a hundred psychiatrists registered at this convention. And the curious among you should cease attempting to figure out who I am and listen to what I say.

He spoke about the fear, the secrecy, and the shame, and he pleaded for them to believe that it need not be this way for "that little piece of humanity called homosexuality." When he finished speaking, he received a standing ovation.[62]

It was hard to go back to the status quo after this presentation. If unknown numbers of its own successful members were homosexual, could psychiatry in good conscience continue to consider it a mental disorder? If not, what were the alternatives?

The matter was referred to Robert Spitzer, who everyone knew was interested in diagnostics. He met with the activists and his colleagues and established a committee to review the literature. And he ultimately came to the conclusion that "for a behavior to be termed a psychiatric disorder it had to be regularly accompanied by subjective distress and/or 'some generalized impairment in social effectiveness of functioning.' "[63] Clearly many homosexuals were neither distressed (except about social discrimination and stigma) nor ineffective in their social functioning. On this basis, they did not seem to suffer from any kind of psychiatric disorder.

In December 1973, at the recommendation of Spitzer, the APA board of trustees voted to remove homosexuality from the *DSM*. When some people—especially the psychoanalytic leadership—protested, the matter was taken to the full membership of the APA, which upheld the trustees' decision by a majority of 58 percent in favor; the vote was 5,584 to 3,810.

In an interview with the *New York Times*, Spitzer made a highly telling admission about why he thought the vote came out the way it did:

> The reason . . . is not that the American Psychiatric Association has been taken over by some wild revolutionaries or latent homosexuals. It is that we feel that we have to keep step with the times. *Psychiatry, which once was regarded as in the vanguard of the movement to liberate people from their troubles, is now viewed by many, and with some justification, as being an agent of social control.* So it makes absolute sense to me not to list as a mental disorder those individuals who are satisfied and not in conflict with their sexual orientation.[64]

Spitzer emerged from the controversy with a reputation as a skillful negotiator who could get things done. In the eyes of Melvin Sabshin, the APA's medical director, he was clearly the man to spearhead the next—third—revision of the *DSM*, which Sabshin felt needed to be (in his words) an "empirically grounded and functional classification system" that would unite the profession. Sabshin successfully lobbied for Spitzer to be appointed chair of the *DSM-III* task force. The NIMH—then in the doldrums for its failed community mental health program—also got behind the new effort. And to a first approximation, Spitzer was the man of the hour.[65]

Around this time, David Rosenhan published his notorious paper, "On Being Sane in Insane Places," in *Science*. Spitzer led the charge among psychiatrists to challenge it, publishing a two-part, blow-by-blow dissection of what he called Rosenhan's "pseudo-science."[66] He later said he considered it was "the best thing I have ever written."[67]

Even as he took Rosenhan down (in his eyes), Spitzer acknowledged that psychiatry did indeed have reason to be concerned about its approach to diagnostics. Reform was needed—but, he stressed, important work was already under way to deliver it. He then referenced the Feighner criteria that had been developed and tested by the Washington University group and, more recently, by himself and his colleagues in New York. He concluded with a meaningful prediction: "It is very likely that the next edition of the American Psychiatric Association's *Diagnostic and Statistical Manual* will contain similar specific criteria."[68]

As Spitzer and his committee plowed on with their work, a recession hit the United States—and it also hit American psychiatry. Some members of Congress argued that in this era of shrinking resources, NIMH funding should be cut because they were not convinced—after a decade or more of relentless critique—that psychiatric research was a good use of taxpayers' dollars. Insurance companies asked why psychiatrists should be reimbursed for their services when the rationale for the expensive care they billed seemed often so unclear. In the early 1970s, the vice president of Blue Cross put it this way: "compared to other types of [medical] services, there is less clarity and uniformity of terminology concerning mental diagnoses, treatment modalities, and types of facilities providing care."[69] In 1977 New York senator Jacob Javits agreed: "Unfortunately, I share a congressional consensus that our existing mental health delivery system does not provide clear lines of clinical accountability."[70]

The pharmaceutical companies, now emerging as a significant funder of psychiatric research, pushed a related point. By the 1970s the FDA required them to demonstrate the efficacy of all new drugs through controlled clinical trials. But if psychiatric diagnoses could not be made reliably, then how could one be sure that the subjects in a clinical trial all really had the same disorder? Such fundamental questions rendered moot the more granular question of whether a particular drug would be effective for a specific condition. Pharmaceutical companies were not interested in Karl Menninger's exhortation to discover "what is behind the symptom." They needed reliable and straightforward ways to decide who was depressed, who was schizophrenic, who was manic-depressive, and so on.

All external conditions now favored a positive reception of Spitzer's diagnostic reform work. It would take a book of its own to tell the entire story of how he set up his task forces, organized his field trials, negotiated with critics, placated the psychoanalysts (somewhat), and managed the multitudes of people seeking to have their favorite disorder included in his new manual. Others have written such books, and they are very much worth reading.[71]

I will cut to the moment when *DSM-III* was completed: it was a remarkable turning point in the history of American psychiatry, in two ways. First, it effectively expunged all, or almost all, psychoanalytic language— talk about "neuroses," "reaction disorders," and more. (To mollify the psychoanalysts, some references to "neuroses" were retained in parenthesis in the final draft.) Spitzer and his co-authors said they dropped these psychoanalytic terms because their retention would have implied a theory about the etiology or cause of disorders. They intended the new *DSM* to be concerned only with descriptive diagnostics and not with etiology. Of course, they were being disingenuous. They believed that biological—not psychoanalytic—markers and causes would eventually be discovered for all the true mental disorders. They intended the new descriptive categories to be a prelude to the research that would discover them. As one psychoanalyst, Richard Friedman, observed after reviewing a draft, "With this book the American Psychiatric Association has withdrawn its claim to psychoanalysis."[72]

Second, *DSM-III* took its cue from the paper by Feighner and colleagues and introduced an approach to diagnostics that used a system of symptom checklists. Within this system, a patient was to be diagnosed as having a particular disorder if (and only if) he or she had a minimum number of the symptoms on the relevant checklist. The idea was to eliminate, as much as possible, the subjectivity inherent in the freewheeling clinical interview. Field tests had documented that when groups of psychiatrists used the checklist system instead of an open-ended interview, many more agreed that a particular patient should be given a particular diagnosis.

Of course, improved rates of what the *DSM* architects called "interrater reliability" did not mean that the disorders themselves were valid. One could easily imagine a group of medieval exorcists all agreeing that certain symptoms—say, convulsions—should lead to a diagnosis of demonic possession. That did not mean that demonic possession really existed. Points like this were made, and the *DSM* architects responded by saying that one had to start somewhere. In due course, research would reveal the biological correlates of mental illness and thereby clarify which disorders in the book were valid and which were not.

Critics notwithstanding, Spitzer and the so-called neo-Kraepelinians got the book they wanted. Too much had gone wrong in recent years for psychiatry, too much was now in crisis. The field needed a clean break with its past projects and ideologies. The new *DSM* offered the prospect of the start of such a break. In 1980 the APA approved *DSM-III*. After the vote was counted, Spitzer received a standing ovation.

For those who had fought so hard for it, the moment was many things, but above all, it was a "victory for science."[73] In an influential general history of psychiatry from 1997, the historian Edward Shorter summed up the 1980s consensus (as well as his own at the time):

> The appearance of DSM-III was ... an event of capital importance
> not just for American but for world psychiatry, a turning of the page
> on psychodynamics, a redirection of the discipline towards a scien
> tific course, a reembrace of the positivistic principles of the nine
> teenth century, a denial of the anti-psychiatric doctrine of the myth
> of mental illness.[74]

The publication of *DSM-III* was indeed of "capital importance" as an effort to bring about greater reliability in diagnostics. But it was not filled with the decisive results of new biological research into mental illness. So what then was actually biological about the 1980s *biological* revolution? To understand, we need now to turn our attention to the historical transformations of psychiatry's most iconic disorders. New approaches to schizophrenia, depression, and manic-depression (bipolar disorder) all contributed to the biological revolution of the 1980s. Each of them, however, did so on different time lines, for different reasons, and in the service of different agendas.

PART II

DISEASE STORIES

CHAPTER 5

Schizophrenia

DIAGNOSTIC CHAOS

In the late 1940s schizophrenia was largely biological or largely environmental. It was incurable or it wasn't. If curable, it was best treated with intensive psychotherapy, or it was best treated with insulin, electric shock, or surgery. If biological, then metabolic and endocrinological research was the most promising direction, or maybe it was genetic research.[1] If environmental, then it was probably caused by a bad mother, except no one could decide what exactly made her bad. Some said she was rejecting, others called her rigid, others thought she was domineering, and still others focused on her anxiety.

People were diagnosed with schizophrenia if their speech was disordered and disconnected, if they were in the grip of some absurd delusion, if they heard disembodied voices, saw things that weren't there, and/or suffered from unstable, inappropriate, or flattened emotions. People could also receive such a diagnosis if they were odd, antisocial, socially isolated, and/or inadequately motivated to work and take proper care of themselves. The diagnosis was applied both to floridly psychotic and to socially isolated patients, and to confused, belligerent, and underachieving adolescents and young adults. Many patients with this diagnosis lived out their lives in mental hospitals. Some got better, even with little or no therapy, while others managed to eke out a life of some sort on the borders of society.

Were they all really suffering from the same disorder? Clinicians dealt with the chaos by slicing and dicing it into subtypes. There were *acute schizophrenic reactions* (catatonic, hebephrenic, paranoid, and undifferentiated sorts that could not be otherwise classified). There were *chronic schizophrenias* that did not resolve. There were people with *schizoid personalities* (eccentrics and shut-ins who were aloof and often daydreamed their lives away). There were less severely impaired people with *latent, incipient,* or *borderline* schizophrenia. Children with so-called *juvenile schizophrenia,* a disorder that looked very different from the adult form, mostly suffered from an autistic withdrawal from reality. There were even conditions such as *five-day schizophrenia* and *three-day schizophrenia.*[2] The whole thing was a giant diagnostic mess, and thoughtful people knew it. In 1946 the endocrinologist R. G. Hoskins—whose career was largely devoted to pursuing the biological basis of schizophrenia—could nevertheless still ask: *What is it?* "Is it an entity, or, mayhap, merely a semantic convention?"[3] Yet the diagnosis continued to be used, because there was nothing better to replace it.

A FAMILY AFFAIR

By the 1950s cacophony was settling into polarization. One "believed" either in a biological approach to schizophrenia, or in a psychoanalytic and social science approach. As the biologically leaning psychiatrist Ralph Waldo Gerard put it in 1955, "Psychiatry is indeed unhappily schizophrenic, rooted in biological science and the body, and fruiting in social science and the nuances of human interaction. Like the mother church, in the speaker's eulogy, 'There she stands; one foot firmly planted on the ground, the other raised to heaven.'"[4]

Of course, the 1950s polarization was weighted: the Freudians and other environmentalists were the high priests of psychiatry's church. The congregation over which they presided may have been intellectually diverse, but they dominated the pulpit. Nevertheless, it was an open secret that all was not well with their project to pin schizophrenia onto the nurturing style of bad mothers. The lack of consensus about how exactly to define her schizophrenia-inducing behavior had begun to jeopardize the entire effort.[5]

What saved the project was a decision undertaken by a group of researchers to broaden their sights. Instead of focusing only on the mother and her schizophrenic child, they began to insist on looking at the whole family. Their idea was that schizophrenia might be a reaction not just to a bad mother but to pathological behaviors—and particularly pathological ways of communicating—within an entire family.[6] This "family systems" approach to schizophrenia was at once—paradoxically—a challenge to classical Freudian approaches *and* a way of giving such approaches a new lease on life. As one of the early architects of family systems theory later recalled, "Psychoanalysis was the force to be reckoned with—the argument to be answered, the invention to be improved upon."[7]

The foundations for the new approach were largely laid by a 1956 paper, written by the anthropologist and systems theorist Gregory Bateson, in consultation with a psychoanalyst, Don Jackson; an expert in communication, Jay Haley; and an engineer turned anthropologist, John Weakland.[8] Entitled "Toward a Theory of Schizophrenia," the paper proposed that people with schizophrenia might have become so because they had grown up in families in which other members (particularly parents) communicated in inauthentic and logically inconsistent ways—generally to cover up the shameful truths of their actual feelings for one another. A mother might say, "Come hug me, sweetie," then flinch or grimace when the child touched her. Systems theory recognized that flinch or grimace as a "meta-level" communication that contradicted the verbal communication. Upon seeing the child's reaction to her flinch, the mother might then challenge the child's (accurate) reading by saying, "What's wrong? Don't you love your mother?"[9]

Bateson's group named the mutually contradictory communication loop at the heart of dysfunctional families the "double bind." The researchers compared double binds to the insoluble riddles, known as koans, that a Zen Buddhist adept is expected to solve. But they then pointed out that while the Zen adept had ways of transcending the koan's dilemma and achieving enlightenment, the schizophrenic patient did not. As a child, he had no way to challenge his family system and still survive.

His only recourse had been (as the Bateson group theorized it) a flight into madness—a break with reality.[10]

The thesis caught on. *Double binding* became an adjective, often attached in one form or another to women. Theoretically, this approach was committed to a neutral moral attitude toward the individual members of the families being studied. The idea was that it was the system—and particularly communication within the system—that was broken, and everyone supposedly suffered from that fact.

In practice, however, attitudes toward the parents—and mothers in particular—remained as harsh as they had been during the heyday of psychoanalytic mother blaming. Family systems literature repeatedly described mothers as domineering and fathers as weak and henpecked. Some therapists went as far as to suggest that such parents were so unpleasant as to almost overwhelm any capacity they had for empathy. Speaking at a symposium in 1962, one clinician was blunt: "These families can confound our rational theories, dispel optimistic planfulness, and plunge us into . . . therapeutic despair."[11]

Jay Haley, a founder of family therapy, concurred: "The greatest challenge to any family therapist is the psychotic family. Whatever difficulties there are in neurotic families, they are exaggerated to the point of parody in the family of the schizophrenic."[12] One of the most challenging things about "psychotic families," many therapists lamented, was their insistence that they were normal. They would say that they were just like any other family and that they could make no sense of the sudden descent of one of their children into madness.

The therapists, of course, thought they knew better. One popular article from 1962 shared the following anecdote from the clinical archives.

> "As I told you," Mrs. Jones declared, "we just don't have any problems." "Except," the doctor noted, "for Judy, who's sitting here worrying about Communists from Mars." "But I explained that she's never acted like that." At that point, eight-year-old Betsy interrupted, "She was too like this before, mother. Remember last Christmas, when daddy didn't come home from his business trip, and you drank too much again and got sick."[13]

Therapists did acknowledge that parents of schizophrenic children suffered tremendous guilt from being told they were ogres who had failed their children. A few even tried to address it.[14] But most seemed to have little sympathy. One 1954 study rather snarkily suggested that such guilt at least motivated parents to pay the therapists' bills promptly: "it would be reasonably adequate to describe the ideal relative as a person who appeared, gave the history precisely, accurately and directly, and disappeared forever, except for paying his bills—by mail."[15] And certainly therapists had no patience with any attempt by guilt-ridden parents to suggest that their children might have something wrong with their brains. This was simply a tactic, conscious or otherwise, to avoid acknowledging their own culpability. One 1956 dissertation even came up with a name for such blame-shirking parents: "dissociative-organic types."[16]

The social sciences were more open to the possibility that some parents could, in all innocence, believe their children suffered from a brain disease simply because they had not been educated otherwise. In one of the most widely cited sociological studies of the 1950s, *Social Class and Mental Illness* (1958), researchers reported finding that a number of lower-class, uneducated families were tempted to suggest that schizophrenia and other serious mental disorders were inherited or had some kind of biological cause. But then, they pointed out, such families also tended to believe that mental illness could be caused by "the evil eye." All the better-educated families, the researchers reported, knew better.[17]

Louise Wilson, a mother in one of these presumably "better educated" families (the name was a pseudonym), sought help with her husband for their mentally ill son, "Tony," and wrote about it in her 1969 memoir, *This Stranger My Son*. She described scenes with doctors like this:

Mother: "And so it is we who have made Tony what he is?"

Psychiatrist: "Let me put it this way. Every child born, every mind, is a tabula rasa, an empty slate. What is written on it"—a stubby finger shot out, pointed at me—"you wrote there."

Wilson also described scenes between herself and Tony:

"I read a book the other day," Tony said. "It was in the drugstore. I stood there and read it all the way through."

We waited, alarmed by the severity of his expression.

"It told what good parents ought to be. It said that people get . . . the way I am . . . because their parents weren't qualified to be parents."

"Oh Tony," I began, but Jack's signal silenced me.

"I'm a miserable wreck, because both of you are, too. You're queers and you never should have had a child. . . . Even the doctor that I've got here agrees! He says nobody's born with problems like mine!"[18]

Tony's behavior became so threatening that his parents were finally forced to put him in long-term residential care. A few years later Tony was admitted to a hospital for a short time for investigation. His parents were told that he was suffering from schizophrenia and that schizophrenia was a biological disorder that was no one's fault. Having lived for years with the nagging fear that they were responsible for Tony's disorder, they were finally relieved of their guilt.

One might imagine that a mother like Louise Wilson would have been emboldened by the rise of feminism. After all, in 1963 the feminist critic Betty Friedan had come out with her groundbreaking *The Feminine Mystique*, which offered an analysis of the "problem that had no name"—that is, the problem of middle-class white women living affluent or at least comfortable domestic lives but feeling miserable. In the course of her analysis, Friedan had also had some choice words for the Freudian "mother blamers." "Under the Freudian microscope," she wrote tartly, "it was suddenly discovered that the mother could be blamed for almost anything. In every case history of a troubled child . . . could be found a mother."[19] In 1970, a group of radical woman psychotherapists—the San Francisco Redstockings—distributed literature to APA colleagues that included the following pointed suggestion: "Mother is not public enemy number one. Start looking for the real enemy."

The problem with the 1960s feminist challenges to mother blaming, though—especially for families struggling to find help for their schizophrenic children—was that while such challenges might cultivate suspicion among educated mothers that they were being scapegoated, they also offered no real, guilt-free alternative explanation for the suffering of the children. Only biology—apparently—could do that, and none of these feminists took an interest in biology.

On the contrary, they all seem to have continued to accept that the roots of mental illness, including schizophrenia, would be found in political and even familial dysfunctions—just not in ones that made mothers responsible for everything. In her 1972 *Women and Madness*, for example, Phyllis Chesler suggested that mothers of schizophrenic patients probably were on some level being accurately described by clinicians. They should not be blamed for the damage they had caused their children, however, because, struggling to survive in an oppressive patriarchal society, they were as psychologically damaged as their children: "Perhaps the mothers are as hospitalized within their marriages as their daughters are within the asylums," Chesler mused.[20] Similarly, the psychologist Pauline Bart, in her 1971 feminist essay "Sexism and Social Science," condemned the mother-blaming tendencies of psychoanalytic psychiatry but went on to welcome the recent moves toward system thinking—because they would finally hold fathers and other relatives also accountable for the problems of children. "Only recently," she noted approvingly, "have psychiatrists been talking about schizophrenogenic families."[21]

PSYCHEDELIA

The arrival of drugs began to change not only calculations of parental guilt but also calculations of the likely role of biological factors in the genesis of schizophrenia. The drug that originally made the biggest difference to these calculations, however, was *not* the drug we might think: *not* Thorazine (chlorpromazine). That drug, as we saw in Chapter 4, initially rubbed relatively peaceably alongside existing neo-Freudian orthodoxy. It was not seen as particularly destabilizing, either because the early psychopharmacologists took care to frame discussions of its action in quasi-psychoanalytic terms, or because it was assumed to merely "tranquilize" the symptoms of schizophrenia rather than to cure an underlying disease.

Instead, the drug that first began to shift thinking about the causes of schizophrenia was one that we associate with a very different kind of social history: lysergic acid diethylamide, or LSD. The Swiss chemist Albert Hofmann first synthesized LSD in 1938, when he was an employee of the pharmaceutical company Sandoz (now Novartis). He had not intended to synthesize a powerful hallucinogenic drug; rather, he was searching for a substance that would reduce the symptoms of migraine headaches. To that end, he investigated the properties of alkaloid molecules found in a grain fungus called ergot, which had long been used to treat throbbing headaches, accelerate labor, and induce abortions. Hofmann also knew it was a toxin that, when taken in excess, could produce hallucinations, irrational behavior, and convulsions. Hofmann synthesized LSD out of two alkaloids that occurred naturally in ergot: lysergic acid and ergotamine.

The migraine project did not pan out, and for several years LSD languished in the vaults. Then in 1943 Hofmann decided to take another look at its potential. While working with it one day in the laboratory, he accidentally absorbed an unknown amount through his fingertips. He began to experience strong emotions and hallucinated (in his later words) "an uninterrupted stream of fantastic pictures, extraordinary shapes with intense, kaleidoscopic play of colors."[22]

Three days later he deliberately ingested 250 micrograms of LSD, thinking that would be the drug's threshold dose. LSD's actual threshold dose, however, is much closer to 25 micrograms, so the dose he had taken was in fact massive. The result was the first bad LSD trip in history:

> My surroundings had now transformed themselves in more terrifying ways. Everything in the room spun around, and the familiar objects and pieces of furniture assumed grotesque, threatening forms.... The lady next door, whom I scarcely recognized, brought me milk.... She was no longer Mrs. R., but rather a malevolent, insidious witch with a colored mask.... A demon had invaded me, had taken possession of my body, mind, and soul.... The substance, with which I wanted to experiment, had vanquished me.... I was seized by the dreadful fear of going insane.[23]

Hoffmann recovered from this drug-induced insanity, but he clearly had to report such an astonishing experience to the company. So he wrote up a report of his sojourn into madness and shared it with his friend Arthur Stoll, head of Sandoz's pharmaceutical department.

As fate would have it, Stoll's son, Werner, had recently secured a position as a psychiatrist at the University of Zurich. Stoll senior suggested that Werner be given samples of LSD so he could study its psychiatric significance systematically.[24] Werner Stoll did so, following a tradition of research going back to the 1920s, in which clinicians attempted to create states of artificial insanity both in themselves and in healthy volunteers, using hashish (from the cannabis plant) and mescaline (the active ingredient of the peyote cactus).[25]

Werner Stoll's study went on for years, stalled several times because of the war. In 1947 he finally published the results, concluding that in fact LSD created bizarre experiences very close to those experienced by psychotic patients in psychiatric hospitals.[26] Given this, the drug appeared to have potential as an experimental tool: by studying willing volunteers under controlled conditions, researchers could learn more about the inner experience and course of schizophrenia. Clinicians might even take the drug themselves in order develop a more empathic understanding of what their patients went through. Finally, Stoll cited preliminary evidence that the drug had therapeutic uses for patients suffering from neurotic disorders; in very small doses, it seemed to open the mind to previously repressed unconscious material. That, he thought, should interest psychoanalysts.[27]

Stoll also reported a particularly tantalizing finding: when he gave the drug to people who were actually suffering from schizophrenia, nothing much happened. This implicitly raised the question of whether schizophrenics' brains were swimming with some endogenous equivalent of LSD.[28] (Unfortunately, results were inconsistent here: some later researchers found that schizophrenic patients given the drug actually suffered an exacerbation of their symptoms.)[29]

Convinced that something of value could be learned from LSD's mind-altering properties, Sandoz gave LSD the trade name Delysid, promoted it as a "psychosis mimicking" drug, and made it available to qualified researchers and clinicians.[30] In 1949, Dr. Max Rinkel, a neuropsychiatrist at the Boston Psychopathic Hospital, was the first person in the United States to request and then work with the drug.[31] His boss, director of research Milton Greenblatt, recalled later, "We were very interested in anything that could make someone schizophrenic."[32]

By the mid-1950s, at least a dozen centers in North America were experimenting with the drug.[33] A few explored its possible therapeutic uses. Humphry Osmond at the Weyburn Psychiatric Hospital in Canada gave it to chronic alcoholics. Ronald Sandison at Powick Psychiatric Hospital in Worcester, England, used it to break down alleged long-standing defenses in psychotic patients. And Lauretta Bender at New York's Bellevue Hospital (shockingly, from our perspective) gave the drug to young children diagnosed with autism (or so-called child schizophrenia) or suffering from less well-defined behavioral problems.[34]

Most researchers, though, focused on using the drug as a tool to make people temporarily crazy—to create a "model psychosis" that could be studied under controlled conditions. To pursue this work, they recruited subjects from prisons, state mental hospitals, VA hospitals, and college campuses—all more or less vulnerable populations. Some of these researchers received secret funding from the CIA, which was interested in the possibility of weaponizing LSD.[35]

One participant in a CIA-funded study was a graduate student at Stanford University, Ken Kesey, on a fellowship in the university's Creative Writing Center. His motivation for participating was almost certainly monetary; the researchers at Menlo Park VA Hospital offered him seventy-five dollars a session, a substantial sum for a graduate student in 1961. For several weeks, he was given LSD, mescaline, and various amphetamines. Remembering the experience in 1988, he compared it to exploring a haunted house. The scientists "didn't have the guts to do it themselves, so they hired students. 'Hey, we found this room. Would you please go inside and let us know what's going on in there?'"[36]

Meanwhile in England, a junior psychiatry resident at St George's Hospital in London, John Raymond Smythies, had been inspired in the early 1950s by the idea that LSD could be used to create a state of temporary schizophrenia in normal people. However, Smythies was more interested in the potential of another hallucinogen—not LSD, but mescaline—to create such states, because the chemical structure of mescaline resembled that of adrenaline. Adrenaline occurs naturally in the body and is known as the "emergency" hormone that mediates the fight-or-flight response. Smythies speculated that adrenaline's functions might be a clue to understanding the biochemistry behind schizophrenia. After all, adrenaline, after it is no longer needed, must be metabolized (chemically broken down or otherwise altered) into something more benign. Smythies knew the body normally did this through transmethylation, an enzyme-mediated transfer of a methyl group (one carbon atom bound to three hydrogen atoms) from one molecule to another.

What, though, if transmethylation sometimes went awry? Perhaps a hallucinogenic molecule akin to mescaline would sometimes result. The person to whom that happened would then experience bizarre changes in his or her perceptions of the world. And the resulting terror might then trigger further surges of adrenaline, which would then be followed by more faulty transmethylation and more production of the mescaline-like hallucinogen. Any person caught in such a recurring biochemical cycle might eventually withdraw completely from reality and be diagnosed with schizophrenia.

Soon Smythies recruited the British psychiatrist Humphry Osmond to help him explore the possibility of using mescaline to illuminate the biology of schizophrenia. Together the two men sought to confirm the transmethylation hypothesis. The first step was to demonstrate that mescaline in fact was capable of producing a robust schizophrenia-like experience. Osmond agreed to be the test case because he had long been keen to better understand his patients' inner lives. He hoped that several hours under the influence of the drug would help him "see with a madman's eyes, hear with his ears, and feel with his skin." Indeed, the experience was transformative. Osmond realized with a shock that when schizophrenics spoke of seeing boiling skies, having strange beasts stare back at them in the mirror, and feeling menace all around, they were not delusional or simply talking nonsense—they were describing the world as it *objectively appeared to them*. In his report on his experiment, he concluded that mescaline, like LSD, "reproduced every single major symptom of acute schizophrenia."[37]

Inspired by these results, in 1952 the two men published a "new theory of schizophrenia" in the *British Journal of Psychiatry*:

We ... suggest that schizophrenia is due to a specific disorder of the adrenals in which a failure of metabolism occurs and a mescaline-like compound or compounds are produced, which for convenience we shall refer to as "M substance." The striking implications of the relationship between the bizarre Mexican cactus drug and the common hormone have, so far as we know, never been recorded before. Psychiatrists appear to have been unaware of its biochemical structure, biochemists to have been uninterested in its production of an artificial psychosis.[38]

By the time this article appeared, Osmond had left his hospital job in London, where he felt his work on hallucinogens was not appreciated, and accepted a new position at Weyburn Hospital, a provincial psychiatric installation in Saskatoon, Saskatchewan, Canada. There he felt he would have a free rein. Smythies joined him several months later, and later still the two men found a third partner, the biochemist Abram Hoffer.

Osmond at this point expanded his research program to include LSD, because supplies were readily available to him from the Toronto branch of Sandoz. In 1953 he and Hoffer experimented with using LSD as a treatment for alcoholism and claimed remarkable results. Working with biochemists, the team also continued to hunt for their hypothesized "M substance" that was supposed to explain the symptoms of schizophrenia. In 1954 they announced that the "M substance" might have been found: an oxidized form of adrenaline known as adrenochrome. When Osmond swallowed adrenochrome, he experienced strange changes in his perception and mood that persuaded him that this substance had the requisite psychosis-making properties.[39] Matters got even more exciting when, in 1958, the Canadian group, now led by Hoffer, announced that they had discovered adrenochrome in the blood of schizophrenic patients. Everything seemed to be falling into place.

But things were actually about to fall apart. The biochemist Julius Axelrod at the NIMH investigated the claims of the Canadian group and was unable to replicate them.[40] A team of researchers from the NIMH then traveled to Saskatoon to investigate the Canadian group's original findings and concluded they had been misinterpreted—the patients' blood samples had been contaminated by ascorbic acid.[41] The Canadians, and Hoffer in particular, refused to retract their original claims. A testy stalemate ensued. As challenges and criticisms mounted, Hoffer and his research team were increasingly denied opportunities to present their work at major conferences and publish in major journals. They also found it more and more difficult to receive funding.[42]

Meanwhile by 1953, Osmond had become friendly with the literary giant Aldous Huxley, and at Huxley's request gave him a dose of mescaline. Huxley experienced the drug's effects, not as a state of transient schizophrenia but as a mystical experience, an elevated state of consciousness that gave him a glimpse into eternal verities. The two books he was inspired to write about these and later experiences, *The Doors of Perception* (1954) and *Heaven and Hell* (1956), went on to become counterculture best sellers.

By 1955, Huxley was also experimenting with LSD and soon introduced it to American counterculture cult figures like Allen Ginsberg and Timothy Leary. (The latter would go on to promote the drug with his infamous call to "turn on, tune in, drop out.") Huxley persuaded Osmond to work with him to challenge the assumption that LSD and mescaline were simply schizophrenia-mimickers: "It will give that elixir a bad name if it continues to be associated, in the public mind, with schizophrenia symptoms. People will think they are going mad, when in fact they are beginning, when they take it, to go sane."[43] Osmond and Huxley together coined a new word to describe the experience of taking LSD: *psychedelic*, which means "mind manifesting." And in 1956, speaking at a major conference of the New York Academy of Sciences in which many new drugs were reviewed, Osmond affirmed for the first time a radical new view on the positive potential of psychedelics:

> If mimicking mental illness were the main characteristic of these agents, "psychotomimetics" would indeed be a suitable generic term. It is true that they do so, but they do much more.... For myself, my experiences with these substances have been the most strange, most awesome, and among the most beautiful things.... These are not escapes from but enlargements, burgeonings of reality....I believe that these agents have a part to play in our survival as a spe-

cies [because] the psychedelics help us to explore and fathom our own nature.[44]

Meanwhile others in the United States were having their own epiphanies and conversion experiences. Ken Kesey, a graduate student at Stanford University who participated in that previously mentioned CIA-funded study of psychedelic drugs, became persuaded that patients institutionalized in mental hospitals were not really crazy but just nonconformists experiencing their own legitimate form of reality. (While the study was going on, he was also working as a psychiatric aide.) His drug-laced experiences of institutionalized psychiatry inspired him to write a novel, *One Flew over the Cuckoo's Nest*, about a rebel who seeks to upend the cruel and hypocritical culture of a repressive mental hospital. *Cuckoo's Nest*, published in 1962, immediately became a counterculture publishing hit (and in 1975, a counterculture film hit).

Kesey didn't stop there. In 1964 he and his friends, calling themselves the Merry Pranksters, bought a 1939 International Harvester school bus with proceeds from *Cuckoo's Nest*. They put a sign on the back that read "Caution: Weird Load" and a destination sign on the front that said "Further," painted it in bright psychedelic designs, and drove it from San Francisco to New York. The idea was to film the journey and produce a feature film that would make them rich. (This idea failed because it proved too difficult technically to sync the film and sound.)[45] Along the way, though, the group made multiple stops to invite ordinary Americans to take the "acid test"—a glass of Kool-Aid laced with LSD. The experimental drug had now gone completely rogue and was being used to blast open the arbitrary boundaries that psychiatry had built between sanity and madness.

Eventually the countercultural embrace of LSD helped put an end to psychiatric research on LSD. By 1966, the Drug Enforcement Administration had reclassified the drug as a Schedule I substance, with a "high potential for abuse" and without any "currently accepted medical use." In short order, all fifty states declared the manufacture, sale, and possession of the drug to be illegal.

"CEREBRAL PELLAGRA"

Even as LSD was losing its status as a clinical research tool, Hoffer continued to defend the adrenochrome hypothesis of schizophrenia, which had been inspired by studies of mescaline. He pushed on, not only because he believed his team was right (and that the investigators from the NIMH were small-minded and wrong) but also because he believed that the adrenochrome hypothesis raised hope for a cure for schizophrenia—a cure rooted in megadoses of B-vitamins.

To understand how, we need to go back to an almost-forgotten disorder, common in the early twentieth century, called pellagra. Pellagra (meaning "rough skin") was initially diagnosed by the appearance of scaly red skin lesions that often darkened over time. Sores in the mouth followed, along with gastrointestinal distress, growing paralysis and nerve damage, mental confusion, emotional lability, and eventually outright dementia. Pellagra was often fatal and seemed to afflict mostly poor rural farm workers, immigrants, and others prejudicially assumed to be of lesser stock. Women were also supposed to be more vulnerable than men. And in the United States, many more blacks than whites tended to succumb.

In 1907 the American physician James Searcy formally described the disease, using records gleaned mostly from the Mount Vernon Hospital for the Colored Insane in Alabama.[46] With germ theory in these years offering a new way of making sense of disease, physicians generally assumed pellagra was an infectious disease brought on by dirty living conditions or perhaps by the moldy corn that was a staple of many poor southern diets.

There was, however, a minority view about pellagra, promoted especially by an immigrant physician from Slovakia, Joseph Goldberger. In the 1910s and '20s, he studied dogs suffering from a canine equivalent of pellagra, black tongue,[47] and became convinced that the disease in humans was caused by a poor starchy diet lacking meat, milk, and vegetables. Few listened, and many, especially in the southern states, were offended by the claim.[48]

Then in the late 1930s, the American biochemist Conrad Elvehjem offered evidence that Goldberger had been right, even though he had failed to understand the specific element missing in the diets of many poor southerners. Pellagra (and its animal equivalents) resulted from a deficiency of nicotinic acid (niacin, or vitamin B3), a nutrient found in liver, meat, and yeast but absent in corn. (He and his colleagues had isolated it from liver extracts). If one gave large doses of the nutrient (either directly or through an improved diet) to affected animals, they recovered.[49] The same subsequently proved true of human patients. All this added up to a success story hardly less stunning than the discovery of insulin as a treatment for diabetes, or penicillin as a treatment for syphilis.

Coming back now to schizophrenia: Hoffer was keenly aware of Elvehjem's work; prior to studying medicine, he had completed a Ph.D. in biochemistry and had written his dissertation on the B vitamins. A further recent finding, that vitamin B3 was a methyl group acceptor, suggested to him a novel treatment strategy for schizophrenia: if the body produced adrenochrome through a pathological transmethylation process, and *if* (Hoffer's hypothesis) the presence of adrenochrome made people psychotic, then one could potentially treat psychosis by using B3 to "mop up" the methyl groups responsible for producing this crazy-making chemical.[50] Put another way, it might be possible to understand schizophrenia as a kind of "cerebral pellagra" and to treat it the way one treated true pellagra.

Hoffer's group at the Weyburn Hospital thus began dosing schizophrenic patients with extremely large amounts (a minimum of 3 grams) of B3 vitamins daily, either nicotinamide or nicotinic acid. In 1957 their formal placebo-controlled clinical trial involving thirty patients claimed a stunning 88 percent success rate in schizophrenia patients who had been put on the B3 vitamin regime, as measured by their ability to stay out of the hospital and find employment. In contrast, only 33 percent of patients in the placebo group improved and remained well one year after treatment.[51]

By 1966, persuaded that their evidence now spoke for itself,[52] Hoffer and Osmond (working with a professional ghost writer) published *How to Live with Schizophrenia* for the general public. The book not only outlined the rationale for treating schizophrenia with vitamin B3 but also attacked the "myth" that mothers and families caused schizophrenia. They pushed instead for families to adopt a regime of vitamin treatment, one that could perhaps be supplemented at the beginning by chlorpromazine to manage the disease's acute symptoms, giving the vitamins a chance to slowly bring the body and brain back into balance.

As luck would have it, the Nobel Prize–winning biochemist Linus Pauling knew several families who had tried Hoffer and Osmond's treatment formula. One day he picked up a copy of *How to Live with Schizophrenia* and found himself impressed.[53] He reached out to the Canadian group and offered his support. They were thrilled to accept it, not least because they were suffering increasing pushback from mainstream colleagues and having trouble finding journals willing to publish their ideas. By 1967, those difficulties had led them to establish their own publication, the *Journal of Schizophrenia*. They now invited Pauling to serve on the editorial board, and he accepted. The following year, in *Science*, Pauling christened the field of megavitamin treatment for mental illness "orthomolecular psychiatry" and called explicit attention to the Canadian group's allegedly remarkable results using vitamins to treat what Pauling himself called "cerebral pellagra" (schizophrenia).[54]

Mainstream psychiatry was far less impressed. In the early 1970s, the APA established a task force to thoroughly review the treatment. Its 1973 report, "Megavitamin and Orthomolecular Therapy in Psychiatry," was about as damning as could be: "The hypothetical structure on which megavitamin therapy is based has little scientific support, and...legitimate empirical attempts at scientific replication have failed." While the authors initially took a measured tone, in the final paragraphs they indulged in some decidedly heated rhetoric: "This Task Force considers the massive publicity which they [the Canadian group] promulgate via radio, the lay press and popular books, using catch phrases which are really misnomers like 'megavitamin therapy' and 'orthomolecular treatment,' to be deplorable."[55]

INVENTING NEUROCHEMISTRY

Meanwhile, dramatic changes were afoot in thinking about brain functioning in general, changes that eventually would set a new direction for approaching the biochemistry of mental disorders. For decades, it had been known that certain chemicals found both inside and outside the body (nicotine, adrenaline, curare, etc.) could be injected into nerves and cause responses similar to the those caused by electrical stimulation. A few people had suggested that this must mean that nerves possessed some kind of chemical "receptor substance" that interacted with the drugs. For decades, though, this kind of talk did not really go anywhere. Up until the 1960s, most people believed that brain neurons communicated with one another through electrical impulses. Neurochemistry as a field barely existed.[56]

It *barely* existed, but it did exist—and to the extent that it did, it was in no small part thanks to the path-breaking work of the English biochemist Henry Dale and the Austrian biochemist Otto Loewi, who in 1936 shared the Nobel Prize for Physiology or Medicine.

Early in the twentieth century, Dale's employer, Wellcome Laboratories, had asked him to investigate the commercial potential of the ergot family of drugs. His efforts yielded a treasure trove of promising synthetic substances, from histamine and tyramine to a substance he called acetylcholine. As part of his effort to discover possible clinical uses for acetylcholine, he injected the drug into the vagus nerve of rabbits. He knew that electrical stimulation of this nerve slowed down the heart rate, and his experiment revealed that the drug slowed down the heart rate just as much. The effect was so striking that Dale wondered whether it was a natural one—whether acetylcholine might actually be produced in the body and then released by the vagus nerve in order to alter the heart rate.

In 1921 his younger colleague Loewi figured out a way to test Dale's idea. The idea came to him, he said, in a dream. As he told the story, he woke up from the dream, leaped out of bed, and conducted the experiment. It involved dissecting the beating hearts of two frogs and perfusing them with saline solution (specifically Ringer's solution, consisting of several salts). One heart still had its vagus and sympathetic nerves attached. Using a battery, he stimulated the vagus nerve of that heart, and its rate slowed down just as he had expected. He then took some of the solution bathing that heart and dripped it into the solution perfusing the second heart, which had been stripped of its vagus and sympathetic nerves. After a brief pause, the second heart's rate also slowed down. Given that the second heart had been stripped of its vagus and sympathetic nerves, this slowing must have been caused by a chemical substance that the first heart had released in response to the electrical stimulation. Loewi called this substance *Vagusstoff* (vagus substance) and strongly suspected it was Dale's acetylcholine (as indeed it would prove to be).

Loewi then carried out another experiment, but this time he electrically stimulated the sympathetic nerve of the first heart instead of the vagus nerve, which caused it to speed up. After again transferring fluid from the first to the second heart, he observed that the rate of the second heart also accelerated. He called this new unknown substance *Acceleransstoff* (accelerating substance), which he suspected was adrenaline, a chemical known to cause heart rates to accelerate. (The substance later proved to be norepinephrine—also known as noradrenaline—a molecule very similar to adrenaline.) Others then continued this line of experiments, eventually showing that acetylcholine affected the whole range of functions carried out by the autonomic nervous system.[57]

All this work persuaded most physiologists that some chemicals could act to reset or alter physiological functions. Most assumed, though, that they were involved only when the nerves communicated with visceral organs such as the heart. There was little thought that the brain itself might use chemical messengers—even after studies in the 1940s showed, tantalizingly, that acetylcholine was present in the central nervous system.

SEROTONIN

In the end, acetylcholine was not the chemical that made people think twice. It was serotonin. This chemical was discovered in the 1930s in gut tissue. Then in the 1940s a group of researchers at the Cleveland Clinic Foundation painstakingly extracted and isolated the chemical from vats of cow's blood. Working with tissue taken from rabbit's ears, this group (Maurice M. Rapport, Arda Alden Green, and Irvine H. Page) went on to show that the substance was capable of causing the smooth muscles that line the walls of blood vessels to contract, raising blood pressure.

By 1949 Rapport had worked out the chemical formula of this powerful muscle-contracting substance. He called it 5-hydroxytryptamine. The American pharmaceutical company Upjohn, which went on to synthesize and market the substance for further research in 1951, chose another name, serotonin (derived from its association with blood serum), and this was the name that largely stuck.

By this time, serotonin's demonstrated capacity to cause blood vessel walls to contract had raised an exciting possibility: maybe serotonin was the cause of at least some forms of high blood pressure. If so, then to find a drug to reduce hypertension in humans, all one needed to do was find a chemical that neutralized serotonin's effects—a serotonin antagonist.

The hunt was on. At the Rockefeller Institute in New York, research-ers Dilworth Woolley and Elliott Shaw noticed that LSD (which everyone was still interested in) had a chemical structure similar to serotonin's. This led to a hypothesis: if serotonin affected the nerves responsible for smooth muscle contraction by attaching to specific receptors (as most biochemists believed), then any substance (like LSD) that resembled serotonin chem-ically might fit into those same receptors well enough to block serotonin from getting into the nerves—acting sort of like an ill-fitting key. Sero-tonin would then be unable to work its effects.[58] Indeed, in 1953 biochemist John Gaddum, working in London, experimentally demonstrated LSD's serotonin-blocking effects.[59]

More generally, the soon-to-be-famous "lock and key" understanding of drug action that Woolley introduced in his discussion of LSD and sero-tonin suddenly allowed researchers to understand how a drug might act on nerves in either of two ways: as a "key" or agonist (something that mim-icked the action of a natural hormone or neurotransmitter) or as a block on the "lock" or antagonist (something that interfered with the ability of receptors to absorb natural hormones). A whole new era of thinking in neu-rochemistry was dawning.

Meanwhile in the United States, the twenty-five-year-old neurochem-ist Betty Mack Twarog and her supervisor Irvine Page overturned all ruling wisdom by discovering that serotonin was present not just in mammals' blood and gut lining but also in the mammalian brain.[60] Woolley and Shaw were fascinated. LSD was the most potent mind-altering substance medicine had ever discovered. It was theorized to make people temporar-ily schizophrenic, and now it had been shown to be a powerful serotonin antagonist. Was it possible that LSD produced states of temporary psychosis by blocking serotonin? If so, serotonin might have an important role to play in preserving mental health.

In a short, straightforward 1954 paper, Woolley and Shaw explained their theory. LSD, they said, "calls forth in man mental disturbances resembling those of schizophrenia." It was also a serotonin antagonist. From those premises, the conclusion followed that the drug-induced mental disturbances caused by LSD could "be attributed to an interference with the action of serotonin in the brain." But what if metabolic disturbances in the body (as opposed to the taking of a specific drug) also interfered with the action of the brain's serotonin? The result might be schizophrenia. If that turned out to be right, the authors concluded, "then the obvious thing to do is to treat patients having appropriate mental disorders with serotonin."[61]

This was a milestone moment. All the earlier discussions about drugs that produced states of artificial psychosis assumed that the effects of LSD (or similar hallucinogens such as mescaline) were due to either the toxicity of the substance itself or its ability to trigger the production of some other toxic chemical (such as adrenochrome). Woolley and Shaw were the first to suggest a completely different approach: that people became schizophrenic, not because their brains were being poisoned but because they suffered from a deficit of a substance (serotonin) that their brains needed to function properly.

It seemed so elegant at first, but it quickly became messy. At a 1956 conference held at the New York Academy of Medicine, several researchers, including Gaddum, raised questions that complicated things. If the schizophrenic-like experiences produced by LSD were a consequence of serotonin depletion, then why didn't all the other active antagonists of serotonin (at least those known to have direct effects on the central nervous system) also produce schizophrenic-like experiences? And why did mescaline—which had no effect on serotonin—also produce schizophrenic-like experiences? One of the participants at the meeting, E. Rothlin, tartly summed things up: "The mere existence of a pharmacological antagonism between lysergic acid diethylamide and 5-hydroxytryptamine . . . no longer provides evidence for the hypothesis that inhibition of the latter in the brain is the cause of the mental disturbances."[62] Seymour Kety, the organizer of the meeting, put matters a bit more diplomatically: "I feel strongly that these data are trying to tell us a story, and I am happy that so many of us appear to be listening."[63]

Researchers went back to their labs and continued to try to "listen." One drug they listened to was a substance then being used to treat schizophrenia (a short-lived alternative to chlorpromazine). It was called reserpine.

Reserpine is derived from *Rauwolfia serpentina*, a plant native to the Indian subcontinent that had long been brewed as a tea and used as a tranquilizing tonic for anxiety, a sleeping aid for children, and even as an aid in quieting the mind for meditation. Gandhi was said to have been fond of drinking it. In the late 1940s, the drug was also studied—initially by researchers in India—as a medication for the management of hypertension.[64] In the United States, a chemist at Ciba laboratories identified the sedative principle of *R. serpentina* in 1952, and called it reserpine.[65] A year later, as Smith, Kline & French was promoting chlorpromazine as the first "tranquilizer" effective in treating schizophrenia, Ciba began marketing reserpine under the brand name Serpasil, hoping it might capture a share of this increasingly lucrative market. In clinical settings, however, reserpine never had the star power of chlorpromazine.

Where reserpine did come into its own, though, was as a research tool. It had earlier been shown to be an effective way to neutralize the symptoms of a bad LSD trip. At the National Institutes of Health, a new generation of biochemists—Bernard Brodie, Julius Axelrod, and Arvid Carlsson—wondered whether that finding had implications for Woolley and Shaw's theory that LSD psychosis was caused by a short-lived serotonin deficit. Maybe reserpine neutralized an LSD psychosis by stimulating the brain to produce more serotonin.

The opposite turned out to be the case. In experiments on both dogs and rabbits, researchers found that reserpine did two things: it had a sedating effect on the animals, and it caused their bodies to dump large amounts of serotonin stores (as evidenced by analysis of serotonin metabolites in the dogs' urine, and direct analysis of the intestines in the case of the rabbits).[66] What this meant, if anything, for understanding the biochemistry of mental illness was initially unclear (but see Chapter 6 for the continuing story).

And so serotonin rapidly declined as the neurotransmitter of the hour, at least so far as schizophrenia research was concerned. By the early 1960s, Woolley, whose pioneering work had sparked these new developments, was struggling to win himself a hearing. By now, he had taken a new tack, suggesting that the agitation and hallucinations of schizophrenia might be caused by "an excess of cerebral serotonin," and depression might be caused by a "deficiency" of this same substance.[67] But by the time he made this suggestion, few were listening. Instead, all attention was turning to a new neurotransmitter called dopamine.

DOPAMINE

A key reason for this development was the work of the Swedish biochemist Arvid Carlsson. As a young man in the 1950s, he had spent five months in the United States visiting Brodie's laboratory. His visit coincided with the period when Brodie's group was striving to nail down the effect of reserpine on serotonin. Carlsson, however, wondered whether serotonin was the whole story. As he recalled in an interview many years later:

> When I was there, I asked Brodie, shouldn't we also look at some other compounds besides serotonin to see whether reserpine could act on those and Brodie said, no, he didn't think so. He was so sure serotonin was the most important compound insofar as psychosis was concerned, he thought it would be a waste of time. So, I thought perhaps I can do that when I get home.... Of course, dopamine was not being discussed at that time.[68]

Carlsson went back to Sweden and convinced his scientist-friend Nils-Åke Hillarp to collaborate in experiments looking at the effects of reserpine on chemical systems other than serotonin. They were successful; when they analyzed brains of the mice they had injected with the substance, they found that reserpine did not just alter serotonin levels; it also led to depletion of the brain's stores of norepinephrine.

Less clear was whether serotonin depletion or norepinephrine depletion was more fundamental in terms of the drug's "tranquilizing" effects.

Carlsson decided to resolve the issue by creating a kind of competition: he would infuse the brains of his mice with each neurotransmitter in turn, and see which one (if either) reversed the tranquilization caused by reserpine.

However, because brain cells create both serotonin and norepinephrine out of simpler precursor molecules, Carlsson did not inject the neurotransmitters directly into his animals. Instead, he injected their precursors: L-DOPA in the case of norepinephrine, and 5-hydroxytryptophan in the case of serotonin.

And at first glance, norepinephrine seemed to win the contest he had set up. "We found a most striking effect when we gave L-DOPA. The animals [who had been sedated with reserpine] started to wake up within ten minutes following an IV injection and, then behaved like normal animals."[69] But when he went to look for all the peppy norepinephrine he expected to find in the brains of the animals, he didn't find any. Disappointed and also puzzled, he decided—"to save face"—to at least look for dopamine in the brain, since he knew dopamine was an "intermediate" between L-DOPA and norepinephrine.

Then things got interesting. After developing a method for measuring dopamine, Carlsson and his colleagues found that the response to L-DOPA was closely related to the "formation and accumulation" of dopamine in the brain. He and his colleagues also found that dopamine was present in the brain under normal conditions (i.e., in brains that hadn't been pretreated with L-DOPA). In fact, levels of dopamine in the animal brains they looked at slightly exceeded those of norepinephrine. "From all these findings," Carlsson recalled later, "we proposed that dopamine is an agonist in its own right in the brain.[70]

So now there was a new chemical, a new neurotransmitter to contend: dopamine.[71] And Carlsson's energized mice made clear that it had behavioral effects. But was it relevant to understanding schizophrenia?

For a while, the question hung in the air. Not until revelations about the role that dopamine played in a completely different disorder—Parkinson's disease—did Carlsson and others see a way to answer it.

Parkinson's disease is a progressive disorder of the nervous system marked by muscular rigidity, uncontrollable tremor, and slowed, imprecise movement. In 1959 two histologists in Vienna, Herbert Ehringer and

Oleh Hornykiewicz, had examined the brains of a number of deceased Parkinson's patients and discovered that an area below the cortex (called the substantia nigra) showed evidence of atrophy.[72] The significance of this became clearer when evidence emerged (thanks to new technologies like the spectrophotofluorometer) that the substantia nigra was a major source of dopamine in the brain and had projections that extended to motor control regions of the basal ganglia. When normal levels of dopamine could no longer reach these critical motor regions (because neurons were dying), it seemed that Parkinson's was the result. All of which strongly suggested that dopamine was critical to normal motor functioning.

It was Carlsson who took it upon himself to determine experimentally if this was the case. He began by injecting mice with large amounts of reserpine, now with the goal of deliberately depleting their dopamine levels. An amazing thing happened: the animals all developed a range of motor symptoms similar to those seen in Parkinson's patients. Carlsson then proceeded to "cure" his animals by injecting them with L-DOPA, dopamine's precursor.[73]

It was beautiful work, and it raised the possibility that human Parkinson's patients might also benefit from L-DOPA treatment.[74] They did (though with many more side effects and limitations than originally appreciated), and in 1970, following various clinical trials, the FDA formally approved L-DOPA as the first pharmaceutical treatment for Parkinson's disease.[75] All these developments, however, had implications for the unanswered question about the role played by dopamine in the genesis of schizophrenia. The fact was, when Carlsson's mice developed reserpine-induced motor symptoms, they did not just resemble Parkinson's patients. Their motoric problems also resembled those of medicated schizophrenic patients on long-term regimens not just of reserpine but (more commonly) of drugs like chlorpromazine and haloperidol.

By the early 1970s, it was becoming clear that chlorpromazine and haloperidol also had the effect of reducing functional dopamine levels in the brain (though it took some time to understand the mechanisms).[76] Was dopamine reduction the reason all these drugs were able to reduce many of the more flagrant psychotic symptoms of schizophrenia? Already by 1967, there was enough circumstantial evidence in support of this idea that one Dutch researcher, Jacques van Rossum, put it forward as a formal hypothesis.[77] In the mid-1970s another group, led by Philip Seeman at the University of Toronto, provided additional confirmatory evidence of the hypothesis by showing that the clinical potency of various antipsychotic drugs for schizophrenia (by now there were quite a few) correlated positively with their capacity to specifically block dopamine activity.[78]

AMPHETAMINES

If lowering a patient's dopamine levels made him less psychotic, did this mean that his original psychosis had been caused by excessively high levels of dopamine? It was tempting to think so, and there was some direct evidence in support of this idea. But it did not come from the studies of the dopamine-blocking effects of the antipsychotics. It came from the dopamine-*enhancing* effects of a quite different class of drug: the amphetamines.

Amphetamines, first synthesized in the 1930s, had been originally marketed by drug companies as nasal decongestants, but it quickly became apparent that they also produced feelings of energy, focus, and euphoria (see also Chapter 6). During World War II they had been routinely given to soldiers to help them stay awake longer, to give them a drug-fueled aggressive edge on the battlefield, or in the case of military pilots, to help them stay conscious longer (because of the elevated blood pressure caused by the drug) in the event they experienced sudden changes in air pressure. In the postwar period, the black market for amphetamines (especially Benzedrine and Dexedrine) flourished. Truck drivers, blue-collar workers, musicians, artists, and students became especially fond of the drug.[79] A once popular jazz piece by Harry "The Hipster" Gibson, penned in 1944, captured the initial buzz: "Who Put the Benzedrine in Mrs. Murphy's Ovaltine?"

> *She never, ever wants to go to sleep,*
> *She says everything's solid, all reet.*[80]

By the 1960s, however, recreational drug users were mainlining the drug (sometimes mixed with heroin) to create an added high. That transformed the culture of amphetamine use, leading to rampant abuse, a new black market economy, and—most relevant to the story here—a new kind of drug addict, the so-called "speed freak."

In 1969 a doctor in Orange County, California, described this new patient for his colleagues. One of the most typical presenting features they might expect to see, he explained, was a kind of psychosis almost indistinguishable from that seen in patients with paranoid schizophrenia: "feelings of persecution, feelings that people are talking about you behind your back (delusions of reference), and feelings of omnipotence." For a while, most speed addicts realized that these symptoms were caused by the drug, and were able to maintain some distance from them. But with time, this awareness could fade, and "the user may respond to his delusional system."[81] A 1970 article in the *New York Times* on "speed freaks" reinforced this emerging perception, explaining that, in many cases "the paranoia causes such eccentricity of behavior that the speed freak is likely to be carted off to Bellevue [mental hospital]."[82]

Were the symptoms of "speed psychosis" relevant, though, for understanding true schizophrenia?[83] The growing assumption was, yes, they were[84]—partly because the 1960s had seen a general transformation in understandings of what schizophrenia "looked like." Through the 1940s and '50s, the typical schizophrenic patient had been confused, docile, and regressed. By the late 1960s, however, new diagnostic criteria increasingly identified schizophrenia with violence and paranoia.

Importantly, as that happened, there is evidence—as historian Jonathan Metzl has argued—that the disorder also became racialized and politicized. By 1970 or so, with the civil rights movement in full swing, the typical case of diagnosed schizophrenia—at least in Michigan, where Metzl studied patient records—was less likely to be a confused white housewife from a rural town than an angry African-American man from Detroit.[85] Certain psychiatrists, consulting on behalf of the FBI, even went so far as to "diagnose" some of the era's more assertive African-American civil rights activists—Robert Williams, Malcolm X—with paranoid schizophrenia, in an effort to stoke public anxiety about them.[86]

All this created a social climate in which the craziness produced by amphetamines seemed to offer a much better model of schizophrenia than the craziness produced by psychiatry's previous favorite street drug, LSD.[87] In the lab, researchers began to use amphetamines to turn rats into small, furry versions of paranoid patients: suspicious, skittish creatures who repeatedly scanned and probed their environment.[88] They also found that when they pretreated their animals with drugs known to block dopamine activity (but still fed them an amphetamine-laced solution), the rats failed to develop these kinds of behaviors. This suggested that the original paranoid behaviors were caused by elevated dopamine levels that must have been caused by amphetamine consumption.[89]

Additional evidence linking psychosis to heightened levels of dopamine was also coming in these years from the world of clinical care for Parkinson's patients. L-DOPA, the new and apparently miraculous drug for Parkinson's patients, sometimes did not work as expected. Sometimes, along with reducing the rigidity and impaired motor capacity associated with the disease, it also drove patients into states of florid psychosis.[90]

One of the earliest—and certainly most vivid—set of cases of L-DOPA psychosis was reported by the neurologist Oliver Sacks. The cases did not involve Parkinson's patients but rather patients who in the 1920s had been stricken with encephalitis and had been "frozen" in Parkinsonian states of immobility ever since. In the 1960s, Sacks accepted a position at a hospital in the Bronx that contained a ward filled with such patients. He decided to give them L-DOPA, even though it was not officially approved for this disorder, and in his 1973 book, *Awakenings*, he described the complex effects. At first, the patients exulted in their newfound alertness and mobility— their "awakening"—but matters then rapidly went in the wrong direction. One patient, Leonard L., had a particularly dramatic fall:

> Mr. L passed from his sense of delight with existing reality, to a peremptory sense of mission and fate: he started to feel himself a Messiah or the Son of God; he now "saw" that the world was "polluted" with innumerable devils, and that he—Leonard L.—had been "called on" to do battle with them. . . . He started to address groups of patients in the corridors of the hospital; to write a flood of letters to newspapers, congressmen, and the White House itself

[Leonard never sent those letters]; and he implored us to set up a sort of evangelical lecture-tour, so that he could exhibit himself all over the States, and proclaim the Gospel of Life according to L-DOPA.

When Leonard L. began to make aggressive sexual advances on the nurses, he was put into a "punishment cell"—described by Sacks as "a tiny three-bedded room containing two dying and dilapidated terminal dements." At this point, Sacks wrote, the patient lost all connection to reality and sank into a state of "suicidal depression and infernal psychosis."[91] Did tragic cases like these have anything to teach psychiatry about the role of dopamine in naturally occurring psychosis?

In 1976 (following a great deal of additional work involving radiolabeling to identify dopamine receptors) the neuroscientist Solomon Snyder finally went for broke and said yes. In his dispassionate words: "If blocking the action of dopamine relieves schizophrenic symptoms, then one could speculate that schizophrenic abnormalities are related to excess dopamine release or perhaps hypersensitive dopamine."[92] (These arguments have now gone through multiple revisions, shaped especially by advances in understanding the roles played by different classes of dopamine receptors in the brain.) That same year in *Saturday Review*, Seymour Kety trumpeted the news—and implied that, with these new developments, the days of the neo-Freudians could be numbered. "There are now substantial indications," he declared, "that serious mental illnesses derive from chemical, rather than psychological, imbalances."[93]

AUTISM

Kety may have declared victory a bit prematurely. The neo-Freudians and family therapists remained largely unmoved. No minds were changed that did not want to be changed. After all, for half a century, a continuing trickle of research had purported to demonstrate the biological roots of schizophrenia, and little of this work had ever seemed decisive or enduring. Why should anyone believe that things were different now? Right up to the mid-1980s, virtually all major psychiatry textbooks still insisted that the origins of schizophrenia were unsettled, while actually giving biological perspectives short shrift.[94]

Not only that, but a whole new industry of psychoanalytic parent blaming actually grew up in the 1960s and '70s, alongside the new biochemistry work that was supposed to put it out of business. It was focused on a kind of schizophrenia that allegedly affected only young children. So-called "childhood schizophrenia" did not look much like adult schizophrenia; it rarely involved hallucinations, strange delusions, or paranoia. It was instead characterized by cognitive decline and withdrawal into a world of fantasy.[95] In 1943 the child psychiatrist Leo Kanner had suggested that childhood schizophrenia was a distinct syndrome of its own and proposed calling it "infantile autism."[96]

Originally, Kanner had suggested that children with this disorder were victims of some kind of inherited, biologically based defect. But he had at the same time been intrigued that most of them also had quite odd parents: "psychometrically superior" but "literal-minded and obsessive." In 1949 he had elaborated: "One is struck again and again by what I should like to call a mechanization of human relationships. . . . They [the parents] were anxious to do a good job, and this meant mechanized service of the kind which is rendered by an over-conscientious gasoline station attendant." The parents, he concluded in a passage he would come to regret, were basically human refrigerators, and they kept "their children neatly in a refrigerator that did not defrost." In 1954 he seemed to suggest that "emotional refrigeration" was probably far more important in the etiology of autism than any inherited predisposition.[97]

It was the psychoanalyst Bruno Bettelheim who helped to translate these ideas into a form that would ultimately cast a terrible shadow over the lives of untold numbers of families with autistic children. In his 1967 book *The Empty Fortress*, Kanner's "refrigerator mother" became more than a cool but conscientious robotic parent; she became a hateful one. "Throughout this book," Bettelheim wrote, "I state my belief that *the precipitating factor in infantile autism is the parent's wish that his child should not exist.*"[98] He and others encouraged children to undergo intensive treatment in special residential centers—such as Bettelheim's school in Chicago—designed to undo the damage caused by such unloving parents.[99]

Many of these allegedly unloving parents turned their children over to the care of the various institutions and treatments because they believed the doctors knew best, and they felt they had no alternatives. "Doctors were gods," one mother recalled much later. "I wanted my child better, so I'd do anything. Parting with my child was the worst thing I did."[100] Most were acutely aware that many of these doctors believed that the parents, particularly the mothers, were responsible for the child's problems. Here is a typical story, recounted many decades later by a mother of an autistic child:

> And in '51, Wendy came. And she was quiet. But when she did cry, she didn't want to be comforted. She much preferred to be by herself. Well, I was confused.... Naturally we want to hold our babies, and make them happy and I just couldn't do that.... I took her to a child psychiatrist. And he called us into his office and he addressed most of his remarks to me. "Hi, Mrs. Roberts, umm... We have noticed that with these children... They seem to reject the mother, they don't want the mother's comforting arms. Now why do you think that is, Mrs. Roberts?" And I thought, "Well, if I knew, I wouldn't be here."... I met another mother, sitting in the hallway... and of course, two mothers always start to talk in the hallway, and she said, "Uh... are you one of the Refrigerator Moms?" And I said, "What do you mean?" She said, "Well, don't you know, that's what we are?"[101]

In the mid-1960s, a number of the parents of these children began to push back. Many found the courage to do so from a rallying cry issued by the psychologist Bernard Rimland, whose son had been diagnosed with childhood schizophrenia or autism. In 1964 Rimland's *Infantile Autism: The Syndrome and Its Implications for a Neural Theory of Behavior* challenged the psychoanalytic perspective on autism, argued in support of a neurodevelopmental alternative, and called for new paths in the care and recovery of afflicted children. In this book, Rimland also included a seventeen-page questionnaire—a kind of diagnostic checklist for parents to fill out—and an address where parents could write to him with their answers. The response was overwhelming. Rimland later learned that some parents were stealing the book from their local libraries and ripping out the final pages to mail to Rimland.[102] In 1965, realizing he had a movement on his hands, Rimland and others went on to establish the Autism Society of America, which soon established chapters across the United States.

Equally significant, during the writing of his book, Rimland began corresponding with Leo Kanner, who gave the book an enormous boost by writing a cordial, complimentary foreword to it. Then in 1969 the original father of the "refrigerator mother" concept stood up at a meeting of the Autism Society of America and apologized. He attacked Bettelheim's *The Empty Fortress* as an "empty book" and explained that he himself had been frequently misunderstood and had never meant to suggest that autism was "all the parents' fault." Then he finished with seven electrifying words: "Herewith I acquit you people as parents." Parents jumped to their feet, and the room burst into applause.[103]

In the course of advocating for reframing infantile autism as a neurodevelopmental disorder that was no one's fault, Rimland made a further move, one that is well-known but whose significance has been largely overlooked: he insisted that autism should be firmly disentangled from all discussions of so-called childhood schizophrenia, a term that had outlived its usefulness.[104] *True* schizophrenia might be biological, or it might have its roots in bad family dynamics. Rimland—and indeed other parents of autistic children—seem to have had no view on that matter. And one unintended possible consequence of the decision to decouple the autism conversation from the schizophrenia conversation was that it short-circuited a possible alliance. None of the autism activists ever seem to have reached out to the equally guilt-wracked parents of adult schizophrenic children, who were also being blamed for driving their children crazy. Not until the late 1970s would parents of adult schizophrenic children finally create their own movement and find their own biologically oriented champions.

GENES

In the years leading up to that new parent-led movement, one significant research development seemed most pertinent to the cause: new evidence that schizophrenia had a significant inherited basis.

For several decades, pursuing research into the heritability of mental disorders like schizophrenia had been close to taboo because of lingering horror over the Nazis' pursuit of such work in the 1930s and '40s. In fact, right through the 1980s, some influential critics continued to insist that any attempt to investigate the genetic basis of schizophrenia must be deemed morally suspect on principle.[105]

Nevertheless some work, here and there, had kept the question of schizophrenia's hereditary basis alive. In the immediate postwar years, the German émigré researcher Franz Kallmann had gained some attention for his work on the incidence of schizophrenia in twins, identical and fraternal. He found that pairs of identical twins (sharing the same genes) were significantly more likely than pairs of fraternal twins to be affected by the disease.[106] (Later critics would question not only his diagnostic methods but his motivation. It later was revealed that, prior to coming to the United States, Kallmann had worked closely with the architect of Nazi sterilization and "racial purity" policies, Ernst Rüdin, and was almost certainly a Nazi sympathizer of some sort, in spite of being half Jewish.)[107]

For a while, an extraordinary case of identical quadruplets, all of whom had received diagnoses of schizophrenia, attracted considerable attention. The children were known to medicine as the Genain quadruplets (a pseudonym to protect the family's identity; the word comes from Greek roots meaning "dire birth"). The fact that all four sisters were considered schizophrenic was widely taken to suggest a genetic component was involved in the disorder. The psychiatrist David Rosenthal, however, who studied the sisters intensively, called attention to the abusive family environment in which these four children grew up. Their common upbringing, he thought, might also be partly or mostly responsible for their mental health problems.[108] Without any way to separate the effects of "nurture" from the effects of "nature," it was almost impossible to say.

Was there a way to separate the two effects? In 1966 the psychiatrist Leonard Heston, working in an Oregon mental hospital, thought he had found one. Studying children who had been born to hospitalized schizophrenic mothers and then been given up for adoption, he compared them to adopted children who had been born to mothers presumed to be without mental illness. If bad family environments caused schizophrenia, then the two groups should have the same incidence of schizophrenia; their biological backgrounds should make no difference. But Heston found that, in fact, of 92 adoptees born to schizophrenic mothers, five also had schizophrenia, but none of the control adoptees did. The chance that this was a coincidence, his team concluded, was 1 in 40.[109]

The biological psychiatrist Seymour Kety, then chief of the Laboratory of Clinical Science at the NIMH, was impressed with Heston's work. He had also thought for some years that the evidence generally presented in genetic studies of schizophrenia was "a bit more convincing" than in other areas of biological research.[110] He certainly recognized that, since the 1940s, it had not been "popular" to "think favorably about genetic factors,"[111] but he thought the time was perhaps finally right to pursue this avenue of research.

He developed a novel strategy for doing so. Instead of starting with schizophrenic mothers and seeing what had happened to the children they had given up for adoption, he began with schizophrenic patients known to have been given up for adoption in infancy or very early childhood, then looked at the incidence of mental illness in their biological families.

To do this, Kety used multiple national population databases, some of which had originally been set up by the Danish government in the 1920s because of eugenicist concern about the effects of inherited mental illness on the fabric of society.[112] He and his group began by identifying all people born in Copenhagen between 1924 and 1947 who had been adopted at birth or in early childhood; there were 5,483 such persons. They then identified 507 adoptees within that group who later ended up in a psychiatric hospital for any reason. Securing the medical records for this smaller group, three clinicians (including two from Denmark) independently scored each of them for definite or possible schizophrenia. Cases in which all three clinicians agreed on a definite diagnosis of schizophrenia were identified as "index cases;" there were 33 such cases. (Thirty-four individuals were actually included in this set, but because two of them were identical twins, they were treated as a single case.)

Having secured its index cases, Kety's team now set out to discover the incidence of mental illness in their biological relatives, all persons with whom the schizophrenic patients presumably had never had any contact.

They searched the Psychiatric Register of the Institute of Human Genetics and of the Bispebjerg Hospital, the psychiatric admissions of the fourteen major psychiatric hospitals, records of the Mothers' Aid organization, police records, and military records.[113]

Kety and his collaborators were surprised by the results. Not a single one of the 463 identified relatives met the rigorous criteria of schizophrenia that had been used to identify the 33 index cases. Many, however, did suffer from eccentricities or milder mental disorders, including what was then commonly known as "inadequate personality" (social ineptitude, unstable moods, difficulty coping with the ups and downs of normal life). The team suggested that such milder disorders were forms of borderline or latent schizophrenia that, while not schizophrenia proper, coexisted with it on an inherited "schizophrenia spectrum."

Even so, Kety and his team were surprised again. More than half the relatives determined to be suffering from a disorder on the "schizophrenia spectrum" were not parents or full siblings. They were the schizophrenic patients' half-siblings on the *father*'s side. The team could not fully explain that finding but did note that it meant that the schizophrenic patients would not have shared any common environment with these half-siblings—not even the same womb.

In 1967 Kety and his colleague David Rosenthal presented their findings at a conference in Puerto Rico, called "The Transmission of Schizophrenia," with the goal of bringing together prominent representatives from the warring perspectives on schizophrenia to see what they could learn from one another.[114] Virtually all the big players involved in debates about the origins of schizophrenia were therefore present when Kety and Rosenthal concluded that the "roughly 10% prevalence of schizophrenia found in the families of naturally reared schizophrenics is a manifestation of genetically transmitted factors."[115]

Many decades later the family therapist Carlos Sluzki recalled how, when the two men stood up and announced their conclusion, the "ground trembled. . . . Schizophrenia manifested itself, apparently, on the basis of a genetic load. Nurture appeared to have lost the battle."[116]

Sluzki's memory might have reflected his own emotions, either at the time or later, but his melodramatic declaration failed to capture the conciliatory intent that was, at least partially, operating at that meeting. In fact, David Rosenthal, Kety's colleague, was at pains to make the point that neither nature nor nurture had won or lost, because both clearly mattered. The real question, Rosenthal said, was how environmental inputs could trigger schizophrenia in someone who had a genetic vulnerability to the disorder.[117]

It was not the geneticists but the advocates for nurture—the analysts and the family therapists—who actually showed little interest in collaboration or in building bridges. In a series of articles written over the 1970s, the family therapist Theodore Lidz was particularly harsh in his criticism of the methods used by Kety and his colleagues in their adoption studies: Commenting on what he judged to be their highly elastic use of the so-called schizophrenia spectrum to diagnose the biological relatives of adoptees, he mused sarcastically: "It must be somewhat difficult to know just who should be categorized as a definite latent schizophrenic," but the fact that the researchers felt they knew "how to judge with any certainty who may or may not be an *uncertain latent schizophrenic* is a rather extraordinary feat."

Lidz insisted that he and his colleagues didn't deny a likely genetic predisposition toward schizophrenia; they just didn't consider it very interesting or relevant. The point he wanted to emphasize instead was that "for a child to grow into a reasonably well-integrated individual, the family, or some planned substitute for it, must nurture, structure, and enculture the developing child."[118]

In response, the defenders of genetic approaches to schizophrenia dug in their heels. They had tried to make nice but had been rebuffed. Besides, they now had other critics to contend with, other battles to fight, like the one with Thomas Szasz, who had become notorious for insisting that the very idea of mental illness was a myth. A dose of hard-nosed genetics seemed like just the ticket for silencing that irresponsible line of reasoning. As Kety himself mockingly noted to his colleagues in 1974: "if schizophrenia is a myth, it is a myth with a significant genetic component!"[119]

Eventually, some advocates for biological perspectives on schizophrenia forgot that they had ever wanted to build bridges. Instead they decided that Kety's work on the genetics of schizophrenia was one of their most effective answers to those who were skeptical of psychiatry's efforts to take back its status as a branch of medicine: antipsychiatric critics, family therapists, and Freudian dinosaurs. As one of his admirers later wrote, Kety's work was the reason that "we no longer hear shrill voices proclaiming that schizophrenia arises from toxic interpersonal family environments."[120]

FAMILIES FIGHT BACK

There is, in fact, another, far more important reason we stopped hearing those "shrill voices": the families of schizophrenic patients finally got mad, got organized, and fought back. And the most important original catalyst for their political awakening was not Kety's work or any other studies of the genetic basis of schizophrenia but rather deinstitutionalization: the decision by state governments across the country to release large numbers of institutionalized psychiatric patients, many in long-term care, back into the community (see Chapter 3).

The original vision behind deinstitutionalization was that, armed with prescriptions for medications that would keep their worst symptoms in check, schizophrenic patients in particular would be able to receive care on an outpatient basis in community mental health centers embedded in friendly neighborhoods. The federal government offered grants to build these centers. And the hope was that the states would save huge amounts of money.

But things turned out to be more complicated. Once released, many patients went off their medications, did not refill their prescriptions, and either lacked access to a community center (many were never built) or failed to show up for appointments at the ones to which they had been assigned. Instead, many cycled in and out of emergency rooms, became homeless, or ended up in prison. By 1986 the psychiatrist E. Fuller Torrey was blunt: "There is now a universal realization that the running down and closing of mental hospitals was a disaster. . . . Half the 'bag ladies' and 37 percent of homeless men are mentally ill."[121]

Some of the discharged patients, though, were relatively lucky: they had middle-aged parents who took them back into their homes and tried to care for them on their own. As they did, they discovered that the gutted mental health care system no longer seemed to have any interest in, or any capacity to deal with, their children.[122] In the words of one: "I feel that closing down the state hospitals has not placed the responsibility back on the community at the local level. It has placed it back on the *parent*. If I am wrong, show me!"[123] Another made clear just how high the stakes were: "We are worried about what will happen to our children after we die."[124]

In 1973 Eve Oliphant of San Mateo County, California, a mother of an adult schizophrenic child, reached out to other parents in straits similar to her own, in an effort to figure out how they could support one another. She was surprised and gratified by the response she received. Parents started meeting in one another's living rooms and eventually decided to organize formally. They called their organization simply Parents of Adult Schizophrenics (PAS). They then began to produce and distribute newsletters to keep themselves informed about developments in the mental health care field. They became increasingly activist. They showed up at county meetings, wrote articles for newspapers, and generally became a force with which the authorities had to reckon. In 1975 they won the right to be represented on every county mental health board in California.

In 1977 Oliphant spoke before the clinicians attending that year's World Congress on Psychiatry in Washington, D.C., about the plight of the adult schizophrenic patients abandoned by the system. In the course of her speech, she called attention to the fact that the family caregivers now working so hard to ensure that their adult schizophrenic children got adequate medical care were precisely the same people who, over the years, had been told by psychiatrists—perhaps some in this very room—that they were "toxic" and "schizophrenogenic." She challenged the psychiatrists at that meeting to explain themselves: "We failed to understand why parents of a child with leukemia were treated with sympathy and understanding, while parents of a child with schizophrenia were treated with scorn and condemnation."[125]

Meanwhile other parent-led movements were developing independently in Maryland and Wisconsin. The Wisconsin group, launched by two mothers from Madison, Harriet Shetler and Beverly Young, had named itself the Alliance for the Mentally Ill (AMI); Shetler liked the fact that the acronym spelled "friend" in French. In 1978 some AMI members saw a PAS newsletter and realized that there was potential to join forces.

Shetler proposed a national conference, and in September 1979, some 250 people showed up in Madison to attend. The participants at the conference then resolved that all the parent networks would combine to form the National Alliance for the Mentally Ill (NAMI).

One important participant at that meeting was the biological psychiatrist Herbert Pardes, who also spoke to the group and told them he supported their goals.[126] He did so not simply because he was sympathetic to their plight (though he almost surely was), but also because it was 1979, and the winds were shifting more generally against the old Freudian establishment. Pardes was not just any old biological psychiatrist: he had just been appointed director of the NIMH on a "back to medicine" platform. He wanted to disassociate the NIMH from its previous preoccupation with "broad social issues" and (as he later put it) make it "a more scientific institute focused on basic biology and behavioral science, major clinical disorders, diagnosis, treatment, and epidemiology."[127]

The families, keen to be absolved as the toxic source of their children's illness, could not have been more receptive to that mission. Biology, both groups were realizing, was a road to redemption not just for psychiatry but for families. As one NAMI member later put it: "schizophrenia is an organic, biomedical condition, and is not caused by bad mothers. Remedicalization is what we families want."[128]

Less than four years later, NAMI had nearly 250 affiliates and was becoming an activist and lobbying force with considerable reach.[129] Its aims were better services for patients with schizophrenia, better (biological) treatments for schizophrenia, better (biological) research into the causes of schizophrenia, and—last but not least—absolution for families.

Not that these families were uncritical cheerleaders for the agendas of mainstream biological psychiatrists. On the contrary, especially in the early 1980s, many NAMI members were actually attracted to the megavitamin treatments for schizophrenia ("orthomolecular psychiatry") still being promoted by Albert Hoffer and his associates in Canada. Having been denounced as frauds and marginalized from the mainstream, Hoffer, Osmond, and others within the orthomolecular community had seen an opportunity in the rise of a large and desperate community of anguished parents struggling to deal with the fallout from deinstitutionalization.

They were among the first to reach out and appeal to this community directly, using vivid language that they hoped would resonate with them.

> In a small prairie town, a young unemployed man with a six-year history of schizophrenia, characterized by numerous admissions to the provincial mental hospital, is watched over by an anxious and concerned mother who supervises her son as he begins to ingest the day's prescription of 30,000 mg of vitamin C and 30,000 mg of vitamin B-3 (nicotinic acid). Conventional psychotherapy, tranquilizers and ECT have been largely unsuccessful in checking the progressive downward swing in his overall personality functioning. Perhaps the vitamins will be helpful.[130]

To a significant degree, such appeals worked. Yes, the families knew that mainstream psychiatry was skeptical of vitamin treatment, but their collective experience had taught them to be skeptical of mainstream psychiatry. They also knew, perhaps better than the psychiatrists, just how problematic so many of the approved drug therapies were for their children. In a 1982 survey of parents about the usefulness of drug treatment, Thorazine (chlorpromazine) was deemed the least helpful of all (only 7 percent rated it as helpful, and more than twice that number judged it as harmful). In contrast, many parents raved about the effects of orthomolecular vitamin treatment: "He's the best he's been for years."[131] One NAMI branch newsletter noted pointedly that those who seemed to do best on vitamin treatment were "some of the most severely and chronically ill patients who have failed other programs."[132]

Orthomolecular psychiatry appealed to families as well because its leaders had signaled their commitment to absolving parents of responsibility for causing schizophrenia long before mainstream psychiatry had begun to search its own conscience on this front. In their popular 1966 book *How to Live with Schizophrenia*, Hoffer and Osmond had not only promoted their own approach to treatment, they had also attacked the dangerous "myths" still surrounding schizophrenia, including the myth that bad mothers caused it—along with perhaps bad fathers, bad husbands, or bad wives. "It is dangerous these days to be the relative of a mentally ill person," the authors noted sharply, "for you will probably be blamed for driving him mad."[133]

Only in the mid-1980s did NAMI families begin to disavow their earlier attraction to vitamins and other alternative therapies. One big reason was the arrival on the scene of the biological psychiatrist E. Fuller Torrey, who became one of their biggest allies. In 1982 Torrey—whose sister suffered from schizophrenia—had published *Surviving Schizophrenia*, a popular book intended not for patients with schizophrenia but for their families. They too needed, Torrey said, a manual to help them "survive" the disorder.[134]

Surviving Schizophrenia opened by making perfectly clear that the debate was over: schizophrenia was "now definitively known" to be a "brain disease." Torrey went on: "Like cancer, it probably has more than one cause. Thus, though we speak of schizophrenia and cancer in the singular, we really understand them as being in the plural; there are probably several kinds of schizophrenia of the brain just as there are several different kinds of cancer of the brain."[135]

NAMI families loved Torrey, and he loved them back. He was convinced that they were, "quite simply, the most important thing [to happen to schizophrenia] . . . since antipsychotic drugs were introduced in the 1950s."[136] When he decided to give all his royalties from sales of the hardcover edition of *Surviving Schizophrenia* to the organization, he became their unofficial spokesman and advocate in the profession. He went on tour across the country, speaking to scores of NAMI groups, in this way shaping new biological understandings of schizophrenia among NAMI families nationwide.[137] Above all, he encouraged the families to look beyond unproven vitamin therapies and invest their efforts instead in lobbying for more and better research into the biological basis of schizophrenia.

And so they did. When Congress allocated an additional $40 million to the NIMH mostly for the support of new schizophrenia research, the institute's newly appointed head, Shervert Frazier, publicly credited NAMI's tremendous lobbying efforts for this decision. Funding triumphs like these began to multiply. By 1986, Herbert Pardes—who had been present at the founding of NAMI—could only marvel at the unprecedented ways in which "citizen groups" were rallying to promote new medical research on mental illness.[138] Not only that: as early as 1981, some of the parents who had set up NAMI also created a new private charity—the National Alliance for Research on Schizophrenia and Depression (NARSAD)—that gave grants exclusively to scientists committed to advancing biological understanding of the major mental illnesses. (NARSAD remains to this day the world's largest privately funded organization dedicated to advancing such research.) Looking back in 1990, one unnamed source within the NIMH quietly gave his assessment: "NAMI is the barracuda that laid the golden egg."[139]

Meanwhile family therapists were growing uneasy. In the mid-1970s a few clinicians began suggesting that, given the changes occurring in the politics of mental health care for schizophrenics, it probably did not behoove family therapists to be so hard on the families of the patients they were trying to help. "Surely," one article gently suggested in 1974, "we can develop a professional lexicon that does not blame anyone."[140]

In 1981 the social workers Carol Anderson and Gerard Hogarty explicitly made the case for a new, nonjudgmental approach to family therapy in schizophrenia that they called psychoeducation. It concentrated, not on identifying the toxic dynamics allegedly operating in a family, but on building emotional alliances with family members. Anderson and Hogarty reported that, when families were approached sympathetically and taught skills for coping better with the profound emotional and interpersonal challenges of being the frontline caregivers of a schizophrenic child, there was a significant reduction in the relapse rates of the children themselves. While the scientific evidence to support the idea that bad families caused schizophrenia was equivocal (and Anderson and Hogarty were in fact skeptical of the idea), it had become crystal clear that blaming as a practical approach—especially in the 1980s, when so many families were directly involved in the care of patients—did not work.[141]

A few years later the community of psychoanalytic psychotherapists committed to treating schizophrenia received bad news, not from one of their rivals within biological psychiatry but from someone within their own ranks: Thomas McGlashan of Chestnut Lodge in Rockville, Maryland. Chestnut Lodge was a small, private psychiatric hospital long known for its pioneering use of psychotherapy in schizophrenia. Frieda Fromm-

Reichman—who coined the term *schizophrenogenic mother*—had been one of its most respected clinicians. In 1984 McGlashan reviewed the case records of some 446 patients there and found that they showed, he said bluntly, that psychotherapy was ineffective for schizophrenia. In his words: "The data are in. The experiment failed."[142]

That same year American public television broadcast a widely viewed five-part documentary on the brain. One episode, titled "Madness," was devoted to explaining to the public the still-novel perspective that schizophrenia was a brain disease—no ifs, ands or buts. The hour-long episode showed psychiatrists—prominently including Torrey—interacting with severely incapacitated schizophrenic patients. It featured interviews with sympathetic mothers and families, sitting in their normal homes, showing family photos of their once-normal and still much-loved children. Strikingly, while drugs were prominently profiled, the feature had very little to say about current scientific research into schizophrenia—nothing was mentioned about either biochemistry or genetics.

Instead, the documentary functioned above all as an extended and very public apology—by psychiatrists—to a generation of scapegoated parents. Once upon a time, various clinicians interviewed in the documentary said, psychiatry had believed that parents were responsible for their children's illnesess, but people now knew that there was not a "shred of evidence" in support of that idea. On the contrary, the clinicians asserted, parents were as much innocent victims of this brain disease as their children. In the words of one of those psychiatrists: "They are like people who have been struck by lightning."[143]

LEGACIES

By the mid-1980s schizophrenia had officially stopped being a disorder of bad families and had become a disorder of damaged brains. And yet this shift did little, if anything, to change the practical care of patients suffering from schizophrenia. In October 1980 a terrified but well-connected father, Dan Weisburd, learned that his brilliant son, enrolled at Harvard, had succumbed to an acute state of psychosis and had been tentatively diagnosed with schizophrenia. Weisburd happened to be friends with Herbert Pardes, then head of the NIMH, and called him to find out where he could find the best doctor and treatment for his son—money would be no object. Pardes told him: "Save your money, Danny. We know almost nothing about the brain. I'll give you a 'least worst' in California."[144]

A decade later schizophrenia was securely established as a poster child disorder for the new biological orthodoxy in psychiatry, but still nothing else had really changed. At a conference in Worcester, Massachusetts, in 1990, and titled "What Is Schizophrenia?," the first speaker paused at the podium to ask for the next slide. It would, he said, show a list of "established facts" about the disorder. The screen then went blank, prompting wry laughter to ripple through the auditorium.[145]

A full generation after that, there was a lot more research, a lot more data, many more claims, but no more certainty. In 2008 a group of researchers launched a multipart project designed to identify and critically assess all "facts" currently established for schizophrenia. They identified seventy-seven candidate facts. Each was graded on a 0–3 scale for reproducibility, relevance for understanding schizophrenia, and durability over time. Some turned out to be more robust than others, but none got full marks.[146] More important, even the most robust individual facts pointed in a range of different directions; they did not, as a group, lead logically to any coherent explanation of schizophrenia. As these researchers reflected in 2011, the field seemed to be operating "like the fabled six blind Indian men groping different parts of an elephant coming up with different conclusions." In fact, they admitted, in the current state of knowledge, one could not rule out another possibility: "there may be no elephant, more than one elephant, or many different animals in the room."[147]

CHAPTER 6

Depression

IN THE 1980s, AS SCHIZOPHRENIA WAS FINDING ITS BIOLOGICAL REGister, depression too came to be presumed to be caused by faulty biochemistry—a "chemical imbalance." By common consensus, it also became the "common cold" of psychiatry. Finally, it became gendered, a disorder that experts felt was more likely to be suffered by women than by men. All these understandings were part and parcel of depression's peculiar biological revolution—a revolution that involved a radical expansion in ideas about what "counts" as depression, and a radical narrowing in ideas about how it should be treated.

WHEN DEPRESSION WAS RARE

After World War II and up through the early 1960s, depression was rare, in two ways. First, it was rarely used as a diagnostic category by psychodynamically oriented psychiatrists. The historian David Herzberg, reviewing the *National Disease and Therapeutic Index* (a medical industries' market survey), found that in 1962 so-called neurotic depression accounted for fewer than one in ten diagnoses.[1] The epidemiologists J. M. Murphy and A. H. Leighton also examined epidemiological work on the prevalence of mental disorders during and after the Second World War. They found that three-quarters of the so-called neurotic patients received an anxiety diagnosis, whereas most of the rest were simply considered "neurotic." Depression as a diagnostic category was *not even included in the summaries*.[2]

To be sure, patients in these years frequently complained to their clinicians about feeling despondent, low-energy, or chronically sad. However, psychoanalytically oriented clinicians (and even many primary care physicians) assumed that these feelings were not primary symptoms but rather a defense against more taboo and fundamental feelings of anxiety, which was supposed to lie at the heart of *all* "psychoneurotic disorders." Depression was just one of its many forms of expression—or more precisely, one of the ways neurotic patients coped with their underlying anxiety. As the Freudian-leaning first *Diagnostic and Statistical Manual of Mental Disorders* (DSM-I), published in 1952, explained: "The anxiety is allayed, and hence partially relieved, by depression and self-depreciation."[3]

That said, all psychiatrists agreed that alongside the derivative "neurotic depressive reaction," a different kind of primary depression also existed, one that was a serious kind of psychosis. It was also—thankfully— quite rare.[4] The same 1952 *DSM* that had dismissed "depressive reactions" as a defense against anxiety described "psychotic depressive reaction" as follows: "These patients are severely depressed and manifest evidence of gross misinterpretation of reality, including, at times, delusions and hallucinations."[5]

For centuries, a disorder akin to psychotic depression was called "melancholy" and was believed to be caused by excess levels of a cold, wet substance in the body (a "humor") known as black bile. It was assumed to be basically a biological disorder that could be triggered by misfortune, guilt, or grief or arise for no apparent reason at all.[6] All through the nineteenth century, the so-called melancholic was a fixture of asylum life: immobile, despairing, wracked with mental pain.

Even after medicine abandoned the term *melancholy* for *depression* in the early twentieth century, American hospital psychiatrists, like their European counterparts, still widely assumed that the disorder had a biological cause. Some called it "endogenous" depression (to highlight its putative

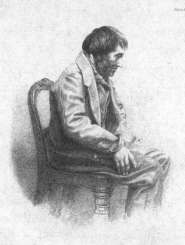

"Melancholy, from a photograph by Dr. Diamond."
Medical Times and Gazette 16 (Feb. 6, 1858), 144.

bodily origins). Others called it "vital" depression (because it seemed to affect the vitality of the whole body).

At the same time, most American psychoanalysts followed variants of classical Freudian theory, which had held that even psychotic depression (Freud had used the older term *melancholia*) had roots not in biology but in unconscious and unresolved grief over loss—often accompanied by unconscious sadistic fantasies toward the object of loss turned inward, and experienced as self-hatred.[7] But most analysts in private practice did not look after patients in states of acute psychotic depression, since such cases almost always ended up being hospitalized. Most of their analyses therefore were offered from a certain degree of distance.

SHOCK

For many decades, those who did look after such hospitalized patients had little to offer them, other than a measure of security against suicide, while they hopefully got better on their own. (And the disorder did often spontaneously remit.)

Then in the 1940s the prospects for such patients began to change. Electroconvulsive therapy (ECT, or shock treatment) arrived in the United States (see Chapter 2). Originally, ECT was seen as relatively nonspecific treatment, useful for all severely distressed or psychotic patients. Not until the late 1940s or so did psychiatrists begin to say the treatment worked best on psychotic depression. No one knew why, but the results seemed incontrovertible. One senior clinician mused late in his career: "Without ECT . . . I would not have been able to tolerate the sadness and hopelessness of most mental illnesses."[8] Some patients agreed. "I don't know, doctor," one patient told his ward physician in 1950, "I had the electric shocks and that's the greatest thing that ever happened in my life."[9]

How did the treatment work? It depended on whom one asked. In 1948 one military medical commentator counted no fewer than fifty "popular" theories, many of them pieces of speculative biology. Ugo Cerletti (the Italian neurologist who came up with the treatment; see Chapter 2) believed that ECT was effective because the body experienced convulsions as a state of emergency. That fact caused the brain to produce a compensatory "vitalizing" substance that had beneficial effects on mental health. Late in his career, Cerletti even tried injecting patients with a suspension made out of electroshocked pig brains, to see if it would produce the beneficial effects of ECT without actual convulsions. (He personally found the results encouraging, but this approach never took off.)[10]

The psychoanalysts (who grudgingly accepted that ECT had a place, especially in hospital psychiatry) also had their theories about it. One popular idea was that ECT worked by satisfying patients' masochistic desires for punishment from a father figure (the physician). Another was that the treatment produced states of regression, which gave patients conscious access to infantile wishes and fears (that could then be explored in therapy).

Still another was that the treatment regressed patients to a childlike state, giving them an opportunity to "rebuild" their personalities.[11]

As they offered these theories, a few psychoanalysts also suggested that clinicians who were willing to perform such a harsh treatment likely had issues of their own—especially unconscious feelings of hostility toward the patients they were shocking. Such hostility was then likely to be accompanied by an unconscious guilty need on the part of the offending doctor for self-punishment. One psychoanalyst was treating a clinician who "regularly experienced back pain on days that he administered electroconvulsive treatment . . . a symptom that patients undergoing shock treatment most frequently complain about."[12]

Regardless of how persuasive all this was, in the 1950s ECT became a staple treatment for severe depression. It was not costly, most standard health insurance plans covered it,[13] and hospitals profited from its use. The Harvard Medical School psychiatrist Alan Stone recalled that as late as the 1960s, "the blue bloods in Boston would go to McLean's [private hospital] and receive psychotherapy. The working-class Irish Catholics would go to St. Elizabeths Hospital and get shock therapy."[14]

A few clinicians, to be sure, worried about the treatment's safety. As early as 1947, *Time* magazine warned that "doctors are beginning to suspect that the 'cure' may be worse than the disease. The treatment . . . causes convulsions that may dislocate the patient's jaw, break his bones, or even kill him."[15] To address such concerns, psychiatrists in the 1950s started giving their patients muscle relaxants (to prevent convulsions) and anesthesia (to reduce anxiety) prior to shock treatment. Patients would then wake up confused, headachy, and sore but generally with no memory of the experience they had just undergone.

Patients' inability to remember the treatment was one thing, but ECT also became increasingly associated with a more general problem involving memory loss. The American psychiatrist Eileen Walkenstein held group therapy sessions for ECT patients in the early 1950s at Kingsbridge VA Hospital in the Bronx. She later recalled that the patients all complained of varying degrees of memory loss and were "furious at their doctors, other staff members, their families, or anyone they thought was responsible for their being shocked. It was only in these sessions that they could safely vent their rage. How they raged and raged!"[16]

Patients' growing fear of side effects associated with this treatment led David Impastato, one of the pioneers of ECT, to recommend in 1957 that hospitalized patients should not be told in advance that they would be getting it. "Of course," he wrote, "the closest relative should know and sign consent for the treatment."[17]

PILLS FOR THE DESPONDENT

Meanwhile, during the first decades of the twentieth century, untold thousands of Americans with "bad nerves" continued to seek remedies for what ailed them (see Chapter 2). In the 1950s, the analysts would make the case that there was no such thing, that all these patients actually suffered from an anxiety neurosis. But for a long time, these kinds of patients generally did not think of themselves as suffering from a "neurosis," or as needing psychotherapy. They just knew they felt despondent ("blue"), achy, and irritable, or they were constantly tired and yet not sleeping well. If they sought medical help, it was more likely to be from their family doctor than from a psychiatrist, neurologist, or psychotherapist. The family doctors in turn would poke and prod them, try to reassure them, and give them bromides (sedatives), vitamins, or sometimes even placebo pills (which could be ordered in various sizes and colors from catalogs).

By the 1940s, however, family doctors learned of an alternative to placebos and bromides. Amphetamines had been developed (see Chapter 5), and the doctors were told that these drugs had a wonderful ability to lift mood and restore "pep" to tired patients who had lost their "zest for life."[18] Benzedrine in particular—originally marketed by Smith, Kline & French as a decongestant—became the center of a new "pep pill" industry. The Boston psychiatrist Abraham Myerson gushed to a reporter in 1936 of their effectiveness in abolishing symptoms of "fatigue and depression without changing the personality or deadening the intelligence." They were also a super remedy for "nervous stomach spasms" and other "nervous ills."[19] They worked, as Myerson explained in numerous lectures, by mimicking the action of "natural chemicals" in the body—especially adrenaline, the energizing hormone that mediates the fight-or-flight response.[20]

The media helped stoke public excitement over the potential of these new drugs. Come experience the "Benzedrine lift," wrote the *Herald Tribune* in 1938, noting that a Harvard Medical School doctor had reported that the drug could help the shy and depressed become "the life of the party" and recover a sense "that life is worth living."[21]

Against a backdrop of reports like these, Smith, Kline & French began promoting Benzedrine as a drug for "mild depression." Tellingly, the company focused most of its advertising budget on reaching family doctors, rather than psychiatrists or psychoanalysts. Although the American Medical Association required the company to state that all treatments for true depression should be done under a psychiatrist's care in a hospital setting, the company found ways to convey its message more widely. Clinicians could consider prescribing Benzedrine, the company suggested, for the many patients who—while of course not *truly* "depressed"—show up in their offices complaining of "vague somatic complaints" with no obvious cause, while also showing signs of exhaustion, apathy, and "low mood."[22]

According to one historian's calculations, by the mid-1940s at least a million tablets of Benzedrine were being consumed daily for depression, and at least as many again for weight loss. (Benzedrine also suppressed appetite.) Sales were so healthy that Smith, Kline & French developed a new amphetamine, Dexedrine, hoping to keep the momentum going after Benzedrine went off patent in 1949. In this same period, the company also reported annual sales of some four million Benzedrine nasal inhalers, which were easily available without a prescription. We can assume that not all of them were being used by people with stuffy noses. Many people had by then discovered that the paper labels in the Benzedrine inhalers could be peeled off and eaten for a quick lift.[23]

Then in 1955, meprobamate arrived on the scene (see Chapter 3), sold under the brand names Miltown and Equanil and known to the public as a "minor tranquilizer." Unlike Benzedrine and Dexedrine, it did not treat depression or fatigue. It treated *anxiety*, now understood to be the problem underlying virtually every neurotic complaint.[24]

That was all well and good, but many family doctors pointed out that their allegedly anxious patients frequently suffered from symptoms of depression as well. They worried incessantly but also felt despondent and had no energy. Some drug companies, responding to this market opportunity, therefore began offering "combination" drugs to doctors. In 1950, before meprobamate came on the market, Smith, Kline & French had already begun selling a drug that combined the lift of an amphetamine (Dexedrine) with the sedative properties of a barbiturate (amylobarbitone). Called Dexamyl, it targeted (in the words of one ad) "the depressed and anxiety-ridden housewife who is surrounded by the monotonous routine of daily problems, disappointments and responsibilities."[25] Within a few years, the drug became a staple of family medicine.

A few years later, after Carter-Wallace realized it had a best seller on its hands with Miltown, it developed a combination drug of its own that it called Deprol, which combined the active ingredient of Miltown (meprobamate) with a muscle relaxant (benactyzine). Like Dexamyl, it targeted the depressed and anxiety-ridden housewife.

It is important to realize that none of these widely dispensed combination drugs were prescribed to cure a specific disease called depression—they were prescribed to treat a *symptom* of neurosis. Depression was still generally assumed, by analysts and family doctors alike, to be a mask that hid something deeper. As one Philadelphia physician, writing about Dexamyl, admitted: "Of course, the ideal treatment would be to discover the causes of the patient's emotional turmoil—the nagging wife or husband; the tyrannical parent; the unsuitable job; the financial burden—and remove it. Unfortunately, this is impracticable. Although dragging a secret worry out in the open—'getting it off one's chest'—is often in itself of benefit, it is not always enough."[26] When it was not practical to try to dig deeper, the pills could help.

THE INVENTION OF ANTIDEPRESSANTS

But even as a wide range of pills became available for patients who suffered from neurotic depression or mixed anxiety and depression, no medication seemed to work on the much smaller group of patients who suffered from psychotic (vital or endogenous) depression. Neither amphetamines nor

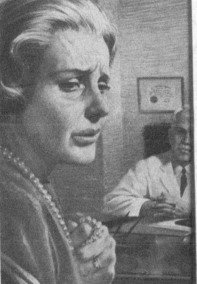

Advertisement for Deprol: "To relieve symptoms of depression and associated anxiety." *American Journal of Psychiatry* 120, no. 9 (March 1964), xviii–xix.

combination drugs seemed to help them. Right into the mid-1950s, shock treatment remained virtually their only option.

Then a new pill came along, quite by chance, as a side effect of an effort to develop a new treatment for tuberculosis.

In the early 1950s, the pharmaceutical company Hoffmann–La Roche had developed an antitubercular drug known as iproniazid (later marketed as Marsilid). During the drug's clinical trials, researchers noticed that some previously moribund and bedridden patients had become energized and even euphoric in ways that doctors could not explain simply in terms of improved health.[27] At the Seaview Sanitarium on Staten Island, patients given the drug literally danced in the halls of the ward. (Photographs of these patients published in *Life* in 1953 became famous.)

Hoffmann–La Roche, however, was not interested in Marsilid's apparent mood-lifting properties. The drug had turned out to be only modestly successful against tuberculosis (its sister drug isoniazid had fared better), and trials had been plagued by reports of a wide range of unwanted side

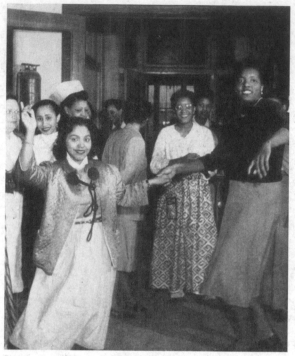

Dancing tuberculosis patients in 1952 responding to iproniazid at the Sea View Sanatorium in Staten Island, New York. *Life* magazine, March 3, 1952, 21.

effects. Company executives initially saw the strange euphoria experienced by some patients as just another one of them.

That might have been the end of it had it not been for the psychiatrist Nathan Kline, director of research at Rockland Hospital in Rockland County, New York. Kline became interested in Marsilid because it seemed like a possible answer to a fantasy he had been nursing for several years. In 1956 he and the psychoanalyst Mortimer Ostow had worked together on a novel neuropsychoanalytic theory which proposed that the new drugs like chlorpromazine reduced the symptoms of schizophrenia by "reducing the amount of 'psychic energy'" (a Freudian concept) available in the mind and brain. With less psychic energy available, they had argued, repressed fantasies, anxieties, and drives lacked the strength to rise to the level of consciousness, and the patients therefore improved.[28]

If this was right, it led to a further hypothesis: even as schizophrenics benefited from having their psychic energy *reduced*, other kinds of patients might benefit from a drug, as yet unknown, that *enhanced* psychic energy. Kline and Ostow called this imagined drug a "psychic energizer" and suggested that, once found, it would be pretty wonderful. It would get rid of the "the sadness and inertia of melancholia," reduce the need for excess sleep, increase appetite and sexual desire, and generally accelerate motor and intellectual activity.[29]

Now with this fond fantasy in his mind, Kline learned through a colleague about the energizing effects of Marsilid on tuberculosis patients. He saw the famous photographs of the dancing patients at Seaview.[30] Then he discovered a study in which laboratory animals were pretreated with Marsilid before being given the tranquilizing drug reserpine (see Chapter 3). Instead of becoming subdued, as usual, the pretreated animals remained alert.[31] Marsilid appeared to have neutralized the usual effects of reserpine.

Was Marsilid the psychic energizer that Kline and Ostow had envisioned? The only way to find out would be to try it on endogenously depressed patients. Kline, joined by several other interested colleagues, persuaded Hoffmann–La Roche to let them test the drug. And at the spring 1957 APA meeting, they reported their results. It had worked—indeed, it had worked startlingly well. And it had worked best on the most "deteriorated, and regressed patients."[32] Psychiatry, these researchers insisted, needed this drug. Hoffmann–La Roche was persuaded, the FDA was persuaded, and the drug swiftly came on the market later that year as the first recognized drug treatment for endogenous depression.[33]

Kline himself, though, did not see Marsilid as a specific treatment for a disorder called depression. It did not act in specific ways on that disease. Instead, he still saw it as the "psychic energizer" about which he had fantasized. It gave new energy to depressives, to be sure, but that did not mean its use had to be limited to them. Kline had taken the drug himself during its clinical trials and found it much easier to tolerate than any of the "psychomotor stimulants" (amphetamines) then on the market. With

Marsilid, he boasted, one got energy with no price to pay later—no hang-over, no letdown, no jitters. To explain the difference, he happily quoted one of his colleagues: "Psychomotor stimulants speed up the pumps—Marsilid fills them."[34]

By 1960, Kline's continuing experiments with self-medication had led him to a further conclusion: Marsilid's energizing properties largely elim-inated the need for sleep, and it did so—he said—without any untoward consequences whatsoever. In the popular press, he reported that during a three-month private trial on the drug, he needed to sleep only three hours a night and was more productive than he had ever been in his life. "I felt abso-lutely fine during the whole time," he bragged. "Usually I slept sometime between 4 and 7am, and woke up feeling fine. No alarm clock was needed." A reporter from *Newsweek* asked Kline whether such a lifestyle was unnat-ural and dangerous. Kline "snorted" at the challenge. "I just can't believe that God made the human machine so inefficient that it has to shut down or be recharged one third of its life span."[35]

By this time, however, most of the rest of the medical community had developed a considerably less sanguine view of Marsilid (and of several copycat drugs that were now also on the market). The drug did help many chronically depressed patients, but many of them were unable to tolerate its side effects, which included constipation, dizziness, difficulty urinat-ing, and neuritis. More worrying, some had come down with jaundice of the liver. If they ate the wrong foods (such as cheese and chocolate), they were at risk of suffering a potentially fatal reaction. Faced with Marsi-lid's association with 53 deaths and 246 cases of hepatitis, Hoffmann–La Roche withdrew it from most world markets in 1961. (It continued to be used in France until 1964.)

By this time, however, a completely different class of drugs, with a com-pletely different chemical structure, had emerged. Originally they were envisioned as a possible new treatment for schizophrenia, but once their mood-lifting properties were discovered, they were reframed as specific treatments for depression—as sober interventions that targeted and cor-rected defects in depressed persons' brains.

It happened like this: by the mid-1950s, chlorpromazine and reser-pine were making lots of money for the drug companies lucky enough to have patented them and other companies wanted to get in on the action. The Swiss pharmaceutical company Geigy was one of these. Its executives instructed their chemists to revisit some of the compounds they had previously developed, to see if any of them might have potential as a drug for schizophrenia.

Meanwhile the psychiatrist Ronald Kuhn, employed at a Swiss public hospital in Münsterlingen (a town near Lake Constance), had previously used chlorpromazine on some of his patients and had been pleased with its effects. His hospital, however, could not afford chlorpromazine in the amounts necessary for all the patients who needed it. In the late 1940s, Kuhn had worked with Geigy on various projects; at the time, he had felt that one of their recently synthesized antihistamines, code named G22150, had shown some positive effects on psychiatric patients. Remembering that now, he asked Geigy to send him samples of the drug for further study, but the new research effort did not go very far—the drug proved too toxic. Kuhn therefore chose a different drug from the Geigy vaults to investigate, one with a side chain identical to that of chlorpromazine and code named G22355.[36]

In 1956, Kuhn's hospital tried this drug—soon to be called imipramine —on three hundred patients with schizophrenia. It was a bust, but a later review of nursing notes revealed that the mood of three patients whose psychoses included severe depressive symptoms had significantly improved.[37] This finding suggested the drug might have potential against depression. In consultation with Geigy, Kuhn tried it on a group of forty severely depressed patients. No one was particularly hopeful that the results would add up to much; after all, no drugs had ever worked against severe depression. Kline's announcement of his "psychic energizer" was still a year away, and the prevailing view in the field was that an effective drug treatment for depression was a pipe dream.

But this drug surprised everyone. In early September 1957, Kuhn reported the results of his first trials:

> The patients get up in the morning of their own accord, they speak louder and more rapidly, their facial expression becomes more vivacious. They commence some activity on their own, again seeking

contact with other people, they begin to entertain themselves, take part in games, become more cheerful and are once again able to laugh. . . . Fits of crying and moaning cease.[38]

It was a remarkable report—and the psychiatric community to whom Kuhn presented it responded initially with considerable skepticism. But he slowly won over his European colleagues, partly by striking a tone markedly different from the one that Kline would soon strike in the United States. This drug, now called imipramine, he said, was not a "super-amphetamine"[39] but a specific treatment that corrected something that had gone wrong in the physiology of depressed patients.[40] It did not "energize"; it "normalized."

So it came about that in 1958, a year after Hoffmann–La Roche began its short-lived run with Marsilid, Geigy began marketing imipramine under the brand name Tofranil. They were two completely different chemical solutions to the same disorder. Other companies began to hope there might be more. In 1959 one company researcher told the *Wall Street Journal* that 1959 "probably will go down as the 'Year of the Antidepressant.'"[41] In the end, though, no radically new alternative drugs were created. Instead, other companies began challenging Tofranil's market share with a range of drugs that were chemically similar, different just by a tweak here or there. Because the chemical structure of imipramine includes three rings of carbon atoms, all drugs in this group came to be known as tricyclic antidepressants.

One of the new tricyclics, amitriptyline (brand name Elavil), did particularly well, not because it worked better than the other tricyclics but because it was far more skillfully marketed. Developed by Merck, it was first promoted as a safe and effective alternative to ECT. But Merck was also interested in broadening Elavil's market beyond hospital-based usage. In 1961 it approached the Baltimore psychiatrist Frank Ayd, who had spearheaded some of the original clinical trials for the drug. Merck suggested to Ayd that he write a book to help other clinicians, especially those in general practice, deal more effectively with patients suffering from depression.

The result was *Recognizing the Depressed Patient: With Essentials of Management and Treatment*. Ayd explained what depression was and discussed how the "chemical revolution in psychiatry" might affect the work of doctors in general practice. The book sold 150,000 copies. "It was a best seller," Ayd happily recalled later.[42] He was right, although one reason was that Merck purchased fifty thousand copies of the book itself, to distribute to general practitioners at no cost.

In 1966 Merck took its marketing strategy a step further by paying RCA to develop a promotional record album called *Symposium in Blues*, which it also distributed to physicians. The album included blues numbers with titles such as "Rocks In My Bed," "I've Been Treated Wrong," "Lonesome Road," and "Blues in My Heart." The company spared no effort in producing an album any jazz aficionado would be pleased to own, one that featured performances by jazz greats Duke Ellington, Louis Armstrong, and Artie Shaw, and liner notes written by the American jazz critic Leonard Feather. When a doctor opened the album, he encountered an insert with the Elavil logo, a strap line that read "therapy often helpful in depression," and notes on the improvements clinicians could expect to see by prescribing the drug for their patients.[43]

A CHEMICAL IMBALANCE

There is no question that many patients given a tricyclic antidepressant experienced profound relief. One patient, interviewed in 1977 by the *New York Times*, felt he had experienced close to a miracle: it was "as if I'd been living in a perpetual fog, a drizzle, or wearing misted glasses for a long time and something had suddenly wiped them clean. . . . Everything shifted back into focus."[44]

That same year the nephrologist Rafael Osheroff voluntarily admitted himself to Chestnut Lodge, a private mental hospital in Maryland, with acute symptoms of anxiety and depression. Chestnut Lodge had a strong psychoanalytic orientation, and Osheroff's clinicians there interpreted his symptoms as evidence of an underlying narcissistic personality disorder. They consequently put him on a course of intensive psychoanalysis. It was ineffective. Osheroff and his family requested tricyclic antidepressants (from which he had previously benefited). The hospital refused, Osheroff's condition deteriorated, and eventually his mother arranged for him to be transferred to a different hospital. There he was given both a new diagnosis and the drugs he had requested. In 1982 Osheroff sued Chestnut Lodge for malpractice. His lawyers and a star-studded cast of expert witnesses argued that because the hospital had failed to prescribe drugs, Osheroff had suffered irrevocable professional and personal losses. Tricyclic antidepressants were of proven efficacy, and all patients had a right to effective treatment. The Chestnut Lodge finally settled out of court for an undisclosed figure.[45]

How, though, did drugs like these affect the brain? Most of the early research on this question was done at the National Heart Institute in Bethesda, Maryland, at the Laboratory of Clinical Pharmacology, run by Bernard "Steve" Brodie.[46] Back in 1955 (see Chapter 4), Brodie and his colleagues had given rabbits some reserpine (a tranquilizer originally developed, alongside chlorpromazine, to treat schizophrenia) and discovered two things. First, the rabbits became sedated in ways that the researchers felt amounted to a reasonable facsimile of depression. Second, upon sacrificing the animals it was found that the drug seemed to cause the brain and body to "dump" its stores of serotonin.[47]

The Brodie laboratory then pretreated the rabbits with antidepressants—both Marsilid and Tofranil. In these experiments, the rabbits' serotonin levels stayed high, and the animals stayed cheerful.

But how did the drugs do this? In the case of drugs such as Marsilid, the answer turned out to involve an enzyme known as monoamine oxidase (MAO). In the 1930s research had shown that MAO breaks down hormones such as adrenaline by means of oxidation, thereby inactivating them. Later research also showed that MAOs were present in the brain, even though originally no one had any idea what they did there. And in 1952 a team at Northwestern University led by the German biochemist Ernst Albert Zeller had also shown that Marsilid could inhibit the body's production of MAO, though the full implications of this finding were not immediately clear.

Once it was shown, though, that MAO was capable of breaking down not just adrenaline but also the neurotransmitters serotonin and norepinephrine (see Chapter 4), it became possible to understand how Marsilid might be affecting brain biochemistry. If Marsilid inhibited the body's production of MAO, this would lead to a slowing down of the oxidation of serotonin and norepinephrine. Brain levels of these neurotransmitters should therefore increase, and *perhaps* higher levels of these neurotransmitters would translate into better mood.

Although the hypothesis was a brilliant piece of inductive logic, it clearly was not the whole story. The tricyclic antidepressants had no inhibiting effects on MAO, yet they still improved mood and (it was shown) also raised levels of serotonin and norepinephrine. For a full decade, no one understood how this was possible. As one researcher, Erik Jacobsen, put it in 1959, "Our present ignorance is such that not even a preliminary hypothesis can be offered."[48]

The person who solved the mystery was Julius Axelrod, who began in Brodie's lab as a lowly technician and went on to win a Nobel Prize for his own research. Unlike Brodie, Axelrod was more interested in norepinephrine than in serotonin. In 1961, using new radiolabeling techniques, and working with colleagues Gordon Whitby and Georg Hertting, Axelrod was able to show that norepinephrine injected into laboratory animals was removed from circulation by being absorbed or taken up at specific sites on nerve cells (or neurons). There it was stored for later use.[49] As his pièce de résistance, Axelrod was further able to show that the tricyclic drugs kept levels of norepinephrine high by blocking access to those absorption sites (synapses at the ends of neurons).[50] In other words, the tricyclic drugs kept norepinephrine levels high by inhibiting (the normally repeated) absorption of norepinephrine into the nerve at the synapses.

Others soon demonstrated that the tricyclic antidepressants blocked the absorption of serotonin as well as of norepinephrine. This led to the question of which neurotransmitter was more important in the relief of depression. Most people, following Axelrod's lead, put their money on norepinephrine. "Norepinephrine is a very potent substance," Seymour Kety explained to a journalist some years later. "And so the way it's kept under control seems to be that the neuron shoots a few drops out—whatever is needed for transmitting the information—and then it pulls the rest right back into the terminal branches of the cell."[51]

Norepinephrine was further enshrined as the favored neurotransmitter of happy moods by the emergence of new tricyclics that selectively affected it. This trend began with amitriptyline, Merck's Elavil, which early on had seemed to block the reuptake of serotonin and norepinephrine, just like imipramine. However, later research had revealed that actually the liver quickly transformed amitriptyline into a related molecule, nortriptyline, which blocked the reuptake of only norepinephrine.[52] Armed with this information, drug companies began developing new brands of antidepressants based on the blocking action of nortriptyline. Maybe serotonin was important for good mental health, and maybe it wasn't, but for now, attention had shifted elsewhere.

In 1965, given how much was now apparently understood about the biochemistry of antidepressants, the NIH psychiatrist Joseph Schildkraut decided the time was ripe for a synthesis. He attempted to put the pieces together in "The Catecholamine Hypothesis of Affective Disorders." (His use of the term *catecholamine* requires a quick word of explanation. Norepinephrine, epinephrine, and dopamine all contain a chemical group known as a *catechol*, and they are also all *monoamines*. For this reason, these neurotransmitters are known as *catecholamines*. Serotonin is a monoamine like these others, but lacks a catechol group.)

In his article, Schildkraut reviewed all the previous research: the animal studies using reserpine, the clinical trials with imipramine and iproniazid, the studies that showed increased catecholamine levels in the blood and urine of people taking antidepressants, and the discoveries of MAO inhibition and the blocking of neurotransmitter reuptake. And he concluded with an important, if tentative proposal:

> This hypothesis, which has been designated the "catecholamine hypothesis of affective disorders," proposes that some, if not all, depressions are associated with an absolute or relative deficiency of catecholamines, particularly norepinephrine, at functionally important . . . receptor sites in the brain. Elation conversely may be associated with an excess of such amines.[53]

Schildkraut's article would become the most frequently cited paper ever published in the *American Journal of Psychiatry*. Two years later he collaborated with Seymour Kety on another article, published in *Science*, that refined the original hypothesis, arguing strongly for seeing norepinephrine—rather than serotonin—as the neurotransmitter that regulated mood states.[54] The hypothesis linking low levels of catecholamine neurotransmitters (especially norepinephrine) to low moods would provide a theoretical focus to pharmacological research for the next quarter century.

Schildkraut always protested that he intended his "catecholamine hypothesis" to be no more than that: a *hypothesis*, a working theory, a tentative way of making sense of all the experimental literature to date. As discussion of the idea spread, though, it began to seem less like a hypothesis and more like a claim. And in the 1970s, the first discussions of depression as a "chemical imbalance" appeared in the popular literature. Publications from *Cosmopolitan* to the *New York Times* explained that depression was caused by deficits in essential brain chemicals, and that antidepressants could fix the problem.[55] One 1977 newspaper headline from *Stars and Stripes*, written during the Thanksgiving season, summed up this new thinking in a particularly pithy way: "No thanks on the holiday? *Check your chemicals.*"[56]

The new proposed linkages between disordered mood and disordered biochemistry even made it into courtrooms. On November 27, 1978, San Francisco was shocked to learn of the murders of a California public official named Harvey Milk and his colleague, Mayor George Moscone. Milk's assassination in particular became a lightning rod for outrage because he was the first openly gay person elected to public office in the country. Both men had been murdered by a disgruntled former police officer, firefighter, and colleague of theirs named Dan White. White had resigned from the board on which all three men sat, partly because he had clashed politically with Milk on various initiatives. He had then changed his mind because he had not been able to get a different career financially off the ground, and so asked Moscone for his job back.

Originally Moscone was inclined to reappoint him, but Milk lobbied heavily for him to hold his ground, and so he had changed his mind. In apparent response to this outcome, White armed himself with a gun and climbed into a window of a government building to evade the metal detectors. He requested and was given permission to see Moscone. They argued over his reappointment, and then White shot Moscone in cold blood. From there, White went directly to Milk's office and shot him five times as well, including twice in the head, execution style.

At White's trial, his lawyers suggested that he had not been wholly responsible for his actions because he was suffering from untreated depression. While he had previously been obsessed with fitness, they reported, he had recently indulged in a diet of junk food, including Twinkies. The psychiatrist Martin Blinder was among several medical experts who testified to White's likely depression. He then suggested—notoriously—that the extreme levels of sugar that White had consumed in recent weeks might have "aggravated a chemical imbalance in his brain."[57] Known in the press, somewhat inaccurately, as the "Twinkie defense," it was arguably one of the most explosive introductions of chemical imbalance language into the public sphere. Combined with other evidence, it was effective. White was convicted of manslaughter instead of murder and received a seven-year prison sentence, of which he served only five. Less than two years after his release, at the age of thirty-nine, he committed suicide.

THE COMMON COLD OF PSYCHIATRY

As depression was being redefined as a chemical imbalance, it was also becoming known as a common disorder, as common, people said, as the common cold.

There are a number of reasons why this happened. Perhaps the most important is that "anxiety"—psychiatry's previous go-to diagnostic category—was running into trouble. By the 1970s, the minor tranquilizers that had once been routinely prescribed for myriad "anxious" patients were increasingly recognized as highly addictive. Newspapers blared the warnings: "A New Kind of Drug Abuse Epidemic," "Abusers Imperil Valium," "Pill-Popping can be Risky."[58] In 1975 government hearings prompted the FDA and the Drug Enforcement Agency to reclassify Valium as a Schedule IV narcotic, meaning that physicians were required to report all the prescriptions they wrote for it, and patients could obtain only limited refills. In 1978 the former first lady Betty Ford publicly admitted that she was both an alcoholic and a Valium addict and checked herself into rehab. A year later, a memoir of addiction by the television producer and documentary filmmaker Barbara Gordon, *I'm Dancing as Fast as I Can*, became an international best seller and in 1982 was turned into a feature film starring Jill Clayburgh and Nicol Williamson. Valium had become a scary, semi-illicit drug. Anxious people would have to find a new solution for their distress.[59]

But what if it turned out that many of those former consumers of Valium had not really been anxious after all but rather depressed, without being recognized as such? Psychiatrists had long observed that many patients presented with mixed symptoms of anxiety and depression, but what if this mix meant that anxiety was actually a symptom of depression? If it was, some began to suggest, then many patients who had previously been told they suffered from anxiety would find that they did just as well— maybe even better—on an antidepressant as on a tranquilizer.[60]

At the same time as anxiety was beginning to be reframed as depression in the United States, something else was afoot. The World Health Organization had undertaken a project to investigate the worldwide incidence of depression. The results were startling. Depression, it seemed, was much more common than people had previously believed. In 1974 the Croatian psychiatrist Norman Sartorius, on behalf of WHO, declared that in the West, as many as "one-fifth of the general population had depressive symptoms." Worldwide, he felt that the disease afflicted upward of 100 million people, or 3 to 4 percent of the global population.[61]

Why had this not been previously known? The answer had to do, in part, with the fact that depression was now being identified and measured through standardized scales.[62] One of the most widely used, the so-called Hamilton Depression Scale (HAM-D), had been developed in 1960 by German psychiatrist Max Hamilton, who worked in the United States. The HAM-D asked patients to rate their level of despondency, the degree to which they engaged in suicidal thinking, the presence or absence of feelings of guilt, the degree of their problems with insomnia, and more.

The scale, however, was not set up to provide insights into the question as to *why* a person might have those symptoms. Some of the cases of depression it registered might have come out of the blue; others might have been triggered by a range of life challenges: profound loss, struggles to survive, experiences of betrayal, and so on. The scale had nothing to say about that. It was capable only of assessing the presence and severity of specific symptoms. For this reason, it had the effect of collapsing previous distinctions psychiatrists had made between the rare endogenous depressions, the common reactive or neurotic depressions, and the even more common "bad nerves" or anxiety disorders of an earlier generation. All these once-different sorts of patients now could potentially be located somewhere on the depression spectrum.

Moreover, scales like the HAM-D were not used just for epidemiological research: they also became critical tools in the new 1960s world of standardized clinical trials. In 1962 the Kefauver-Harris Amendment to the 1938 Pure Food and Drug Act required that all drugs sold to the public demonstrate "substantial evidence" of safety and efficacy. From now on pharmaceutical companies would have to demonstrate that any new medication being brought to the market actually improved outcomes for the specific disease it claimed to treat. And that requirement, in turn, meant that researchers had to ensure that all the patients involved in their clinical trials actually suffered from the target disease in question. (This may seem like an obvious requirement to us, but prior to 1962, physicians had sometimes carried out open trials of new medications on patients with a range of diagnoses. That way they could see which symptoms were affected most by a particular medication.)

Clinical researchers used rating scales like the HAM-D to create the homogenous groups of patients now required for clinical trials. They used them first as diagnostic tools and then to track the hoped-for improvement over time. Again, some participants in these trials might have been depressed because of something going on in their lives, and some might have been depressed for no reason that anyone could pinpoint. However, because medication seemed to help all patients regardless, in the eyes of growing numbers of researchers, the conventional distinctions between the two kinds of depression began to feel unimportant.[63] Thus, by the late 1970s, when the revision process for *DSM-III* was under way, the decision was made to drop all reference to life story, family history, triggering factors, and the like, and to simply provide a checklist of symptoms designed to allow clinicians to locate patients on a spectrum of "affective disorders."

And so depression, once rare, became very common.[64]

NOT JUST ABOUT CHEMICALS AFTER ALL?

Some felt that there was another reason depression had become so much more common. It had to do less with changes in diagnostic practices and more with changes in the world. We were under greater *stress* than ever before, some began to say, and our stress levels put us at a heightened risk of depression.

In the 1970s, the concept of stress was still relatively new. It had emerged after World War II out of a marriage between interwar laboratory science and attempts to make sense of the mental breakdown of soldiers. Postwar anxieties about the cost of prosperity on American's emotional and physical well-being had then encouraged interest in the idea that some people—especially overworked (white, middle-class, male) Americans— might be at particular risk of suffering from excess stress. The classic stressed worker was believed to be, above all, at risk of heart attack, but there was also concern about the effects of stress on mental health.[65]

An important technology in focusing the conversations about stress and ill health in general was the Social Readjustment Rating Scale. Designed in the mid-1960s by the psychiatrists Thomas H. Holmes and Richard H. Rahe, the scale aimed to measure the cumulative effects of stress on health. It presented individuals with forty-three more or less common life events and asked them to check the ones they had experienced in the previous twelve months. Each event on the list had been given a "stress" score, calculated in "life change units" or LCUs, ranging from 0 to 100. "Death of a spouse" was considered the most stressful thing a typical person might experience, so it was scored a full 100 LCUs. "Taking out a big mortgage" was scored at 31 LCUs, and going through the Christmas holidays was scored at 12 LCUs. Some events on the list were not intrinsically negative (e.g., getting married) but were still judged to be stressful because they required adaptation.[66] A person who racked up more than 200 LCUs over the course of a year was considered to be at significant risk of depression. More than 300 LCUs, and the risk became grave.[67]

It all made so much sense: a person could obviously only cope with so much. A 1974 article from *Better Homes and Gardens* explained the argument to readers this way:

Dr. Beck [a psychiatrist] found that before the onset of the depression, all [his patients] had suffered episodes of stress—an average of four per patient—and most commonly these were sexual and marital problems. Dr. Beck suggests that the problems have a cumulative effect. He recalls one patient who weathered the death of her husband and the death of her dog, only to collapse when the canary died.[68]

Then the argument took a gendered turn. Research from the early 1970s showed that worldwide, women were more than twice as likely as men to score high on depression scales. Moreover, considerably more women than men consistently participated in clinical trials of antidepressants. Were women more prone to depression than men, and if so, why? Maybe fluctuating hormones associated with menstruation, oral contraception, pregnancy, and childbirth could explain the difference.

Or maybe women had higher stress levels. Globally, researchers observed, women tended to be more socially disadvantaged and disempowered than men and were therefore potentially subjected to more stress, which might lead to a greater frequency of feelings of hopelessness and low mood.

In the mid-1970s the Yale epidemiologist Myrna Weissman and her Harvard psychiatrist colleague Gerald Klerman were among the most prominent researchers of gender differences in depression.[69] One of Weisman's most alarming early findings was that high rates of depression among women were bad not only for them but also for their children. Depressed mothers failed to communicate well with their children and had more trouble expressing (and feeling) affection. Their children, in turn, had trouble in school, got into fights, and otherwise acted out.[70]

Weissman and others were persuaded that, perhaps ironically, recent efforts by women in the United States to empower themselves could be aggravating their tendency to depression. The problems they faced came, not from their desire for liberation, but from the resistance of a society not ready for them to be equals. "Does Liberation Cause Depression?" *Harper's Bazaar* asked in 1976.[71]

In 1979 the Association of Black Psychologists met to discuss the tragic increase in suicide among urban African Americans. They made the stakes very clear. "There is a direct correlation between stress and depression," the association's chair, Dr. Malisha Bennett, reminded her colleagues. "Severe depression can lead to a variety of self-destructive behaviors including suicide and homicide."[72] The African-American community was in the midst of an epidemic of depression, in need of urgent attention.

What could be done about the ways stress was driving people into states of depression? A society-wide commitment to fighting racism and sexism would presumably be one answer—and, indeed, such a commitment had, a decade earlier, inspired the founding of the Association of Black Psychologists (1968), the Association for Women in Psychology (1969), and the Black Psychiatrists of America (1969). In the late 1970s, however, some began to argue for a different, more politically quiescent approach.. Evidence was accumulating that individuals seemed to respond to the same stressors in different ways. Some seemed to be remarkably resilient, while others crumpled under what would appear to be only modest provocation. Such findings led the psychologist Richard Lazarus, in the mid-1950s, to point out what should have been obvious: people are not engineered systems that can absorb only so much load; they are thinking organisms who appraise their situation and whether or how they can cope with it. Teach people coping strategies, and they will be able to navigate life's stressors (and society's inequities) with greater resilience.[73]

One person who read Lazarus's work was the psychiatrist Aaron Beck. In the 1960s, he had worked with depressed patients, where he was particularly interested in testing the psychoanalytic assumption that depression was a form of unconscious anger or hate directed against oneself. To his surprise, he found little evidence for that assumption. What he saw instead was that depressed patients tended to judge themselves as unworthy and helpless. Lazarus's ideas helped Beck make sense of his findings, suggesting that depression might occur not because the external world inevitably drove a person to emotional collapse, but because a person believed that he or she was helpless or undeserving of a better life.

Meanwhile a colleague of Beck, Martin Seligman, was conducting research on dogs that also impressed Beck. The dogs were given a large number of electric shocks and no way to escape from them. Seligman found that after a while, they ceased to struggle and passively accepted their fate. Their state of "learned hopelessness" persisted not only in the original experimental setting but also in new settings where their struggles might have been more effective. In other words, they had learned (wrongly) that things were always hopeless and they were always helpless.[74]

On the basis of these experiments, Seligman, Beck, and others suggested that many patients were depressed because they had learned that they were helpless. Their faulty beliefs told them that they were unworthy and inadequate. Perhaps, though, beliefs could be challenged and changed. Perhaps what had been learned could be unlearned.[75] Thus emerged what would become the most widely adopted new genre of psychotherapy since psychoanalysis—a cluster of therapeutic approaches known variously as cognitive therapy or cognitive-behavioral therapy (CBT).[76]

What did the rise of CBT mean for the argument that depression was caused by a chemical imbalance best treated with medication? That question hung in the air in 1977, when psychiatry resident Augustus Rush encouraged Beck to conduct a twelve-week clinical trial that would compare the effects of CBT and antidepressants on patients with severe depression. The outcome was a stunner: cognitive therapy *outperformed* imipramine, the standard medication for depression. The depressed patients who underwent CBT not only showed significantly greater improvement (as gauged by their scores on various rating scales), they were also more likely to remain well longer. After six months, 68 percent of the medicated group were back in treatment, while only 16 percent of the CBT group were.[77]

If depression could be so effectively treated simply by changing people's negative beliefs about themselves, did it still make sense to think of it as resulting from a "chemical imbalance"? For a brief time, a space for uncertainty opened up.

NEW BIOCHEMICAL LIFESTYLES

Then Prozac arrived. And while this new antidepressant did not quite change everything, it did throw such a bright spotlight on the chemical imbalance theory that other ideas found themselves rather left in the shadows.

With Prozac, the chemical that was presumed to be out of balance was serotonin rather than norepinephrine. Serotonin had briefly been American psychiatry's favorite neurotransmitter (see Chapter 4), but Axelrod's Nobel Prize–winning work on norepinephrine reuptake systems in the early 1960s had shifted the field's focus. Indeed, Axelrod once scoffed that serotonin's presence in the brain was probably just "a remnant of our marine past." (Serotonin was first discovered in mussels.) So even though research had shown that the tricyclic drugs affected both norepinephrine and serotonin, most work into the 1970s was focused on the former.

To be sure, some researchers, particularly in Europe, had not been sure that norepinephrine was the whole story. In 1960 a team in Edinburgh led by the psychiatrist George Ashcroft presented evidence from autopsy findings and cerebrospinal samples that seemed to show that patients with major depression (including depression resulting in suicide) had abnormally low levels of serotonin. (In 1970 Ashcroft withdrew this claim, saying the team had misinterpreted the findings.)[78] A few years later the London-based psychiatrist Alec Coppen and his team found that pretreating patients with the naturally occurring amino acid tryptophan (a precursor of serotonin) markedly improved the effect of an MAO-inhibiting antidepressant. The team went on to claim that tryptophan, used alone, often "was as effective as ECT in treating depressive illness."[79] This suggested that serotonin might play a significant role in mood regulation (though Coppen himself wanted to be cautious about jumping to premature conclusions).[80]

In Sweden, the biochemist Arvid Carlsson also decided to take a second look at the role played by serotonin in antidepressant efficacy. He knew that tricyclic antidepressants had varied effects on the symptoms of depression (as measured on rating scales). He had also reviewed evidence suggesting that the drugs that did the best job of specifically lifting mood also seemed to have the strongest blocking effects on the brain's serotonin reuptake mechanisms. This led him to imagine a theoretical drug that would selectively block the reuptake of only serotonin. Such a drug might allow one to offer depressed patients an effective drug treatment without putting them at risk of the cardiovascular side effects often associated with drugs that strongly blocked norepinephrine reuptake. By 1971, financed by the Swedish firm Astra Pharmaceuticals, Carlsson and his team had come up with a prototype drug that selectively blocked serotonin reuptake. They called it elidine. Astra tested it on Swedish patients, found adequate reasons to believe it effective, and received approval in 1981 to market it in Europe under the brand name Zelmid. In the United States, Merck became interested in Zelmid and submitted an application to the FDA to license it for testing and eventual commercial use.

Unfortunately, some European patients on Zelmid began to report a flu-like condition that came to be known as "zimelidine syndrome." Other patients were diagnosed with Guillain-Barré syndrome, a sometimes-fatal neurological disorder. While it wasn't clear that the drug was responsible for those illnesses, the cost of resolving the issue was prohibitive. Astra consequently withdrew Zelmid from the market in September 1983, and Merck abandoned its application with the FDA soon afterward.[81]

Meanwhile the pharmaceutical company Eli Lilly had also begun, in the early 1970s, to investigate the possibility of developing an antidepressant that would not have the cardiovascular risks associated with many of the tricyclic drugs on the market. The Eli Lilly team synthesized several chemicals that were derived from an antihistamine called diphenhydramine (the active ingredient in over-the-counter sleeping aids such as Sominex and Tylenol PM).[82] One member of the team was the Hong Kong–born biochemist David Wong, who knew about the European research suggesting that serotonin might play a role in regulating mood. Wong encouraged the team to screen their newly synthesized chemicals for any that might selectively inhibit reuptake of serotonin, and on July 24, 1972, they found one. Eli Lilly originally identified the chemical as "Lilly 110140" but in 1975 renamed it "fluoxetine." In 1977 the company filed an application with the FDA to investigate this chemical's clinical potential as an antidepressant that selectively boosted serotonin levels.[83]

Expectations were modest. In 1983 the *Wall Street Journal* reported that Eli Lilly was testing fluoxetine's potential as an antidepressant alongside two other products: a drug that increased milk production in dairy cows and one that might be useful in treating symptoms of Parkinson's disease. None of the products, according to a company spokesperson, were expected to be major hits. Yet stockholders need not worry; the company's fortunes could still get a boost from its Elizabeth Arden cosmetics line and its medical instruments business.[84]

With the collapse of Zelmid, however, Eli Lilly suddenly saw a new market opportunity for fluoxetine. It seemed much safer than either Zelmid or the existing tricyclic drugs on the market. In December 1987 the drug was approved by the FDA as an antidepressant, and the company began marketing it a month later under the trade name Prozac.[85] Within months, Prozac sales outpaced those of the former market leader, the tricyclic Pamelor that (unlike Prozac) principally targeted norepinephrine receptors. Clinicians began prescribing Prozac by preference, primarily because of the perception that it was safer than all the other brands on the market. In addition, many patients on Prozac lost weight, whereas one of the more annoying side effects of the tricyclics had been unwanted weight gain.

And because Prozac was assumed to be so safe, clinicians also began to prescribe it for patients with milder symptoms of depression, patients to whom they might have hesitated to prescribe a tricyclic. By 1988, doubtless to Eli Lilly's surprise, Prozac had become the best-selling antidepressant in history. By 1990, the company was filling an estimated one million prescriptions a month.

It was not all good news for Eli Lilly. In the year 1990 the company found itself facing a first slew of lawsuits that suggested Prozac might not be as safe as all that, after all. Pointing to research spearheaded by the Harvard psychiatrist Martin Teicher, the plaintiffs in the cases argued that Eli Lilly had suppressed evidence that the drug was capable of sparking violent or suicidal behavior in a fraction of patients who had never previously acted that way.[86] Lilly denied all charges, settled out of court, and more or less righted the ship for the moment.

Then in 1993 the Prozac story took a controversial turn with the publication of a book called *Listening to Prozac*. Its author, the psychiatrist Peter Kramer, suggested that Prozac was not working in the ways one would expect if the drug were simply correcting a chemical imbalance. No,

Prozac was also enhancing people's personalities. This made it both more seductive and potentially more worrying than any other antidepressant on the market.

To explain what he meant, Kramer told stories from his own psychiatric practice. A woman he called Tess was the oldest of ten children, born to an alcoholic father and a depressed mother. She grew up in one of the poorest public housing projects in her city and suffered childhood sexual abuse. After her father died, she raised her brothers and sisters, steering them all into stable jobs and marriages. She then finished school and began a successful business career. Her personal life, however, remained troubled. She had a series of unhappy relationships and fell into a deep depression. Kramer prescribed Prozac, and it worked—not only by lifting her depression but also by seeming to turn her into a new kind of person. She said she felt "clearheaded" for the first time in her life. Men found her more attractive because she was more relaxed, self-possessed, and able to handle challenging situations. She formed a new circle of friends, moved out of her old neighborhood, and received a substantial pay raise.

After about nine months on Prozac and clearly no longer depressed, Tess went off the medication and remained free of symptoms for a time. Then about eight months off medication, she called Kramer and said, "I'm not myself." She meant, of course, that she was no longer that new, more self-confident self she felt herself to have been while on the drug. Business pressures were mounting, and she felt she could use "the sense of stability, the invulnerability to attack, that Prozac gave her." She wanted Prozac not because she had a mental disorder but because she believed it would give her an edge in her professional life and restore bounce to her personal life. Kramer hesitated, then wrote her the prescription. In a remarkable sentence that would be quoted in countless articles, he explained his decision this way: "Who was I to withhold from her the bounties of science?"

Back on the drug, Tess did become her "better" self again. She was able to negotiate with union leaders without becoming defensive or doubting herself. As her troubled company settled down, she was given another substantial pay raise, "a sign that others noticed her new effectiveness." The fact that she was a woman who had used Prozac to get ahead in her career did not escape Kramer's notice. As he put it, "There is a sense in which antidepressants [such as Prozac] are feminist drugs, liberating and empowering." And he concluded, "The way neurochemicals tell stories is not the way psychotherapy tells them. If Tess's fairy tale does not have the plot we expect, it is nonetheless happy."[87]

What had been true for Tess was, Kramer went on, true for countless others who had taken the drug—far more than the profession had been prepared to admit. "Prozac seemed to give social confidence to the habitually timid, to make the sensitive brash, to lend the introvert the social skills of a salesman." And that meant that we faced a future in which doctors would find themselves under pressure to prescribe pharmaceuticals not to cure diseases but to enhance lifestyles—to brighten a dull personality, to give a a shy student new confidence in the classroom, or to facilitate the ambitions of an employee looking to climb the corporate ladder. Kramer called this emerging trend "cosmetic psychopharmacology." Although he harbored personal ambivalence about using drugs in this way, he also questioned his own hesitancies. After all, people changed their hair color without embarrassment. Why not their personalities? "Since you only live once, why not do it as a blonde; and why not as a peppy blonde?"[88]

Throngs of people took notice. *Listening to Prozac* was on the *New York Times* best seller list for twelve weeks in 1993. And even though critics were up in arms, decrying the drug as a cheap chemical fix for real-life problems, sales of Prozac increased that year by 15 percent. The growth was so remarkable that an independent commission in France felt compelled to investigate the possibility that Kramer had been hired by Eli Lilly to write *Listening to Prozac* with the intent of boosting profits. (He hadn't.)[89]

During the first half of the 1990s, Prozac was responsible for 29 percent of Eli Lilly's revenues. By 1996, however, revenue had begun to slow as new SSRIs entered the market. In 1992 Pfizer introduced Zoloft. One year later SmithKline Beecham (successor to Smith, Kline & French) introduced Paxil. It was SmithKline Beecham that coined the now familiar term *selective serotonin reuptake inhibitor* (SSRI) to describe the new antidepressants. The moniker was designed to underscore the idea that these were "clean" drugs that targeted only the parts of the brain responsible for depressed people's pain.[90]

Worried about its shrinking market share, when the FDA relaxed regulations over direct-to-consumer marketing in 1997, Eli Lilly leaped at the opportunity to reach out directly to potential customers. The company hired the Chicago-based advertising firm Leo Burnett, and in late 1997, a print advertising campaign called "Welcome back" launched in some twenty general-interest magazines, including *Family Circle*, *Good Housekeeping*, *Sports Illustrated*, *Cosmopolitan*, *Men's Health*, *Newsweek*, *Time*, *Parade*, and *Entertainment Weekly*.

The ads were nothing if not powerful. They underscored the message of the new biological psychiatry, that disorders like depression were real diseases requiring real medical solutions: "Some people think you can just will yourself out of a depression. That's not true." Visual imagery suggested the stark contrast between a life with depression and a life after recovery: rainclouds versus sunshine, a broken vase versus a vase with flowers. "Prozac has been prescribed for more than 17 million Americans. Chances are someone you know is feeling sunny again because of it. Prozac. Welcome back."[91]

It was not Eli Lilly, however, but Pfizer—the manufacturer of Zoloft— that first based a direct-to-consumer ad campaign specifically on the idea that depression was caused by a deficiency of certain biochemicals in the brain—a "chemical imbalance." Early print ads for Zoloft included a simple cartoon of neurons emitting different amounts of small circles (representing neurotransmitters) before and after treatment.

Several years later, as television ads largely displaced print ads, the advertising firms for Pfizer and others again chose to make use of the "chemical imbalance" theory, crafting a range of messages designed to convey the impression that depression was now known to be caused by too little serotonin, and these drugs had been scientifically designed from the ground up to target the problem:

> Just as a cake recipe requires you to use flour, sugar, and baking powder in the right amounts, your brain needs a fine chemical balance in order to perform at its best.

Normally, a chemical neurotransmitter in your brain, called serotonin, helps send messages from one brain cell to another. This is how the cells in your brain communicate.

Scientists believe people with depression could have an imbalance of serotonin in their brain.[92]

And so the public was again schooled to think about depression as a chemical imbalance—but now with the twist that serotonin, not norepinephrine, was the specific brain chemical that one was supposed to need in abundance in order to be happy. Thus in her 1996 memoir of life on Prozac, the author Lauren Slater claimed—with a touch of bravado and self-deprecating irony—to have come to terms with the fact that she was, after all, "a purely chemical being, mood and personality sweeping through serotonin."[93]

Ironically, just as the public was embracing the "serotonin imbalance" theory of depression, researchers were forming a new consensus that all the simplistic "chemical imbalance" theories of depression—whether focused on serotonin or some other neurotransmitter—were deeply flawed and probably outright wrong.[94]

Not until the second decade of the twenty-first century, however, did public skepticism toward "chemical imbalance" theories of depression finally began to catch up with growing scientific skepticism. And when it did, it was not so much because the public had reviewed the relevant scientific literature but because public (and media) enthusiasm for SSRIs as a quick fix for one's unruly biochemistry had begun to dim. The drugs remained widely used, but with greater awareness that they did not always work, that they did not work forever, and that taking them was not without risks.[95]

Thus in her 2018 book *Blue Dreams* (part memoir and part history), Lauren Slater no longer imagines herself as a "purely chemical being" and is far more realistic about the flaws in the science behind the mood-altering drugs on which she had been dependent for most of her adult life. Her skeptical turn was clearly driven not just by sifting through the literature but by her long personal experience with these drugs. Her thirty-plus-year diet of mood-altering medications had taken its toll on her body. "A single warning from a single doctor when I was in the depths of despair," she reflects, "could not adequately convey the message that by swallowing this new drug I was effectively agreeing to deeply damage the body upon which I rely to survive." And yet it is not clear that she could or would have made different choices, even had she fully understood. "I am unhealthy, and this is largely due to psychiatry's drugs," she concludes. "And yet, I cannot live without these drugs."[96]

CHAPTER 7

Manic-Depression

IN THE ERA BEFORE THE ARRIVAL OF DRUGS, MANIC-DEPRESSION AS A diagnosis was a kind of clinical no-man's-land, bounded by schizophrenia on the one side and depression on the other. It was given to patients who had bouts of agitation such that they did not seem to suffer just from depression yet who also, for whatever reason, did not seem quite ill enough to receive a diagnosis of schizophrenia.[1] Such patients were then generally subjected to any and all the treatments used for schizophrenia or depression—psychotherapy, electroshock treatment, lobotomy—and the outcomes were generally less than ideal.[2]

THE INVENTION OF MANIC-DEPRESSION

It was not supposed to be like this. Manic-depression was the "other" psychosis in Emil Kraepelin's bipartite division of the psychoses. The diagnostic category had been his attempt to synthesize and bring order to the whole vexed subject of mood disorders, including (but not limited to) disorders that fluctuated between pathological agitation (with or without elation) and despondent listlessness.

The roots of the confusion he was sorting out, in his view, were old indeed. For centuries, a disorder called "mania" and a disorder called "melancholy" had divided the world of mental illness into two halves. Mania was any form of madness in which a person was furious, raving, or agitated, whereas "melancholy" was any form of madness in which a person brooded unceasingly over imagined slights or sins, was wracked by despondency, or was immobilized by indecisiveness. To reinforce the consensus, for 150 years (from 1676 to 1815), visitors to the gates of London's Bethlem Royal Hospital (widely known as Bedlam) were greeted by two giant statues, Mania and Melancholy, carved by the Danish sculptor Caius Gabriel Cibber. Melancholy was shown lying on his left side, placid and despondent. Raving Madness, by contrast, was shown on his right side, straining with clenched fists against the chains restraining him.[3]

In the mid-nineteenth century, though, a small number of clinicians, mostly based in France, began to say that some patients were neither exclusively manic nor exclusively melancholic but had periods in which they were one or the other. They gave this condition various names: circular insanity, intermittent insanity, periodic insanity, and insanity of double form. It came to be considered a serious form of madness. Each new round of attacks was believed to progressively weaken the mind in ways that ultimately led to dementia. No one was supposed to ever recover from the mental scars of circular insanity.[4]

In 1882, however, the German asylum physician Karl Ludwig Kahlbaum proposed the existence of at least one type of circular insanity that was different from the ones highlighted by the French. It affected *only* moods and did not lead over time to permanent dementia. He felt it needed a new name, and so he proposed to call it "cyclothymia" (a combination of the Greek *kuklos*, "circle," and *thūmós*, "temper/disposition"). He further proposed calling the excited states of this new disorder "hyperthymia" and the depressive states "dysthymia."[5]

By the late nineteenth century, the conversation about mood states had become pretty complicated. Many clinicians still referenced the original circular insanity described by the French, in which patients cycled between acute attacks of mania and melancholy and ended up mentally impaired. Others had adopted Kahlbaum's new syndrome, cyclothymia, in which the cycling seemed to affect only moods and did not cause intellectual degeneration. These periodic sorts of mood disorders coexisted alongside a wide range of other recognized disorders that were believed to be variants of mania or melancholy, each of which in turn was said to present in a "simple" form that affected mood alone, or in a "chronic" form that involved delusions and mental confusion.

In 1899 Emil Kraepelin took stock of all this and declared it incoherent. Forget circular insanity, he said. Forget cyclothymia, and all the various categories of mania and melancholy, be they simple or chronic. Having undertaken a longitudinal study of these syndromes, he had come to the conclusion that beneath their dramatic surface differences, all these disorders were different expressions of one and the same disease, which he proposed to call "manic-depressive insanity."

> Manic-depressive insanity... includes on the one hand the whole domain of so-called periodic and circular insanity, on the other hand simple mania, the greater part of the morbid states termed melancholia and also a not inconsiderable number of cases of amentia (confusional or delirious insanity). Lastly, we include here certain slight and slightest colourings of mood, some of them periodic, some of them continuously morbid, which on the one hand are to be regarded as the rudiment of more severe disorders, on the other hand pass without sharp boundaries into the domain of personal predisposition. . . . I have become more and more convinced that all of the above-mentioned states only represent manifestations of a single morbid process.[6]

By creating the category of manic-depressive insanity, Kraepelin was proposing a distinction between this disorder and dementia praecox or schizophrenia (a distinction that he later confessed was sometimes less clear than he had originally proposed).[7] But he was also, with the stroke of a pen, proposing to eliminate the centuries-old category of melancholy (depression) as a distinct disease. Persuasive as he was on so many fronts, Kraepelin ultimately could not persuade all his colleagues to accept this second proposal.

So it happened that, in the early twentieth century and beyond, depression (vital, endogenous, psychotic) persisted as a diagnostic category that was used alongside manic-depression (see Chapter 6). The first *DSM*, published in 1952, described "manic-depressive psychosis" as a disorder a bit like schizophrenia (in that it sometimes included hallucinations and delusions), and a bit like depression (in that it generally included episodes of deep despair and listlessness)—but distinct from both. It was distinct above all because it was "marked by severe mood swings, and a tendency to remit and recur." Care needed to be taken in particular, the *DSM* authors made clear, to distinguish this disorder from a "psychotic depressive reaction," which was marked by an "absence of history of repeated depressions or of marked cyclothymic mood swings."[8]

THE PATIENTS NO ONE LIKED

As the diagnostic category "manic-depressive insanity" found its somewhat unstable place in the lexicon of American psychiatry, a consensus also took hold that people with this disorder were distinctively difficult to treat—partly because they were so unlikable. Classical Freudian theory had described them as developmentally stalled somewhere between the "second biting oral phase" and the "first expelling anal phase." This had made them prone to fantasies focused on feces, death, and cannibalism.[9]

When psychoanalytically inclined clinicians paid attention to the family backgrounds of these patients, they focused less on the maternal roots of these patients' psychic wounds (as they did with their schizophrenic patients) and far more on the extent to which these patients were as much a problem to their families as their families were to them.

> The manic-depressive patient is frequently the best endowed member of the family. He often occupies a special position in the family as a result of his own strivings, or because of some fortuitous circumstance such as being the eldest child or an only son. This leads him to guard his special position enviously and subjects him to the envy of the other siblings and the parents.[10]

Even Frieda Fromm-Reichmann, who was willing to accept gifts of feces from her schizophrenic patients (see Chapter 5), seems to have had difficulty mustering much compassion for manic-depressive patients. In the early 1950s, she summed up her view of the typical patient with this disorder. He was "a good manipulator, a salesman, a bargaining personality." He was invariably hungry for "prestige" and became hugely anxious when "his manipulations failed." Ultimately, she concluded, this kind of patient was dominated by "feelings of emptiness and envy."[11]

THE WONDER DRUG THAT EVERYONE (ORIGINALLY) IGNORED

In the end, the reputation of manic-depressive patients would be salvaged—dramatically. But the decisive factor in their rehabilitation was neither a new psychodynamic understanding of their personalities nor a new commitment to embracing them with unconditional regard. It was a new biological treatment—a drug called lithium.

The path by which lithium emerged as a treatment for manic-depression has the feel of a shaggy dog story. During World War II, the Australian psychiatrist John Cade had been held as a prisoner of war by the Japanese on Singapore, where he witnessed bizarre manic behaviors among his fellow prisoners. He wondered whether they were a form of intoxication caused by some kind of endogenous toxin. Later, as a practicing psychiatrist in Australia, he tried to find evidence for the existence of such a toxin. If mania was caused by a toxin, he reasoned, then the urine of manic patients would likely contain a metabolite of it. So he collected urine from manic, schizophrenic, and control patients, and injected the samples into the abdomens of guinea pigs. All the guinea pigs went into convulsions and died, but Cade had the impression that those that had been injected with urine from manic patients did worse. That suggested to him that he was on the right track.

Cade next faced the challenge of isolating the presumed toxic metabolite in the urine of his manic patients. Family members later recalled the vials of "manic urine in the family fridge," as he pursued this work.[12] He began by isolating salts of pure urea taken from the urine of the manic patients. He also took urea from the urine of schizophrenic and mentally healthy subjects to act as controls. He dissolved the salts and injected the solutions into guinea pigs. They all suffered fatal convulsions, and none of the groups seemed to do any better or worse than the others.

This avenue having failed to yield insights, Cade turned his attention to uric acid, another component of urine. But uric acid presented him with a problem: he could not prepare an injectable solution of it because it does not readily dissolve in water. Some physiologists at the University of Melbourne then informed Cade that combining uric acid with a lithium salt would produce lithium urate, and lithium urate would readily dissolve in water.

Cade took their advice, performed the injections, but then was startled by the results. This time none of the guinea pigs convulsed or died; it was as if the addition of lithium had somehow been protective. He then tested whether lithium salts injected on their own (he used lithium carbonate) had any effects. The results were even more striking: the normally skittish animals became lethargic and placid. When placed on their backs, instead of frantically trying to right themselves, they just lay there, apparently content.

The striking sight of "chilled out" guinea pigs led Cade to wonder if lithium salts were the treatment for the "manic" toxin that he had been trying to find. As he would later conclude in a 1949 publication, "It may seem a long way from lethargy in guinea pigs to the control of manic excitement, but as these investigations had commenced in an attempt to demonstrate some possibly excreted toxin in the urine of manic patients, the association of ideas is explicable."[13]

Wasting no time, Cade ingested some lithium carbonate himself to determine its safety and was soon satisfied on that score. He then conducted an open clinical trial in which either lithium carbonate or lithium citrate was given to ten patients with mania, six with schizophrenia, and six with chronic major depression. Only the manic patients improved, he reported, and some very dramatically. His first case, identified only by the initials W.B., was "restless, dirty, destructive, mischievous and interfering" and "had long been regarded as the most troublesome patient in the ward." After completing a course of treatment, W.B. was a changed man. He left the hospital on July 9, 1948, and was "soon back working happily at his old job."[14]

The results of Cade's lithium experiments were published some three years before the first open trials of chlorpromazine as a treatment for schizophrenia led to an explosion of interest in the use of pharmaceutics in psychiatry. Cade's astonishing claims about the antimanic effects of lithium, however, were passed over almost in silence. Another twenty-five years would go by before lithium would truly come into its own and usher manic-depression into the new world of biological psychiatry.

To understand the decades-long delay, we must understand a few things about lithium. Unlike all the other psychoactive drugs of the 1950s and '60s, lithium compounds were not developed in commercial laboratories. They exist naturally. Discovered in the early nineteenth century, lithium is the lightest metallic element, akin to other alkali metals—sodium, potassium, and three other less-familiar elements. Like them, it is malleable, a good conductor of heat and electricity, and highly reactive with the halogen elements fluorine, chlorine, bromine, and iodine. Salts of alkali metals are also readily soluble in water.

Over the years, lithium's properties and relative abundance enabled it to become an ingredient in many useful products that had nothing to do with mental illness. Combined with other elements and compounds, it improved the performance of ceramic glazes, batteries, and lubricating greases. In the 1950s it was a secret ingredient used to help fuel the first atomic fusion bombs.

But lithium's most time-honored use, perhaps tellingly, was as a medication and health tonic. In the mid-nineteenth century, its various compounds were used to dissolve bladder stones and gallstones, and to treat migraines, epilepsy, and eczema. Some clinicians used it to treat gout, a disorder caused by pathological levels of uric acid salts. Believing that some uric acid deposits could infiltrate the brain, the English physician Sir Alfred Baring Garrod used lithium compounds to treat what he called "brain gout," but that psychiatrists today would probably consider to be symptoms of depression. The Danish brothers Carl and Fritz Lange also believed that unusual levels of uric acid in the blood could cause mental problems and that lithium salts could help.[15] Although Cade never mentioned that he was familiar with the nineteenth-century literature that touted lithium as a remedy for "brain gout," there is at least circumstantial evidence that he was, and that this familiarity shaped his interest in its possible use as medicine for mood disorders.[16]

By the late nineteenth century, lithium lost its status as a medication prescribed by physicians for specific disorders; it became instead a popular health tonic with commercial value. Famous mineral water companies such as Vichy and Perrier promoted the high lithium content of their waters, which they insisted was particularly beneficial for people with "bad nerves." In 1929 the American entrepreneur Charles Leiper Grigg made lithium the central selling point of a new soft drink he developed for the Howdy Corporation, "Bib-Label Lithiated Lemon-Lime Soda." A doctor who endorsed the beverage testified that it provided customers with "an abundance of energy, enthusiasm, a clear complexion, lustrous hair, and shining eyes." Grigg later came up with a punchier slogan for his soda, "You Like It, It Likes You," and he rebranded it "7 Up." No one is sure why Grigg chose that name, but one theory is that it had to do with lithium: 7 is the rounded-up atomic mass of lithium (6.9), and "up" might allude to the element's alleged power to lift spirits.[17] Be that as it may, lithium remained an ingredient of 7 Up until 1950, when it was removed.

At about this time, the reputation of lithium as a health tonic took a decided nose dive, because of a scandal over its use as a salt substitute for patients with high blood pressure. Lithium chloride, one of the many compounds of lithium, happens to have a salty taste, and in the 1940s certain American companies had begun to market lithium chloride as a salt alternative, under such brand names as Westsal, Foodsal, Salti-salt, and Milosal.

In early 1949, scandal broke when *Time* magazine ran an article, "Case of the Substitute Salt," and quoted various clinicians who believed that the products were not safe, especially for patients with high blood pressure or heart disease—precisely the patients who might be tempted to use a salt substitute.[18] Several weeks later the *Journal of the American Medical Association* published corroborating letters and reports from other clinicians. Some patients using the products, they reported, had developed tremors, weakness, blurred vision, and unstable gait. In at least two cases, lithium poisoning was believed to have contributed to death.[19] The FDA now issued its own warning: "Stop using this dangerous poison at once."[20]

All this happened the same year Cade published his article touting lithium as a safe and effective antimanic drug. And again, his claim was almost completely ignored.

THE GREAT "MOOD NORMALIZER" DEBATE

Nevertheless a few years later, Erik Strömgren, head of the State Hospital for Psychiatric Research at Aarhus University in Denmark, attended a conference in Paris, where Cade's work on lithium as an antimanic treatment was mentioned. His interest was piqued not only by Cade's original study but also by a report that a pair of clinicians in Australia, Charles Noack and Edward Trautner, had verified Cade's claims more systematically using a much larger patient pool. These two researchers had also tackled the problem of lithium's potential toxicity by showing that the risks of poisoning were minimized if patients' blood serum levels were monitored throughout treatment.[21]

Strömgren asked his research assistant, Mogens Schou, to look further into the matter. Schou happened to have a younger brother who, since the age of twenty-five, had suffered recurrent, debilitating attacks of cyclical depression (seen by some as a variant of manic-depression). Schou was thus personally motivated to explore even implausible treatment options if they showed any promise at all.

And Schou did find Cade's claims in the original paper to be implausible. The experimental design, as he later recalled, was "not particularly clear." The conclusions seemed likely unsound: "Those guinea pigs probably did not just show altered behavior; they were presumably quite ill."[22]

Nevertheless, Noack and Trautner's follow-up work led Schou to conclude that Cade might have stumbled onto something profoundly important, perhaps despite himself. Over the next two years, he and his colleagues in Denmark investigated lithium, using a method very familiar today but quite novel back then: a double-blind, placebo-controlled trial. Some thirty-eight manic patients were randomly allocated into two groups. One group received treatment, the other a placebo. No one, including the evaluating clinicians, knew which was which. The results, published in 1954, found an 84 percent likely or possible effect: 14 of the 38 patients responded strongly to the drug, and a further 18 improved, "but a spontaneous cessation of the mania could not be excluded." Only six patients showed no appreciable response.[23]

This study—like Cade's original report—initially attracted little attention. Manic-depression was just the "other" psychosis, the afterthought psychosis. Nevertheless, while attention was focused elsewhere, a colleague of Schou's, Poul Christian Baastrup, quietly carried out a further clinical trial of his own. It was designed simply to confirm that lithium's effects were specific to mania (i.e., that the drug did not simply suppress states of excitation in general). It did not seem earth shattering, until matters took an unexpected turn.

Baastrup's protocol required him to follow up with patients who had been discharged from the hospital after a successful course of lithium treatment. Because lithium's potential toxicity was a real concern, all these patients had been ordered to cease taking lithium immediately upon discharge. Years later Baastrup recalled the "hair-raising" discovery that not only had eight of the patients continued to take lithium, against all orders, but two of them had even handed out these "miracle pills" (as they saw them) to relatives with the same disease. They told him, "Their reason for continuing the treatment in spite of our agreement was . . . that continuous lithium treatment *prevented psychotic relapse*."[24]

Something was wrong, Baastrup thought. His manic-depressive patients were claiming that the same drug, a simple element, was acting to prevent both psychotic manic attacks and psychotic descent into depression. It made no sense to him. Drugs either tranquilized or energized, it was thought—a single drug could not do both.

Unless that thinking was wrong. Baastrup discussed the situation with his colleague Schou. The two men agreed that, whether it made sense or not, the evidence, at least anecdotally, seemed strong. Schou even decided to put his own brother, still struggling with cycles of crippling depression, on a preventive course of lithium treatment. The brother seemed to stabilize. Urged on by a now enthusiastic Schou, in 1964 Baastrup published a short observational study involving eleven patients. In this report, he asserted for the first time that lithium was not only a useful drug for mania; when taken on a long-term basis, it could also act as a prophylactic, suppressing both the ups and the downs of manic-depression.[25]

Such an unprecedented claim was not going to be an easy sell. Baastrup's article came out during a time when concern was growing about the potential for long-term abuse of some of the popular mind-altering drugs on the market—especially the amphetamines and minor tranquilizers. He and Schou thus undertook to demonstrate that lithium did not have the same potential for abuse. To that end, the two men and at least one other colleague ingested therapeutic levels of lithium to see what effect the drug had on what they called "normal minds." The answer was, very little. They all felt some initial nausea, and their hands developed slight tremors. Some also reported a certain muscular heaviness and a slight sensation of "slowing." One of the unnamed participants in this informal study reported that his family found him more congenial. Another wryly reported that his family thought he had become "too dull." But if the changes were real, they were subtle. And the results strengthened the Danish researchers' view that lithium was different from other drugs on the market. It did not alter the mind. It simply stabilized and normalized it.[26]

By 1967, convinced that the evidence now warranted taking the research to the next level, Baastrup and Schou collaborated on a study that incorporated more than six years of data. It involved close to ninety Danish female manic-depressive patients who had undergone lithium treatment for at least twelve months. Using hospital records, Baastrup and Schou were able to show that prior to long-term lithium treatment, relapses within this group had occurred on average every eight months. Once the patients were on lithium, relapses occurred only once every 60 to 85 months and were of notably shorter duration.[27]

Nevertheless, the results failed to persuade skeptics, least of all an influential group of psychiatrists at London's Maudsley Hospital. Given the known dangers of lithium, the hype about its miraculous benefits was, they insisted, a dangerous "therapeutic myth."[28] Two of the Maudsley clinicians, Barry Blackwell and Michael Shepherd, further summed up their position in a pointed letter to the *American Journal of Psychiatry*, where they compared advocates of lithium to "the honest, well-intentioned enthusiasts who championed the ducking stool, purging, bleeding, and even insulin." No one should be using a treatment like this, they concluded, absent "proper controlled evaluation."[29] Nothing less than a double-blind, placebo-controlled trial would do.

These attacks mortified Schou and Baastrup.[30] If prophylactic lithium treatment stood any chance of surviving, they realized, they would have to subject it to what was increasingly recognized as the most rigorous approach to clinical testing: a placebo-controlled trial. But the thought of such a trial left them highly distraught, because it meant some of their patients would have to go off the drug and onto the placebo. That prospect seemed unconscionable, as by now they were personally convinced that the drug was all that stood between their patients and insanity—even suicide. Even naysayer Blackwell later ruefully admitted that, in calling for a placebo-controlled trial of lithium treatment, he and his colleagues had "underestimated the understandable concerns about safety and suicide."[31]

Nevertheless, Schou and his colleagues bit the bullet and designed the trial. Patients who had been on a course of continuous lithium treatment for at least a year (some as long as seven years) were now randomly and blindly allocated to one of two equal groups, one to receive lithium, the other a placebo. The 1970 report of the five-month trial noted that twenty-one of the approximately forty-two patients who were taking placebos relapsed, while not one of the patients taking lithium did.[32]

So much effort, so much pain, and yet in the United States at least, little changed. Even after the results of Schou's placebo-controlled trial were published, a very cautious FDA failed to budge. Eventually it did approve lithium as treatment, but only for acute mania, the original use for which it had been tested. It was a small step and much overdue. The United States was the *fiftieth* country to grant such approval.[33]

The question then became how American patients would access lithium. Pharmaceutical companies were not very interested in producing and marketing it because it could not be patented and so would not make them the significant profits they were now accustomed to getting from psychopharmaceutical products. Only after a personal appeal from members of the American College of Neuropsychopharmacology did a few relent.[34] Smith, Kline & French was one of the companies that agreed to sell lithium carbonate (under the brand name Eskalith), but only because its big moneymaker, Thorazine, was going off patent in 1970 and the company was reorienting its entire operational strategy anyway.[35] Pfizer also agreed to sell lithium salts (under the brand name Lithane). It then seems to have decided to integrate its promotion of this less lucrative drug with the marketing of one of its patented drugs for schizophrenia, called Navane. A 1970 ad, which appeared in the *American Journal of Psychiatry*, reproduced *The Creation of Adam*, the fresco painting by Michelangelo, over two pages. The text on the left, above Adam, described Navane as "an important psychotherapeutic agent that helps schizophrenic patients to communicate." Paired text on the right introduce Lithane as "the new psychotherapeutic agent that helps control manic episodes in manic-depressive patients." The word "new" was used an additional two times in the continuing explanatory text to describe this drug.[36]

THE LITHIUM UNDERGROUND

Even as lithium slowly made its way into the market as a treatment for controlling manic episodes, most clinicians who had followed the literature knew that the drug's real interest lay in its ability to normalize patients' moods over the long term. Lithium had not formally been approved for use as a mood normalizer, but clinicians found ways to work around this fact. Some filed Investigational New Drug (IND) applications that, once approved, allowed them to legally use the drug for uses other than those approved by the FDA. Others simply ignored the FDA regulations. In 1969 the *New York Times* reported on the rise of a "lithium underground" of rogue physicians who had decided to circumvent the law and do what they thought best: "Many psychiatrists, both in private practice and on hospital staffs are bringing in capsules from foreign drug houses or getting their corner pharmacists to buy some lithium from local chemical supply houses, and dispensing the medication to patients."[37]

Some of these doctors took their case to the public. In 1974 one clinician, for example, urged the advice columnist Abigail Van Buren ("Dear Abby" writer Pauline Phillips) to tell a worried wife that medications were now available that might stabilize her suddenly erratic and moody husband.[38] Others like Nathan Kline and Frederick Goodwin contributed to popular articles on lithium's mood-stabilizing effects in publications ranging from *Good Housekeeping* to the *New York Times*.[39] Some of the most compelling articles drew on dramatic personal testimonials. The title of a 1974 *Newsday* piece reads like a true confession potboiler: "How a Long Island Woman, Tormented by Wild Swings of Mood for 10 Years, Was Restored to a Normal Life by a Simple Drug Called Lithium."[40]

The biggest public relations coup during these years, however, was scored by the psychiatrist Ronald Fieve. In the early 1970s, he persuaded his patient Joshua Logan (who began lithium maintenance treatment in 1969) to testify on television and in other public forums about his positive experiences with the medication. Logan's testimony was riveting not only because of what he said but because of who he was: the brilliant playwright and director-producer of such Tony-winning musicals as *Annie Get Your Gun*, *Camelot*, and *South Pacific*. The climactic moment of his career as the human face of the benefits of long-term lithium treatment came in June 1973, when he spoke at a panel organized by the American Medical Association. As the *New York Times* reported his testimony:

> Mr. Logan said he had previously been treated over 20 years for "several 'nervous breakdowns' that were really manic elations—I would be going great guns, putting out a thousand ideas a minute, acting flamboyant—until I went over the bounds of reality" and was then caught up in a profound "wish to be dead without having to go through the shaming defeat of suicide."
>
> Speaking quietly, with his fingers carefully interlaced and twiddling his thumbs, he said that the "aggravated agony" of the depression phase was "terrifying" and that "elation, its non-identical twin sister, is even more terrifying—attractive as she may be for a moment. You are grandiose beyond the reality of your creativity."
>
> "It's a little as though you got too close to the microphone and you blasted, and so nobody could understand what you said," he suggested. He said he had been "tempered" by continuing dosages of lithium four times a day.[41]

As doctors and patients alike worked the court of public opinion, we also see, more and more, claims being made that the effectiveness of lithium also demonstrated the failure of the Freudian approach to mood disorders. The 1974 *Newsday* article about the Long Island woman with manic-depression explained that she had spent "thousands of dollars" on psychotherapy, and it had all been "money down the drain." Lithium, in contrast, had been a "miracle drug," the "savior" of an entire family.[42]

A year later, in 1975, Ronald Fieve came out with *Moodswing*, the first book specifically devoted to explaining manic-depression to the general public. It declared that the "lithium breakthrough" was helping to usher in a new revolutionary era in psychiatry—one based on biology rather than unproven psychological constructs:

> The lithium breakthrough . . . has clarified the fact that major mood disorders—which may at times be advantageous and productive— are stabilized by a simple, naturally occurring substance. Further- more, findings point to the fact that mania and mental depression must be due to biochemical causes handed down through the genes, since they are correctable so rapidly by chemical rather than talking therapy.[43]

Some, picking up on this theme, suggested more specifically that manic-depression resulted from a kind of chemical "imbalance" in which neurotransmitter deficits first "damp down the circuits" to cause depres- sion (in Nathan Kline's words), while "surplus" neurotransmitters "pro- duce the opposite manic effects."[44]

The problem was that there was no evidence from laboratory studies or anywhere else in support of the idea that the highs and lows of manic- depression were caused by alternating deficits and surpluses of neurotrans- mitters. More to the point, the observation that a single drug could put the brakes on both highs and lows was hard to square with conventional "imbalance" talk.[45]

Even though no one really understood how lithium worked, it unques- tionably helped turn manic-depression into a biochemical disease that could be treated pharmaceutically. In so doing, it also helped rehabilitate the character of patients who had previously been so often disliked. Tamed by lithium, they became sympathetic, appealing, even brilliant people who had simply been betrayed by their unruly biochemistry. As one patient told a *New York Times* journalist in 1978, "It's not *me*, you see; it's my biochemistry."[46]

BIPOLAR DISORDER

Even while the precise biochemistry of manic-depression remained mysterious, champions of manic-depression's 1970s biological revolution could find comfort in the disorder's inheritance patterns. Beginning in the 1960s, various twin studies had shown that the identical twin siblings of patients with manic-depression had close to a 70 percent chance of also suffering either from manic-depression or from another mood disturbance. The likelihood of fraternal twins both suffering from manic-depression was only about 20 percent. Adoption studies showed that the biological parents of adopted manic-depression patients had a 30 percent chance of also suffering from some kind of mood disorder (major depression or manic-depression), whereas the incidence within the pool of adoptive parents was only 2 percent.[47]

The most influential studies on the inheritance of manic-depression did more than simply confirm that the disorder was inherited in some way. In the eyes of some, they also provided significant new evidence that depression and manic-depression were different disorders and that Kraepelin had in fact overreached when he included depression within his capacious diagnostic category of manic-depression. In the late 1950s, the East German psychiatrist Karl Leonhard published evidence that the frequency of manic attacks was greater in the families of patients who were affected by the classical "circular" form of the disease than in patients who simply presented with depression.[48] Because manic-depression had originally been used to categorize *all* the mood disorders, Leonhard felt the time was right to introduce some new, more useful terms to better capture the distinctions he believed he had demonstrated. He therefore proposed dropping the term *manic-depression* altogether and using the term *bipolar* to refer to mood disorders that cycled, and *unipolar* to refer to those that did not.[49]

Leonhard was soon in good company. In the late 1960s Jules Angst in Switzerland and Carlo Perris in Sweden found differences in the family histories of patients who cycled and in those of patients who presented with only depression.[50] The first American studies with conclusions similar to Leonhard's were published in 1969 by three researchers at Washington University: George Winokur, Paula Clayton, and Theodore Reich.[51]

These studies are particularly important for our story because of their impact on the *DSM-III*, published in 1980. Influenced by their findings, this was the version of psychiatry's diagnostic manual that got rid of the expansive and fraught Kraepelinian term *manic-depression* and replaced it with Leonhard's alternative, *bipolar disorder*. The committee recommending this change had considered using Leonhard's term *unipolar disorder* for depression, but ultimately decided against it because, according to notes taken by committee members, the term *unipolar* "perturbed" some psychotherapists involved in the conversation. They worried that it "carried an implication of biological etiology." Strangely, these same psychotherapists seem to have had no problem changing the name *manic-depression* to *bipolar disorder*.[52] Did they think that term *failed* to carry any implication of biological etiology? Perhaps they did not care in the same way—as we know, most had never much liked, or had much success with, bipolar patients.

As time passed, advocates and clinicians alike also increasingly felt that the term *manic-depression* was not just a relic of an older, excessively capacious understanding of mood disorders, but was also stigmatizing and misleading, not least because the term *mania* evoked images of wild-eyed, dangerous "maniacs." Thus in August 2002, the National Depression and Manic Depression Association (NDMDA) officially changed its name to the Depression and Bipolar Support Alliance (DBSA). On their website, they explained that they wanted to align their terminology with that of the *DSM*, and to create a name that was easier to remember. But their most important reason, they admitted, was that "many people are frightened by the term 'manic-depression' and this keeps them from contacting us for help."[53]

THE HUNT FOR MOOD GENES

While manic-depression was slowly morphing into bipolar disorder, the search for its genetic basis continued. This story begins in the 1960s when a sociology graduate student, Janice Egeland, formed an unlikely friendship with a community of Old Order Amish in Lancaster, Pennsylvania. The Old Order Amish are an extremely private religious community that eschews most contact with outsiders ("the English"). But in 1962 one family allowed Egeland to move in with them. Her plan was to do a Ph.D. dissertation on their health beliefs and behaviors.

Egeland soon became vaguely aware that one of the women in her host family suffered from manic-depression, even though at the time she knew little about the disorder. As she told an interviewer three decades later:

> One morning, I saw this woman doubled up in pain, moaning and sobbing. When I asked her what was wrong, she responded, "I don't have a physical pain. It's the pain of the thoughts I'm having that is doing this to me."[54]

At a picnic soon afterward, a grandmother explained to Egeland that they were all very familiar with the disorder she had witnessed, since it ran in the family—or as she actually put it, *siss im blut* ("it's in the blood").[55] That remark "made such an impact on me," Egeland later recalled, "that I shifted gears right there—that was about thirty years ago—and said, 'That's it. My life's work will be with this condition.' "[56]

Egeland now looked for collaborators who might be interested in joining her in a study of the heritability of manic-depression among the Amish. Her first connection was to the physician Abram Hostetter, who had been raised in a Mennonite family on a farm in southeastern Pennsylvania. More collaborators joined them, eventually coming from eight schools of medicine in the United States and Canada. In 1976 "The Amish Study" was launched with grant support from the NIMH.

Despite the Amish's well-known commitment to privacy and aversion to engagement with modern technologies, the study subjects seem mostly to have cooperated willingly with the protocols: they gave blood for DNA samples and allowed probes into their family medical backgrounds. Talking to a journalist many years later, one of them explained why: "This disease has torn our family apart. I was 17 when my mother came to me and spoke of not being able to face the day—I didn't know what she was talking about. At the time none of us knew anything of the illness, but Janice has changed that."[57]

Egeland and her collaborators soon realized, however, that studying manic-depression among the Amish was likely to do more than produce information that would be helpful to this community. The community itself had the potential to function (in Egeland's words) as "an ideal type of human laboratory for behavioral and medical genetic studies."[58]

This was so for a number of reasons: the Amish rarely married outside their community; they tended to have very large families; and they kept extensive genealogical records. In fact, members of the Amish community with whom Egeland worked could trace their ancestry back to a group of thirty-two immigrants who came to Pennsylvania in the 1750s from a province in what is today Germany.

Moreover, the Amish lived according to traditions that had changed little over the generations. This meant, as the researchers saw it, that any changes in disease patterns over time were unlikely to be caused by social change but could be assumed to be genetic in nature.[59]

Finally, the task generally of identifying people with manic-depression among the Amish was made much easier, it was felt, by the fact that the Amish lived according to values of simplicity, humility, and personal modesty. Any members who deviated markedly from those virtues—for example, because they were in the throes of a manic attack—would (in the words of a later newspaper article) "stand out like sore thumbs."[60] And because the Amish abstained from alcohol and drug use, there was little risk that researchers' ability to diagnose manic-depression would be obscured by behaviors associated with substance abuse.

By 1983, the team had identified 112 cases of manic-depression within the Amish community, out of a population of 12,500 based in fifty Amish church districts. Many of these cases were concentrated in a clan of 236 individuals who spanned four generations. Some 71 percent of these individuals had experienced either major depression or manic-depression. The inheritance pattern suggested that the disorder was inherited as a dominant gene but with incomplete penetration. For an individual to inherit the gene, only one of that individual's parents needed to have carried it, and those who inherited the gene had a roughly 60 percent chance of suffering from manic-depression. By examining old family records, the team tracked the source of the illness for this clan back to a single individual who had been born in Europe in 1763.

The team then made the then-novel move of collecting DNA samples from their subjects' blood to perform what is called a linkage study. This form of gene hunting takes advantage of the fact that genes that sit close together on the same chromosome are often inherited together (because they remain linked during meiosis). In a linkage study, researchers therefore first screen DNA for the presence of a genetic marker: a segment of DNA with a known physical location on a chromosome. They then see whether that genetic marker is consistently found in the DNA of individuals suffering from an inherited disease—but absent in individuals who don't suffer from that disease. If the researchers do find such a linkage, then there is a plausible case to be made that the unknown gene for the target disease is being inherited along with the known genetic marker and likely sits somewhere very close by to that marker.

Egeland's linkage study found that within the clan (code-named Pedigree 110), nearly 80 percent of those who had inherited a particular genetic marker near the tip of the eleventh chromosome also had manic-depressive illness or major depression. Nothing like this had ever been found for schizophrenia, for major depression, for any other mental disorder, or indeed for any other clinical disorder whatsoever. In 1987, with great fanfare, the results were published in *Nature*:

> For the first time the application of a generalized strategy for scanning the human genome has provided convincing evidence for the localization of a gene that is implicated in the etiology of a com-

mon clinical disorder. These findings have broad implications for research in human genetics and psychiatry.[61]

Psychiatric research was setting a new standard for medicine as a whole! As a neuroscientist active in 1987, Steven Mark Paul, recalled many years later, "For a year or two, it was probably the most exciting and interesting finding in psychiatry."[62] Newspapers across the country heralded it as "one of the most profound discoveries" and "the strongest evidence yet" that serious mental illness had a genetic basis.[63]

Unfortunately, within a year, new evidence had cast serious doubt on the linkage claims. Two people from the original group who had shown no previous signs of mental disorder and who shared the genetic pattern of those who did not have the illness began to develop manic-depressive symptoms. Then, when researchers looked for a similar linkage pattern on chromosome eleven in *non*-Amish patients with manic-depression, they found none. Egeland and her collaborators co-authored a second paper in *Nature* in 1989, bravely reporting this failure to confirm.[64]

Disappointment at the failure to nail down the specific gene or genes involved in manic-depression lingered for years. In 2001 the psychiatrist David Dunner admitted to the American College of Neuropsychopharmacology:

I am disappointed that we have never identified the "bipolar gene." ... I realize now how complicated it is and how naïve we were. Very good people are now looking for the genes, not a single gene. I am not going to be the one to find them, but it would be nice to know that there really are genes when patients ask, "Is this a genetic disorder?" and [right now] I can only say, "Well, we think so."[65]

A GLAMOR DILEMMA

For decades, it had been appreciated that many manic-depressives were extremely gifted and intelligent people, at least when they were not ill. Before the 1970s, however, no one had gone so far as to suggest that whatever (possibly inherited) biological quirk was responsible for the illness might play a role in facilitating their intellectual and/or artistic gifts. This first began to change during the public campaign to promote lithium as a mood stabilizer. In his 1975 book *Moodswing*, Ronald Fieve had celebrated not only the birth of a biological revolution in psychiatry but also the creative, impossible, maddening, and brilliant patients who were, in his view, on the front lines of that revolution. "People who suffer from . . . [manic-depression] . . . in its milder forms of mood swing tend to be magnificent performers, magnetic personalities, and true achievers. Many forms of manic elation seem to be a genetic endowment of the same order as perfect pitch, a photographic memory, great intelligence, or artistic talent of any sort." Many "super achievers in business, the arts, and especially in politics," owed a debt to a "superior energy" that, Fieve said, was "specifically biochemical and hereditary." Yes, he conceded—perhaps in a nod to the older Freudian judgment of these patients—super achievers such as these were "manipulators par excellence," but they were "also the people who get things done. Without them society would be much impoverished."[66]

These were, of course, mere clinical impressions. Was there any independent evidence linking manic-depression to "super achievement"? Over the course of the 1970s and '80s, a series of attempts were made to answer this question. In 1974 a medical resident named Nancy Andreasen (who ten years later would help announce the 1980s biological revolution with her book *The Broken Brain*) was interested in the relationship between creativity and familial mental illness. She studied a large sample of writers and found that as many as 80 percent had experienced at least one episode of major depression, mania, or hypomania, whereas only 30 percent of a control group of "noncreative" people had. Relatives of writers also had a higher incidence than expected of mood disorder. "The data support Aristotle's dictum," she concluded, "that . . . there *is* an association between genius and psychiatric disorder."[67]

In 1987 Andreasen returned to her original pool of writers and controls and made an even stronger claim: thirteen years later no fewer than 43 percent of them had received a diagnosis of bipolar disorder, compared to only 10 percent of the control group and 1 percent of the general population.[68] It seemed that it was not quite right to say that there was an association between genius and mental illness in general. The association seemed to be primarily limited to *bipolar* forms of mood disorder.

Two years later the clinical psychologist Kay Redfield Jamison published an article that made even more ripples. "Mood Disorders and Patterns of Creativity in British Writers and Artists" analyzed forty-seven British authors and visual artists who were members of the British Royal Academy and found that 38 percent had been treated for a mood disorder, particularly the bipolar variety. Jamison concluded by suggesting that the remarkable and apparently inherited connection between creativity and bipolar disorder raised important ethical issues. "Genetic research," she wrote, "is progressing to the stage where ethical issues will, in due course, arise about amniocentesis and early identification and treatment of individuals at high risk for affective, especially bipolar, illness." Would parents be encouraged to abort fetuses at risk for bipolar disorder—but also perhaps with the potential to be unusually creative? If so, at what cost to society?[69]

In 1993 Jamison pushed this point further in her widely noted book *Touched with Fire*.[70] By this time, she had been appointed a professor of psychiatry at the Johns Hopkins University School of Medicine and had co-authored, with Frederick Goodwin, an authoritative textbook on manic-depression (see page 239).[71] *Touched with Fire* celebrated the brilliant contributions made by many people born with this disorder, even as it asked readers to appreciate the enormous burden of suffering under which they labored.

Jamison's interest in the positive side of manic-depression turned out to have roots in personal experience. Two years after *Touched with Fire*, in her memoir *An Unquiet Mind*, she announced that she herself suffered from the disorder and described her own experiences with it. She focused especially on her struggles to reconcile herself to the price of submitting to effective treatment. Lithium was a lifesaving drug, she knew, but it also damped her down, made her less creative, less interesting, and less productive. "When I am my present 'normal self,'" she mused wistfully, "I am far removed from when I have been my liveliest, most productive, most intense, most outgoing and effervescent. In short, for myself, I am a hard act to follow."[72]

An Unquiet Mind made Jamison a celebrity and a role model, even as others worried that it painted a glamorous picture of a deadly serious mental illness. Edwin Fuller Torrey, a prominent schizophrenia researcher (see Chapter 5), told the *Washington Post* in 1995, "I think there's a real danger in what Kay does. The danger is the romanticizing of serious mental illness. . . . Our tendency is to romanticize Sylvia Plath or someone like that without asking whether, if they hadn't had the disease, they wouldn't have produced better things over time."[73]

All the same, by the 1990s, the public had absorbed the new message: if you had to suffer from a serious mental illness in the age of biological psychiatry, manic-depression was the one to have. In the early 1990s, Robert Boorstin, a journalist and aide to President Bill Clinton, was hospitalized for manic-depression. He arranged to have a sign put over his bed that read simply: "Thank God I'm not schizophrenic."[74]

THE BIPOLAR SPECTRUM

This destigmatizing of manic-depression coincided with—if it did not necessarily directly create—a steady broadening of the criteria for being diagnosed with bipolar disorder. By the late 1990s, many more people than before were being diagnosed with the disorder, especially newly established milder variants.

In 1980 *DSM-III* had laid down quite strict criteria for a diagnosis of bipolar disorder. It drew a clear line between bipolar disorder and major depression. It advised clinicians not to make diagnoses of bipolar disorder unless the patient showed evidence of psychotic behavior, including symptoms of full-blown mania. It told clinicians they might sometimes see patients with milder cycles of "mood disturbance" with no psychotic features; they should diagnose such patients not with bipolar disorder but with "cyclothymic disorder." Some researchers, the authors of this section of the book conceded, thought cyclothymic disorder was on a continuum with bipolar, but they took the view that there was not yet adequate consensus that this was the case.[75]

In the years following the 1980 publication of *DSM-III*, however, some of these researchers started to win their argument. One of these was David Dunner from the NIMH, who had been arguing since the early 1970s for expanding the category of bipolar disorder to include patients who suffered from depression and mild mania but not severely enough to require hospitalization. "It turned out," he told a later interviewer, "that those patients had a very high suicide attempt and suicide rate."[76] Another was the Armenian-American psychiatrist Hagop Akiskal, director of one of the country's first specialized mood disorder clinics, based in Memphis, Tennessee, who had also been arguing since the mid-1970s for seeing "cyclothymia" as a mild form of bipolar disorder.[77]

Fourteen years later, in 1994, the fourth revision of the *DSM* told clinicians that psychiatry now believed there were two kinds of bipolar disorder. Bipolar I was the classical, psychotic form of bipolar, and Bipolar II was a milder form in which episodes of depression alternated with experiences of either elevated mood or anger and irritability (positive or negative hypomania).

But if bipolar disorder could have two subtypes, then why not more—maybe even a lot more? Akiskal soon proposed that, beyond Bipolar I and II, there were also Bipolar III and IV (and possibly still more intermediate versions between these four). More generally, his point was that bipolar disorder was best seen, not as a narrowly defined category, but as a fluid "spectrum" of disorders.[78] A spectrum approach to bipolar, he said, was actually consistent with Emil Kraepelin's original expansive vision of manic-depressive insanity—even though the authors of *DSM-III* had abandoned it (while, ironically enough, allowing themselves to be called "neo-Kraepelinians).[79] "I have no use for the DSM," Akiskal cheerfully told a blogger who came to interview him in 2011.[80]

Meanwhile 1990 saw the publication of a monumental textbook, *Manic-Depressive Illness*, jointly authored by Frederick Goodwin and Kay Redfield Jamison and widely acclaimed as a definitive synthesis of the literature.[81] In the course of their decade-long study of the literature, the authors had become convinced of something else: that *DSM-III*'s sharp boundary between bipolar disorder and depression (what some called unipolar disorder) just didn't hold up. "We became more and more convinced that isolating bipolar illness from other major depressive disorders prejudges the relationships between bipolar and unipolar illness and diminishes appreciation of the fundamental importance of recurrence."[82] A bit like Akiskal, they insisted that, in rejecting sharp and categorical distinctions between bipolarity and depression, they were returning to the original vision of that master diagnostician Emil Kraepelin.

A lot was a stake. If bipolar disorder was actually a spectrum of disorders—and if that spectrum encompassed some kinds of depression—then a lot of patients might require a different sort of medication than they had been getting. And some who might have struggled their whole lives without realizing they suffered from bipolar disorder might finally get the medication they needed. A disorder that was once assumed to affect only about 1 percent of the population might now (according to some calculations) affect as much as 6 percent.[83] And all these sufferers needed help.

Something else may have been at stake, at least for some players in these discussions: profits. As a number of critics soon pointed out, the push to expand the category of bipolar disorder happened during exactly the same years when the pharmaceutical industry finally found a way to make significant money from medications targeting it. Lithium had never been profitable, but in 1995 the pharmaceutical company Abbott gained FDA approval to market the proprietary drug Depakote for symptoms of mania.[84] Depakote was not a new drug; Abbott had been selling it since the 1960s to stabilize epileptic convulsions. However, the company had then run some trials that suggested it might also be effective in "stabilizing moods"—they called it a "mood stabilizer." It was a breakthrough moment for the industry, and other "mood stabilizing" drugs followed in short order. (They in turn would then be partly supplanted by so-called atypical antipsychotics; see Chapter 8.) Were the drug companies simply meeting an unmet need that clinicians had identified, or were they—as the psychopharmacologist David Healy, among others, insisted—cynically working behind the scenes to push the agendas of researchers whose clinical understanding of bipolar disorder aligned with their own financial interests?[85]

The question took on added ethical urgency when children emerged as the fastest-growing group of newly recognized bipolar patients. Before the 1990s, it had been very rare for children and adolescents to be diagnosed with bipolar disorder. Between 1994 and 2003, however, the number increased a remarkable *forty*-fold, from about 20,000 to about 800,000 cases per year.[86] Some said this happened because the bipolarity of children had not previously been recognized. Bipolar children did not "cycle" the way that adults did. Instead, they were chronically irritable, hyperactive, angry (or sad), and prone to bouts of explosive rage.[87] For this reason, they had previously been seen just as problem kids, or had been (inaccurately) diagnosed with attention-deficit disorder (ADHD). Realizing that many of these children actually had juvenile bipolar disorder, the argument now went, absolved their families of guilt and offered the children new pharmaceutical options.

The argument for the existence of a hitherto unrecognized form of bipolar disorder in children (some as young as two or three) was given huge visibility by the publication in 1999 of *The Bipolar Child*, authored by a husband-and-wife team (Demitri Papolos was a psychiatrist at Albert Einstein University, Janice Papolos an author and family advocate). The reassuring book they co-authored was designed to help parents identify the telltale signs of juvenile bipolar disorder in their own troubled kids, and get them the help they needed.[88] While the book talked about ways to support such children in schools and at home, it foregrounded the importance of getting them on a course of "mood stabilizing" medication. And thousands of distraught parents welcomed its advice with open arms, especially after *The Bipolar Child* was featured on television shows like *Oprah* and *20/20*. The testimonies of some of the parents in question, left on the review page of the online bookseller Amazon, are moving:

> I ordered this book. I got just a few pages in before I started to cry, because for the first time, I knew that I wasn't the only one going through this. I wasn't imagining it or making it out to be worse than it was as many people have told us.[89]

The pain and despair were real, but critics like Healy argued that profligate use of this new diagnostic category was having the effect of putting countless young children on powerful medications (mood stabilizers and antipsychotics) that had not been tested and approved for them.[90] These medications might reduce the irritability and outbursts seen in such children, but they also often caused serious side effects (especially significant weight gain, with the risk of diabetes and heart problems later in life).

The matter got sufficiently controversial that in 2013, the APA intervened by introducing a new—but inevitably also controversial—diagnostic category into the fifth revision of the *DSM*. "Disruptive mood dysregulation disorder (DMDD)" was intended to provide clinicians with an alternative diagnosis to juvenile bipolar disorder. It was classified as a form of depression rather than bipolar disorder.[91] The problem was, no one knew if DMDD was a real disease, with its own biology. Perhaps it was just a new way of talking about the same highly disruptive behaviors that had previously led to so many diagnoses of juvenile bipolar disorder. Nevertheless, the once solid-seeming boundaries around bipolar disorder were now so soft that something, it seemed, had to be done.

PART III

UNFINISHED STORIES

CHAPTER 8

False Dawn

RALLYING 'ROUND

In the 1970s lead-up to the biological revolution, psychiatrists had rallied around biology and the "medical model" as a way of exorcising the specters of psychoanalysis, antipsychiatry, and radical social science. In the 1980s they continued to rally around that model, but largely for a different reason: to assert guild privilege. "We use the term 'medical model,'" one clinician admitted in 1981, "to rally the troops," while announcing "to the world that we are doctors, medical specialists."[1] This had become necessary because other mental health workers were knocking at the gate of mental health care with increasing energy. Clinical social workers, psychiatric nurses, counselors, and clinical psychologists had, to a significant degree, taken over the field of psychotherapy.[2] Now they wanted Medicare reimbursement, hospital privileges, and above all, the right to prescribe drugs.[3]

Not surprisingly, the psychiatrists pushed back hard. Prescribing drugs, they said sharply, must remain a privilege granted exclusively to medically trained clinicians such as themselves. Any other conclusion would have been an abdication of responsibility to patients.[4] The psychologists and social workers responded to this ostensibly altruistic rationale with distinct skepticism. "It's [actually] a question of turf," a spokesman for the National Association of Social Workers, Ray Hamilton, told the *New York Times* in 1985. "Whenever a new mental health profession vies for payments, it cuts down the number who can get that same therapy dollar."[5]

Doubling down on their assertion of professional privilege, many psychiatrists suggested that, having reclaimed biology as the foundation of its work, their field's best days lay just over the horizon. Hopes for a bright future were further stoked when, in 1990, the U.S. Congress and President George H. W. Bush declared the coming years to be the "Decade of the Brain." This declaration facilitated the flow of federal dollars (though not as many as had been hoped) into research, especially new neuroimaging technologies.[6]

Psychiatrists had some reason to believe that these technologies could be a game changer for them. As early as the 1970s, an older technology called computerized axial tomography (CT) scanning, had allowed researchers to produce anatomical images of the brain *in vivo*. And in 1976 the Scottish neuroscientist Eve Johnstone had fanned early hopes for CT scanning as a research tool in psychiatry when she used it to support her claim that the ventricles, or cavities, in the brains of schizophrenics were larger than those of people without the disease. Over the next several years, other labs confirmed this finding, but what did it mean? In the mid-1980s, even Johnstone admitted the answer was unclear.[7]

In the 1980s and '90s, though, newer imaging technologies, such as positron emission tomography (PET) and magnetic resonance imaging (MRI), did more than just take pictures of the static brain; they allowed researchers to create colorful images of the brain's activity levels—snapshots, so to speak, of the "brain in action." Naturally, this sparked the hope that psychiatrists would soon be able to look at the brains of their patients the way cardiologists use angiograms to identify blockages to blood flow—to "see" what was wrong. In her 1995 memoir on bipolar disorder, the psychologist Kay Redfield Jamison confessed to sharing in the excitement:

> There is a beauty and an intuitive appeal to the brain-scanning methods, especially the high-resolution MRI pictures and the gorgeous multicolored scans from the PET studies. With PET, for example, a depressed brain will show up in cold, brain-inactive deep blues,

dark purples, and hunter greens; the same brain when hypomanic, however, is lit up like a Christmas tree, with vivid patches of bright red and yellows and oranges. Never has the color and structure of science so completely captured the cold inward deadness of depression or the vibrant, active engagement of mania.[8]

The infusion of new funds into still more impressive imaging technologies like functional magnetic resonance imaging (fMRI) failed, however, to move knowledge of mental illness forward in the definitive ways that so many psychiatrists had hoped. There were plenty of findings, but they varied across studies and proved hard to replicate and interpret.[9] Above all, the new neuroimaging work failed to have any appreciable impact on how the overwhelming majority of patients were diagnosed and treated. As Tom Insel, director of the NIMH, soberly concluded in 2010, "During the so-called Decade of the Brain, there was neither a marked increase in the rate of recovery from mental illness, nor a detectable decrease in suicide or homelessness—each of which is associated with a failure to recover from mental illness."[10]

EMBRACING BIG PHARMA

This is not to say that the new era of biological psychiatry failed to touch the lives of ordinary patients. On the contrary, this was the time when drugs began to dominate virtually all conversations about how to handle mental suffering, certainly among psychiatrists (as opposed to psychologists and social workers). This new consensus, however, did not happen simply because everyone now "believed" in the medical model, or because prescribing privileges were one of the few things that still allowed psychiatrists to assert their identity as physicians, or because Freud the man and psychoanalysis as a movement continued in the 1990s to suffer an onslaught of steady blows to their reputations.[11] All three of these factors were true and relevant, but they were dramatically amplified by a fourth: by the late 1980s, a critical mass of clinicians and researchers had aligned their professional interests with the commercial interests of the pharmaceutical industry.

To understand how this happened, we need to realize that 1980 was not just the year that saw the publication of *DSM-III*, and a slew of proclamations celebrating psychiatry's return to the medical model. It was also the year that Ronald Reagan won the presidency of the United States on a pro-business, prosperity platform. Previously academic medicine had jealously defended its autonomy from industry, but Reagan's election began to change this situation. Desiring to lift constraints on business and encourage profitable innovation, the U.S. Congress enacted a series of laws to speed the translation of basic research into useful new products— sometimes referred to as "technology transfer."

In particular, the 1980 Bayh-Dole Act (named after its chief sponsors, Senators Birch Bayh and Robert Dole) allowed universities and individual scientists to patent any potentially profitable discovery resulting from medical research, even federally funded research (i.e., they could retain private ownership of valuable products developed with tax dollars). They could then strike lucrative deals with industries interested in developing the commercial potential of that discovery.[12]

As relations between academia and industry became closer, pharmaceutical companies began offering clinicians and researchers the opportunity to work for them directly: to join "speakers' bureaus," and act as "key opinion leaders." Key opinion leaders were paid handsomely for providing advice on designing clinical trials, for authoring study results, for fielding questions from the media, and for talking up new drugs to colleagues at conferences and company-sponsored dinners. For psychiatrists feeling like the poor relations of the medical world—and financially pinched by the incursion of psychology and social work onto their turf—the siren call of industry consulting work was difficult to resist. In 2008 disclosure reports filed by 273 speakers at the annual meeting of the APA revealed that, among them, the speakers had signed 888 consulting contracts and 483 contracts to serve on so-called "speakers' bureaus" for a drug company.[13]

One drug company representative who worked for many years with such clinicians was frank about the rationale for these contracts: "Key opinion leaders were salespeople for us, and we would routinely measure the return on our investment, by tracking prescriptions before and after their presentations. . . . If that speaker didn't make the impact the company was looking for, then you wouldn't invite them back."[14]

Clinicians were not the only ones who were targeted: drug companies also advanced their goals by supporting the work of family advocacy groups, such as NAMI, that were resolutely committed to the "medical model" of mental illness. In 2004 a "veteran pharma marketer" was frank about why this was done:

> I have witnessed that the most direct and efficient tool for driving long-term support for brands has been, and continues to be, a well-designed, advocacy-based public education program. . . . Working with advocacy groups is one of the most accomplished means of raising disease awareness and enhancing the industry's image as deliverer of new and tangible value to patients.[15]

By 2010, as much as 75 percent of NAMI's budget came from the pharmaceutical industry.[16]

All this alliance building might have been forgivable if it had led to innovative and effective new treatments, even empirical ones based on trial and error. But no such treatments emerged. Instead, the 1990s and early 2000s were widely deemed (in the words of one *Nature Review* article) a "barren time for the discovery of novel drugs for psychiatric disorders, in particular those that could revolutionize disease treatment."[17] A couple of new antidepressants were developed that targeted norepinephrine instead of serotonin—so-called SNRIs, such as venlafaxine (Effexor) and nefazodone (Serzone)—but they were only moderately successful. Most research in this period managed, at best, to make incremental improvements to classes of drugs that had been in use since the 1950s and '60s.

Ironically, however, this period was nevertheless a halcyon time for psychiatric drug sales. Marketing was the critical reason. In 1997 the FDA agreed to dramatically relax the rules regulating direct-to-consumer (DTC) advertising of prescription drugs, which thereafter exploded, increasing from less than $800 million in 1996 to $2.5 billion in 2000, and peaking at $4.9 billion in 2007. Psychiatric drugs were among the most heavily advertised; as late as 2014, two of the top-ten most heavily adver-tised drugs targeted mental health conditions.[18]

The numbers seem to say it all: between 1987 and 2001, the amount of revenue generated by (not so new and not so innovative) psychiatric drugs increased sixfold, twice the rate generated by sales of prescription drugs overall.[19]

Key to understanding these numbers, however, is the extent to which the drug companies did not just market the heck out of drugs already approved for specific disorders (like depression). They also actively sought new markets—that is to say, new disorders—for those same drugs. And to do so, some looked to *DSM-III*, with its 265 disorders, some of which had not yet been claimed for pharmacology.

PANIC DISORDER

One early effort of this sort targeted the newly established DSM diagnos-tic category "panic disorder." This disorder had been distinguished in the 1970s from more general forms of anxiety through a process that the New York psychiatrist Donald Klein had called "pharmacological dissection." The antidepressant drug imipramine, he said, uniquely "blocked spon-taneous panics (manifested by desperate appeals for help) in patients in whom long-term intensive psychoanalytic psychotherapy had failed." But it failed to work on the patients' so-called anticipatory anxiety, their fears of succumbing to a panic attack. For this second kind of (neurotic) anxiety, a benzodiazepine like Valium (or even psychotherapy) was more useful, Klein felt. Put another way, Klein understood panic disorder to be a dis-crete, biological disease that was best treated with antidepressants, while seeing anticipatory anxiety more as a psychological reaction to be managed with benzodiazepines.[20]

The authors of *DSM-III* went even further than Klein in slicing and dicing anxiety into different discrete disorders. Alongside panic disorder (a form of anxiety marked by episodes of irrational panic), they also recog-nized phobic disorder (with several subtypes, including social phobia, the fear of being humiliated in front of others); obsessive-compulsive disor-der, post-traumatic stress disorder; and finally generalized anxiety disorder, a residual category for patients who did not seem to quite fit into any of the others.

Klein, however, was most interested in panic disorder. In 1981, a year after the authors decided to include it in *DSM-III*, he and his colleague Paul Wender co-authored an article for *Psychology Today* in which, among other things, they aimed to introduce the general public to this unfamiliar disorder that was different from garden-variety anxiety. Consider, Wender and Klein asked readers, the case of patient Mary J., a "23-year old unmarried buyer for a department store who was stricken by a series of panic attacks." Mary J. "would suddenly be overcome by dizziness, a pounding heart, and an inability to catch her breath while walking down the street or riding on public transportation." Mary J.'s doctors initially chalked up her symptoms to "nerves" and put her on a course of rest and Valium, but it had, of course, been unsuccessful. She had then tried lengthy and expensive psychoanalysis, followed by behavior therapy, also to no avail.

Mary J.'s luck finally changed when she joined a clinical trial for people with conditions like hers. She went on a course of a new medication (a tricyclic antidepressant). Her symptoms stopped—and she remained symptom free, even after going off the medication six months later. Mary J. could now look ahead to a bright future, including "a possible marriage." Targeted medication had hit the spot for her in ways that no amount of talking, behavior coaching, or even old-school sedatives like Valium had been able to do.[21]

Klein clearly thought panic disorder should be treated with antidepressants, not benzodiazepines. However, in 1981 the Upjohn Company received a long-awaited approval from the FDA to sell a new benzodiazepine that it called Xanax. Upjohn had manufactured alprazolam, the active ingredient in Xanax in the early 1960s, the heyday of the minor tranquilizer boom, and had envisioned it at that time as a faster-acting successor to Valium; it would treat "anxiety neurosis" with fewer side effects.[22] While the company was awaiting its long-deferred FDA approval, though, *DSM-III* was published, abolishing the old concept of anxiety neurosis. Not only that, but the use of Valium and other benzodiazepines was in decline. The future for Upjohn's newly approved drug therefore did not look bright.

Then David Sheehan, a young psychiatrist at Massachusetts General

Hospital who had been hired by Upjohn as a consultant, had a brilliant thought. What if it could be demonstrated that Xanax was an effective treatment for the new *DSM*-approved category of panic disorder? Yes, Klein had been skeptical of using benzodiazepines to treat panic, but Sheehan had become convinced that Klein's was not the last word here. Through trial and error in his own clinical practice, he had come to the conclusion that benzodiazepines were actually quite helpful in quelling symptoms of panic. He didn't think that Xanax was likely to be *more* effective for panic than the other benzodiazepines on the market, but he worked for Upjohn, and Upjohn needed an angle for its new drug. As he told the psychiatrist David Healy years later, he and the Upjohn executives therefore decided "to create a perception that a drug had special and unique properties that would help it capture market share and displace [Valium] from the top position."[23]

The effort to transform Xanax into the first specific treatment for panic disorder commenced in the summer of 1982. The heart of the effort was a two-phase clinical trial that tested the drug first against a placebo, then against the antidepressant imipramine, which Klein preferred.[24] The new drug seemed to perform well in both phases.[25] In fact, as Sheehan later revealed, the first group of patients in the trial were so impressed by the drug that they concluded it would be a blockbuster—and a few of them pooled their money and bought stock in Upjohn. The FDA granted approval in 1990, and almost immediately Upjohn took out eight-page color ads in psychiatric journals, trumpeting the good news: "Xanax: the First and Only Medication Indicated for Panic Disorder."

But since Xanax worked on everyday anxiety as well, the FDA was also persuaded to approve it as a short-term treatment for the *DSM* category "generalized anxiety disorder."[26] In this dual capacity, Xanax became a blockbuster drug of the 1990s; in 1993, the year it went off patent, it was the fifth most widely prescribed drug in the United States—America's favorite new *DSM*-approved "chill pill."[27] With a much shorter half-life than Valium, it produced less of a "hangover" than that older standby. Most consumers believed it to be much safer. Not until well into the new millennium were concerns about addiction and abuse, of the kind that had led to Valium's downfall, finally raised about Xanax.[28]

SOCIAL ANXIETY, PTSD, GENERALIZED ANXIETY

Meanwhile the drug companies that had gotten rich from SSRI anti-depressants were looking for new markets for these drugs before they went off patent. If the companies could persuade the FDA to license their SSRIs as an effective treatment for some disorder other than depression, they could potentially look forward to years of renewed profits. The obvi-ous place to turn their attention was the anxiety market, which the suc-cess of Xanax had made clear was major. It had long been known that SSRIs could also alleviate the symptoms of anxiety frequently seen in patients diagnosed with depression. Why not therefore seek to remake SSRIs into treatments for specific forms of anxiety? Never mind that the drug companies had previously marketed them as specific treatments for depression.

In 1999 SmithKline Beecham sought and received a license from the FDA to sell Paxil not just as an antidepressant but as a treatment for a then little-known disorder that the *DSM* called "social phobia" or "social anx-iety disorder." Since few people had ever heard of this disorder, the com-pany realized it needed to sell the disease before it could sell the drug, so it launched a public advertising campaign called "Imagine Being Allergic to People." The campaign included the "cobbling together" of a patient advo-cacy group called the Social Anxiety Disorder Coalition. A public relations firm hired by SmithKline Beecham, Cohn & Wolfe, "handled all media inquiries on behalf of the group."[29]

One analyst, looking back in 2009, assessed the results of this campaign:

> The PR campaign resulted in more than a billion media references to social anxiety disorder, up from roughly 50 in previous years, almost all of which mentioned that Paxil was the only approved treatment for the condition. Seven months after its launch, the campaign had made the Paxil brand name one of the most recognized prescription drugs in the United States, and the drug was responsible for a size-able increase in the anxiety medication category.[30]

That same year, 1999, Pfizer won FDA approval to market its SSRI, Zoloft, as a treatment for post-traumatic stress disorder, or PTSD. This was also quite a coup, because when PTSD debuted as a diagnostic category in *DSM-III* in 1980, it had not seemed like a disorder that would be best treated biochemically. The term had been coined specifically to convey the idea that people sometimes break, *not* because they suffer from a medical disorder, but because the world breaks them. For this reason, psychother-apists and psychologists—not psychopharmacologists—were originally conceived as the front-line caregivers for victims of PTSD.[31]

Undeterred, Pfizer used the Chandler Chicco Agency, its public rela-tions firm, to help create another new "advocacy group" that it called the PTSD Alliance. The alliance developed educational material that explained how PTSD could affect "anyone who has experienced extreme trauma, been victimized or has witnessed a violent act, or has been repeatedly exposed to life-threatening situations." PTSD, this material explained, was incredibly common: one in thirteen people was likely to suffer from it at some point in their lives.[32] However, "once properly diagnosed," the firm concluded, "PTSD is treatable with psychotherapy, medication, or a combination of both."[33]

In September 2001 terrorists attacked the World Trade Center in New York City and the Pentagon in Washington D.C. In the aftermath Pfizer ran "public service" ads on TV, showing heartbreaking images of emer-gency services personnel rescuing victims of the attack near the downed buildings, intercut with images of weeping people, flags, and candles. A narrator explained that Pfizer had given generously to relief services and urged viewers to do the same. A male voice then reflected compassionately: "We wish we could make a medicine that would take away the heartache." Of course, on some level, they wanted to persuade people that they had already done so.

While all this was happening, GlaxoSmithKline (successor to the merger of Glaxo Wellcome and SmithKline Beecham) received permis-sion from the FDA to market Paxil for another anxiety disorder—so-called "generalized anxiety disorder."[34] In December 2001, three months after the September 11 terrorist attacks, its advertising agency rolled out a series of commercials that showed strained-looking people looking into the camera and sharing their thoughts: "I'm always thinking something terrible is going to happen." They never directly mentioned terrorism or 9/11—they didn't need to.

The strategy of repurposing old drugs for new disorders (that, in many cases, people had not known they had) was highly successful. U.S. sales of SSRIs picked up again dramatically, peaking in 2008 with revenues of $12 billion.

"BETTING THE FARM" ON ANTIPSYCHOTICS

The period after 1980 was not completely bereft of breakthroughs in psycho-pharmaceutical treatments. The one exception was a treatment for schizophrenia: the so-called atypical antipsychotics. For the pharmaceutical companies that produced and marketed these drugs, however, the challenge would be to ensure that they were profitable enough.

The story here goes back to the late 1950s, when the Swiss pharmaceutical company Wander AG (later acquired by Sandoz) created the drug clozapine, based on the chemical structure of the tricyclic antidepressant Imipramine. Clozapine was initially envisioned as an antidepressant also, but in early trials it failed to impress on that front. To everyone's surprise, however, some early animal tests showed that it had sedating effects similar to those associated with chlorpromazine, the standard treatment for schizophrenia. Had the chemists at Wander accidentally created a new antipsychotic? By the late 1960s, researchers were cautiously optimistic: their drug seemed especially effective in patients who had not responded to other antipsychotics.

Then it was discovered that clozapine, unlike all previous antipsychotics, did not seem to cause extrapyramidal side effects (twitching, restlessness, Parkinson's-like forms of motor retardation, etc.). The German psychiatrist Hanns Hippius, who was involved in the early trials, later talked about how "almost unbelievable" this discovery had felt: "At that time it was a part of psychopharmacological dogma that extrapyramidal effects went in tandem with antipsychotic efficacy."[35]

It turned out that clozapine did not cause these side effects because it acted only weakly on dopamine receptors. It was a much stronger blocker of serotonin receptors. Recall that, back in the heady days of LSD research, there had been considerable interest in the idea that schizophrenia might be caused by too much (or maybe too little) serotonin. In the 1970s, though, excess dopamine was supposed to be the problem in schizophrenia. The field seemed to know a lot less than it sometimes claimed about the functions of these neurotransmitters.[36]

Despite not knowing why it worked, Wander AG put clozapine on the market in Europe in 1975. It did not stay there long. Reports emerged from Finland that patients on the drug had developed a disorder called agranulocytosis (in which the body's white blood cell count drops precipitously), and some had died. The drug was withdrawn from use in Europe, and in the United States, Sandoz (which had by now acquired Wander) decided in 1976 to stop all further clinical trials.

Even so, the drug remained available for "compassionate use," and by 1982 new blood test protocols had been developed that allowed clinicians who prescribed the drug to monitor their patients in ways that would reduce their likelihood of developing agranulocytosis. Cautiously encouraged, Sandoz undertook a new multisite clinical trial that compared the drug head-on to the standard of care, chlorpromazine. Clozapine came out squarely ahead: it was as effective as chlorpromazine in reducing active symptoms of schizophrenia. It also seemed helpful in reducing so-called "negative" symptoms (withdrawal, apathy), and it did not lead to extrapyramidal side effects.[37] This all seemed like a real treatment advance. So it came that clozapine entered the market in 1990 under the brand name Clozaril and was billed as a second-generation or "atypical" antipsychotic.

Not all the news was good. Clozaril was extremely expensive, not least because Sandoz initially insisted that all blood monitoring be carried out through its own designated vendors. (Eventually, the company was pressured to relent on this front.) Early reports of extreme weight gain also presaged problems to come. Nevertheless, many press reports from the early 1990s were glowingly enthusiastic: "You go from hating the sunshine in the mornings to loving it," said a schoolteacher, Daphne Moss. A psychiatrist from Emory University, Samuel Risch, sounded almost in awe of the drug: "In 15 years of practice, I've never seen anything like it."[38]

With press like that, other drug companies soon wanted a piece of the action. In short order, they introduced a number of copycat atypical anti-psychotics to the market: risperidone (Risperdal), olanzapine (Zyprexa), quetiapine (Seroquel), and (a bit later) aripiprazole (Abilify). Many outside observers, understandably, assumed this fresh bounty was a product of all the new neuroscience research of the 1990s.[39] Few were aware that the pro-totype antipsychotic, clozapine, was actually a "failed" antidepressant that had been first synthesized in the 1950s.

Be that as it may, as company chemists created new variations on the prototype, executives plotted how to make their new drugs as profitable as possible. They decided they would have to redefine what it meant to prescribe an antipsychotic. One way or another, antipsychotics would have to become drugs that were no longer exclusively targeted to people with schizophrenia. In 1995 one California researcher, William Wirshing—hired by Eli Lilly to oversee clinical trials on Zyprexa—was driving to the airport when a story came on the radio about Zyprexa. As Wirshing listened, a company execu-tive explained how Eli Lilly saw its marketing potential.

"He says it's got the potential to be a billion-dollar-a-year drug," Wirshing recalled. "I almost pulled off the road and crashed into the side rail." At the time, the entire market for atypical antipsychot-ics was only $170 million. "How the hell do you make $1 billion?" Wirshing thought. "I mean, who are we gonna give it to? It's not like we're making any more schizophrenic brains."[40]

The answer, of course, was that Eli Lilly had no intention of limiting the market for Zyprexa just to people with "schizophrenic brains." It had made a tremendous amount of money from Prozac, but that drug was due to go off patent within six years (in 2001). So the company decided (in the words of internal company documents, later made public) to "bet the farm" on Zyprexa. It planned to aggressively market it as a treatment for bipo-lar disorder (for which it received FDA approval in 2004). It also hoped physicians could be persuaded to prescribe it for depression and behavioral problems associated with dementia. In addition, it planned to train its sales representatives to promote the drug to primary care physicians as a non-specific treatment for moodiness, irritability, and insomnia.

We have this information because in 2006 hundreds of sealed documents, submitted to a court in the course of litigation against Eli Lilly, were leaked to the *New York Times* reporter Alex Berenson, who published a multipart exposé of Eli Lilly's practices in December of that year.[41] The internal documents also revealed the extent to which Eli Lilly had actively downplayed or buried evidence showing a strong link between Zyprexa and medication-induced obesity, high blood sugar, and diabetes. It was very common (and well known to the company) for patients to gain well over twenty pounds during their first year on the drug, and a significant number gained more than one hundred pounds.

By 2007, Eli Lilly had paid at least $1.2 billion to settle lawsuits involving some 28,500 people who claimed to have developed diabetes or other disorders after taking Zyprexa. Alex Berenson, who reported this development, noted that an additional twelve hundred cases were still pending.[42] In 2009 the company reached a further settlement for $1.4 billion with the U.S. Department of Justice for illegal off-label marketing of Zyprexa, including a scheme to persuade doctors to prescribe Zyprexa to elderly nursing home patients and disruptive children, for whom the drug was not federally approved.[43]

None of this should lead us, looking back, to disregard the perspective of the patients whom these drugs were originally intended to help. In late December 2006, shortly after Berenson's multipart exposé, the *New York Times* published the following poignant letter to the editor:

To the Editor:

Zyprexa is a miracle drug for some of us. That should not be forgotten in light of all that is coming out about Eli Lilly's marketing practices. It opened up the world, allowed me to read and feel a crackling enthusiasm for life for the first time in years, and it cut down drastically on the voices and strange thoughts.

Zyprexa was also the worst drug I have ever taken, making me gain 65 pounds, adding 100 points to my cholesterol, and raising my triglycerides sky-high. I was both ecstatic to be involved in the world and miserable, obese, and unhealthy.

The problem is to solve the difficulties with Zyprexa, not simply take it off the market. It is too helpful a drug, especially for those who can tolerate it. I could not.

I now take three different antipsychotics that are effective but not as miraculous.

I miss Zyprexa.[44]

PSYCHOPHARMACOLOGY IN CRISIS

By now, pretty much every thoughtful person had heard (whether or not they fully believed) that "big pharma"[45] cared only about profits and had deceived and harmed us all. In 2004 Marcia Angell, former editor of *The New England Journal of Medicine*, authored a book called *The Truth About Drug Companies*. There she argued that the industry "in some ways is like the Wizard of Oz—still full of bluster but now being exposed as something far different from its image." It had become less an "engine of innovation" than a "vast marketing machine" that benefited from government-funded research even as it claimed monopoly rights on its products. "We get nowhere near our money's worth," she concluded. "The United States can no longer afford it in its present form."[46] By 2018, her book had been cited almost 2,500 times.

In the next several years, a veritable library of whistle-blowing books elaborated on this litany of grievances against the pharmaceutical industry. Their titles speak for themselves: *Side Effects: A Prosecutor, a Whistleblower, and a Bestselling Antidepressant on Trial*; *Our Daily Meds: How the Pharmaceutical Companies Transformed Themselves into Slick Marketing Machines and Hooked the Nation on Prescription Drugs*; *Shyness: How Normal Behavior Became a Sickness*; *Let Them Eat Prozac: The Unhealthy Relationship Between the Pharmaceutical Companies and Depression*; *Comfortably Numb: How Psychiatry Is Medicating a Nation*; and *Anatomy of an Epidemic: Psychiatric Drugs and the Astonishing Rise of Mental Illness in America*.[47] Once celebrated for giving hope to patients long deemed hopeless, the psychopharmaceutical industry had become a target of moral outrage.[48]

This did not mean, though, that most people wanted—not really—to return to a world of mental illness before drugs, or failed to acknowledge drugs' positive effects on clinical care, even if those effects came at a price. When word trickled out that the psychopharmaceutical industry might be losing its moxie—indeed, might be in trouble—even some of the field's critics responded with an uncertain mix of Schadenfreude, surprise, and ultimately, unease.

The dearth of genuinely innovative new products, already discussed, partly explains the industry's new woes, but only partly. The industry was also increasingly struggling with a placebo effect problem that it saw no easy way to solve. Since the 1960s, randomized, placebo-controlled clinical trials had been de rigueur for any company wanting to bring a new drug onto the market.[49] Everyone knew that patients in the placebo group—the patients who received an inert dummy pill rather than the experimental treatment—often improved. The assumption had long been that this fact was of no clinical interest but simply noise in the system. Ever since they were developed as a method, the question in clinical trials was always whether the experimental drug resulted in more improvement than a fake (placebo) drug. If it did, then the trial had succeeded. If it did not, the trial was deemed to be a failure.

Even if the researchers running clinical trials were not particularly interested in unpacking what might be causing the improvement in patients taking placebo pills, in the 1990s some psychologists, brain scientists, and clinicians began to suggest that the placebo effect was actually worth studying in its own right.[50] One of them was the psychologist Irving Kirsch. In the late 1990s, he and his graduate student Guy Sapirstein decided to use antidepressant clinical trial data to study the magnitude of its effect. Depression seemed like a good place to look for placebo effects, since (as Kirsch later recalled) "one of the prime characteristics of depression is the sense of hopelessness that depressed people feel." Their thought was that simply receiving a promise of effective treatment in itself should help people feel more hopeful and in this way reduce depression.[51]

Kirsch and Sapirstein used a meta-analytic method to see whether this was the case. A meta-analysis uses statistical methods to analyze the results of multiple studies of a common phenomenon in an effort to increase confidence in the conclusions drawn from those studies. In their depression study, much as Kirsch and Sapirstein had predicted, the placebo effect in clinical trials of antidepressants turned out to be substantial. Patients in these placebo groups experienced substantial relief.

What surprised the researchers was that patients in active treatment groups did only marginally better than those in placebo groups. In fact, some 75 *percent* of the improvement seen in people taking the active medication could be attributed to the placebo effect. As they put it in their first 1998 report, they had "listened" to Prozac, then realized they were actually "hearing" placebo.[52]

The report in which Kirsch and Sapirstein laid out the evidence for all their claims received an extremely testy reception, to put it mildly. It simply could not be true, many critics said. The efficacy of antidepressants was so well established that it was suggested that the researchers must have cherry-picked among the clinical trials they analyzed (intentionally or not) or made some other kind of fundamental error in their methods. (Meta-analyses were in any event viewed with some skepticism in these years.) The psychopharmacologist Donald Klein summed up the sense of outrage: the paper was, "a trenchant example of a tendentious article whose departures from any critical standard has not precluded publication and has been foisted on an unsuspecting audience as a 'peer reviewed' contribution to the literature."[53]

Deciding that these critiques could not go unanswered, Kirsch recruited additional colleagues to undertake a far more comprehensive analysis. This time they used the Freedom of Information Act to compel the FDA to send them the data it had received from pharmaceutical companies seeking approval for the six most widely prescribed antidepressant drugs: Prozac, Paxil, Zoloft, Effexor, Serzone, and Celexa. Now they had data not just on published trials but on all trials, published and unpublished, that the drugs' owners had submitted as part of the FDA approval process.[54]

In 2002 the Kirsch group reported what they had found. First, only 43 percent of the trials had shown that the drugs provided any statistically significant advantage over placebo. Put another way, 57 percent of the trials had failed.[55] Second, even in trials where the drugs outperformed the placebo, the placebo effect's magnitude was even larger than Kirsch and Sapirstein had reported in 1998: "82 percent of the drug response was duplicated by the placebo response." In other words, a mere "18 per-

cent of the drug response is due to the pharmacological effects of the medication."[56] The difference was significant statistically but probably not
clinically significant—that is to say, the difference between taking a drug
and taking a placebo would probably have not been readily apparent to a
patient or his or her doctor outside an experimental trial setting.

By this time, Kirsch's was not the only study to draw devastating conclusions like these from the FDA archives. In 2000 the psychiatrists Arif
Khan and Walter Brown, looking at data on 19,639 depressed patients in
clinical trials, found no statistically significant difference for suicide risk
between those taking active medication and those merely swallowing a placebo each day. Beyond that, there was only about a 10 percent difference in
general symptom reduction between the two groups.[57]

Around this time the pharmaceutical company Merck had to abandon its efforts to bring a promising new antidepressant (MK-869) onto
the market, because, try as it might, it was unable to get the drug to outperform placebos. Yes, many subjects in the active treatment group felt
considerably better, reporting less hopelessness and less anxiety, but so
did nearly the same number of subjects taking the look-alike pill. This
failure was a terrible blow for Merck, especially because it was facing the
expiration of patents on some of its most profitable drugs. It was also a
huge embarrassment, because Merck's executives had been imprudent
enough to hype the drug in advance of these disappointing results, even
bragging in 1997 that they expected Merck, in the next years, "to dominate the central nervous system."[58]

Meanwhile the psychiatrist William Potter, head of early clinical
development at Eli Lilly throughout the 1990s, was struck by the fact that
his company seemed to have increasing difficulty mounting trials in which
psychiatric drugs outperformed placebos, especially when they were medications that targeted symptoms of anxiety and depression. Potter decided
to look more systematically into the matter.

What he found challenged the industry's basic assumption that medicines are equal-opportunity substances, that they work the same way
in the human body, regardless of whether the patient is in a hospital in
the United States or in a clinic in India. On the contrary, Potter found
that geographical location made a huge difference in the performance

of drugs. In the late 1990s, for example, diazepam (Valium) was outper-
forming placebos in France and Belgium, but in the United States, it no
longer did. In contrast, Prozac performed considerably better against placebo in trials in the United States than in trials in western Europe and
South Africa.[59]

What was going on? One analyst, Christopher Lane, suggested that
the problem, at least in the United States, might have been largely of the
pharmaceutical industry's own making: the intensive marketing of drugs
in the previous decade, especially marketing directly to consumers, might
have raised the expectations of patients participating in clinical trials in
ways that significantly enhanced their placebo responses. Others pointed
to the length and elaborate nature of U.S. clinical trials.[60] No one, though,
knew for sure.

The question that loomed for the drug companies, in any event, was,
what next? By 2009, Potter—now vice president of translational neuroscience at Merck—persuaded a number of companies to fund a massive
(and semisecret) data-gathering effort called the Placebo Response Drug
Trials Survey. Overseen by the Foundation for the National Institutes of
Health, the goal was to get to the bottom of the whole situation. Funding
came from Merck, Lilly, Pfizer, AstraZeneca, GlaxoSmithKline, Sanofi-
Aventis, and Johnson & Johnson, all the big companies.[61] Meanwhile some
of them started hiring consultants to train their research scientists to avoid
doing things that might inadvertently enhance placebo effects in trial participants: there must be no "inappropriately optimistic" body language, no
looking patients in the eye, no shaking patients' hands.[62]

About this same time, a further problem emerged. When researchers
looked below the aggregate data in their trials to the patient-level data (the
"raw" data), they discovered that the placebo effect, while real, was not the
only problem they faced. It turned out that individual patients in the active
treatment groups also had profoundly different responses to the drugs.
Some responded strongly, others barely at all.[63]

The reason, they concluded, lay in the industry approach to diagnostics. All patients in clinical trials are supposed to be suffering from the same
disorder. All are diagnosed using rating scales that, since the 1960s, had
been the industry standard for creating supposedly homogenous groups of

trial participants. But it now turned out that all along, there had been a big problem with using rating scales or *DSM* checklists: two people could be diagnosed with depression—the "same" disorder—without sharing a single symptom. Small wonder, one might think, that they might not respond to a drug the same way.

The problem, though, was that companies had no idea which patients were more likely than others to respond to one drug or another. The rating scales were clearly unable to do the sorting, and the individuals lacked any biomarkers (reliable biological aberrations found in some patients but not in others) that would allow researchers to create useful subtypes.[64] Some efforts were under way to develop a new framework for this kind of work— beyond rating scales and *DSM* checklists—but they had not yet yielded firm results.[65] The situation looked increasingly grim.

One of the last straws came when the European Medicines Agency told drug companies that, going forward, any new drug proposed for their markets would no longer just have to outperform placebos: it would either have to outperform existing standard of care drugs on the market, *or else* the company would have to clearly identify subgroups of patients (ideally with a predictive biomarker) who were likely to respond well to it.[66] It was all too much. As Steven Hyman, director of the Stanley Center for Psychiatric Research at MIT and Harvard, explained in an email to me, after reviewing an earlier version of this manuscript: "When companies were told they had to compare new drugs not only to placebo but to an existing drug known to be efficacious, or have a predictive biomarker to gain approval in Europe—their response was: 'we don't know how to do that.' . . . In essence the EMA called their bluff."[67]

So they began to give up. For decades, they had struggled to create novel drugs using molecular targets discovered in the 1950s and early '60s.[68] They had then marketed what they had in their vaults, while innovating around the edges. But now the difficulties of meeting even the basic requirements of new clinical trial protocols were defeating them. They had "run out of brainy ideas," as a 2010 article put it, and were beginning to think about cutting their losses.[69] One after another AstraZeneca, GlaxoSmithKline, and other big companies abandoned the field of psychiatry altogether.[70] Many turned their attention to developing new cancer treatments. Journalists and commentators watched the companies go in a mood that was wistful, confused, and defiant. "Watch out big pharma," one blogger called out in 2017, "we're not giving up on psychiatry just yet."[71]

PSYCHIATRY LOSES FAITH IN THE *DSM*

Meanwhile in 2013, the APA released a fifth edition of the *DSM*—the first fully updated edition since 1994. And then something quite extraordinary happened. The director of the NIMH, Dr. Tom Insel, drew a clear red line between the new edition and the institute's research activities: "NIMH," he stated, "will be re-orienting its research away from *DSM* categories . . . to begin to develop a better system."[72]

For years Insel had been critical of the *DSM*, insisting that the so-called "bible of psychiatry" had "100 percent reliability and 0 percent validity."[73] Now as director of the NIMH, he could do something about his convictions: he could reject this book. "As long as the research community takes the *DSM* to be a bible, we'll never make progress," he told a *New York Times* journalist. "Biology," he concluded firmly, "never read that book."[74]

How could this be? Hadn't the radical 1980 edition, *DSM-III*, been a foundation for the whole biological turn? In the 1980s, this had certainly been almost everyone's understanding. By the 1990s, however, unease had already been building. Many had noticed that each new *DSM* revision increased the number of ways a mental illness could be diagnosed. The original *DSM*, published in 1952, had recognized 106 forms of mental illness. *DSM-II*, in 1968, had tallied up 182. The paradigm-changing *DSM-III*, in 1980, recognized 285. With the fourth revision in 1994, the number stood at 307. Were all these new categories really novel discoveries driven by rigorous scientific inquiry? Were there really so many different ways to be mentally ill?

Some thought it unlikely. The year 1997 saw the publication of an influential polemic against the *DSM*. In *Making Us Crazy*, social workers Herb Kutchins and Stuart A. Kirk argued that this so-called bible of psychiatry had to be exposed for what it was: a guide created through the wheeling and dealing of many disparate insider interests; a document whose categories, in many instances, bore traces of gender and racial bias; a vehicle to allow mental health professionals to be reimbursed by insurance companies and drug companies to sell drugs; and a weapon that politicians and psychiatrists used to "assassinate character and slander the opposition."[75]

To be sure, reviewers in 1997 could dismiss Kutchins and Kirk relatively easily—especially reviewers who were psychiatrists—as ill-informed and biased. After all, the authors were professors of social work and therefore arguably people with no love for the "medical model" and with a clear professional ax to grind.[76]

With the passing of ten years, however, efforts to dismiss and marginalize critics of the *DSM* became harder to do. The hardest-hitting critiques were no longer being penned by angry outsiders but by some of the very people who had initially been most enthusiastic about the manual and its role in ushering in a new era. In 2007 Nancy Andreasen, whose 1984 book *The Broken Brain* had been one of the first to announce the arrival of a new chapter in psychiatry, now wrote that *DSM-III*, with its checklist approach to diagnosis, had unintentionally led to a decline in "careful clinical evaluation," a loss of interest in rich descriptive psychopathology, and even "the death of phenomenology in the United States," more generally.[77]

Two years later Allen Frances, who had spearheaded the revision that resulted in *DSM-IV*, cautioned that efforts then under way to revise the book again were only going to make an imperfect situation considerably worse: the newest revision process, he observed, "started with a grand ambition to provide a 'paradigm shift' in psychiatric diagnosis, based initially on the identification of biological markers." But that goal had proven "clearly unattainable," so efforts were now under way to create new syndromes likely to result in diagnoses for more and more people who were not really sick—leading to "false positive 'epidemics' with harmful excessive treatments."[78] When, in late 2012, the APA voted to approve *DSM-5* (it changed to Arabic numerals with this edition), Frances declared the moment "a sad day for psychiatry"—more, "the saddest moment in my 45 year career of studying, practicing, and teaching psychiatry."[79]

Herein lies the irony of Tom Insel's denunciation of *DSM-5* as a book that "biology had never read." The fifth edition had originally been imagined as the *DSM* revision that would finally realize the aspirations of the 1980 revolutionaries and put psychiatric diagnostics on a firm biological basis. It clearly failed to do so. Hyman, a former NIMH director, recalled that he assumed from the beginning that it wouldn't work. He knew the biological foundations weren't there to justify a new edition.[80]

The APA went ahead anyway,[81] but the results of the *DSM-5* process were as Hyman had predicted. The science that was necessary to support its grandiose ambitions was not on hand. The biomarkers were not found. So the architects of *DSM-5* had instead turned to revising and refining criteria for a range of disorders—or as Allen Frances bitingly put it, to "rearranging the furniture."[82]

When the book made its public debut at the May 2013 meeting of the APA in San Francisco, the mood was somber rather than celebratory. I attended this meeting and can personally testify to this fact. Frances's sorrowful critiques and Insel's biting rejection of the new manual hung in the air. People hovered uncertainly before the display exhibits. At a May 18 news conference held to announce the book's unveiling, reporters were allowed to submit questions only in writing; they were not allowed to pose them directly or to ask any follow-up questions.[83]

Reflecting on the situation in 2013, Hyman acknowledged that back in the 1980s, no one could have anticipated such a decisive downward spiral. The original authors of *DSM-III* "were real heroes at the time. . . . They chose a model in which all psychiatric illnesses were represented as categories discontinuous with 'normal.'" But, he went on, they were "totally wrong in a way they couldn't have imagined. So in fact, what they produced was an absolute scientific nightmare. Many people . . . get five diagnoses, but they don't have five diseases—they have one underlying condition."[84]

Two years after *DSM-5* made its forlorn debut, Insel left the directorship of the NIMH to work for Google's research arm, Alphabet. In 2017, he left Alphabet to cofound and lead a new digital technology startup called Mindstrong. He had decided that the quest to put diagnosis and treatment of mental illness on a biological basis was futile, at least in any useful time frame that would help patients. But he had become persuaded that a wholly new approach—one grounded in digital data analytics—might succeed where biology had failed:

I spent 13 years at NIMH really pushing on the neuroscience and genetics of mental disorders, and when I look back on that I realize that while I think I succeeded at getting lots of really cool papers published by cool scientists at fairly large costs—I think $20 billion—I don't think we moved the needle in reducing suicide, reducing hospitalizations, improving recovery for the tens of millions of people who have mental illness. I hold myself accountable for that.[85]

In 2017 Insel's predecessor at the NIMH, Steven Hyman, is still more sanguine, or perhaps more stubborn, about the potential of psychiatry to ultimately make good on promises to advance biological understanding of mental illness. In the second decade of the new millennium, much of the focus of the Stanley Center has been on novel forms of big data analysis designed to reveal patterns of complex interactions among genes that may play a role in disorders like schizophrenia. Yet even as the Stanley Center's researchers express excitement to the press about what they are doing, they acknowledge that "it may take decades before genetic research on schizophrenia yields new treatments."[86]

Afterthoughts

THE 1980s BIOLOGICAL REVOLUTIONARIES WERE NOT THE FIRST GROUP in the history of psychiatry to make audacious promises on which they could not deliver. The nineteenth-century mental hospital has failed as a therapeutic institution? All right, forget about therapy, and focus on learning what you can from the brains of your patients after they die. The anatomical research program has been a disappointment? No problem: focus instead on collecting all possible relevant facts and pursuing any and all somatic therapies, because times are desperate, and one can never have too much data. All those diverse facts have turned out not to add up to very much? The Wild West world of shock and surgical treatments has likely caused more harm than good? That's okay: the postwar world is in crisis and needs the insights provided by psychoanalysis and social science. Things haven't worked out with the Freudians' expansive social agenda? Psychiatry is on the brink of losing all credibility as a profession? Not to worry: let the biologists take over!

The bold 1980s venture to bring about a "biological revolution" has now run into the sand as well. Far from flocking to psychiatry, many pharmaceutical companies have recently been fleeing it, as the prospects for new and potentially lucrative psychiatric drugs have dimmed. The manual on which the profession has rested so much of its biological authority has come under sharp attack, not just by outsiders but by insiders committed to the mission. Too many of the severely mentally ill remain shamefully underserved. Mental illness still is stigmatized in ways that other kinds of illness are not.[1] Racial bias and inequities in care persist.[2] And of course, firm understandings of psychiatry's illnesses, of their underlying biology, continue to elude.

There is some good news. Recent decades of hard-nosed critique have begun to have an effect. Psychiatrists are now required to report any ties they might have with the pharmaceutical industry; and awareness of the potential for conflicts of interest is widespread. The restless ex-patient and psychiatric survivor movements from the 1970s and '80s have morphed into consumer advocacy groups that have won for patients a voice in their own care. There is greater consensus than we saw in the 1980s about the role that not just drugs, but also psychotherapies—especially variants of cognitive-behavioral therapies—can have on the well-being of many patients. Some are finding cautious hope in very recent efforts to treat acute depression using variants of old drugs like ketamine and certain psychedelics, though it is much too early to say now (in 2019) where this will lead. The field's mainstream imperfect drugs continue, not just to cause harm, but to save lives.

Above all, more and more people are starting to talk honestly about the current stalemate, the current state of crisis. This is good news, not bad. Times of crisis are times of opportunity.

So where should the profession go from here? Can today's biological psychiatry resist the temptation to lurch into yet another chapter of overpromising that is likely to end in tears? Can it appreciate that trashing all rivals generally means that everyone becomes more ignorant? Can it acknowledge and firmly turn away from its ethical lapses—and especially the willingness of so many in recent decades to follow the money instead of the suffering?

As we consider these questions, we should keep in mind one very basic fact. Among the very many people who present with a mental affliction, some are (almost certainly) suffering from a real illness, one that is understandable (in principle) like any other medical complaint. By the same token, others are (almost certainly) not. Mental suffering takes many forms, only some of which have roots in disease. The suffering of those who are not really ill in any meaningful medical sense can still be acute. I have only to look at the struggling students I teach and advise to know how true this is. If there is to be a future biological psychiatry, more effective than those that have come before, how will it deal with this fact?

A century ago some of those who suffered mentally but were not really sick received fictive diagnoses from their doctors like "bad nerves" or "neurasthenia." By the early twentieth century, most of the doctors who treated such patients knew there was nothing literally wrong with their "nerves." The patients may or may not have known, or they may or may not have cared. They may not have cared, because the labeling process, when it worked well (and sometimes it was used coercively), was a way of acknowledging the gravity of their suffering. It provided a coherent explanation for real symptoms. Regardless of the (doubtful) validity of the diagnostic terms employed, the very act of naming allowed patients to find support and (perhaps) feel relief under a doctor's care.[3] Given the motives and outcomes, did it matter that virtually everything in play here was likely fictive, save for the suffering and the care? Were these nerve doctors wrong to do what they did?

The question is not of merely historical interest, because today many general practitioners and psychiatrists play a similar game. Patients present with acute mental or emotional distress, and doctors look for a *DSM* diagnosis that will make sense of their suffering. They prescribe drugs because that is what insurance companies will pay for, and because they believe the drugs will take the edge off their patients' distress. Often, they do. By acting this way, general practitioners and psychiatrists perpetuate the fiction that the drugs they are prescribing are correcting biochemical deficiencies caused by disease, much as (say) a prescription of insulin corrects a biochemical deficiency caused by diabetes. Is this wrong? Is it inconsistent with our understanding of the ethics of the doctor-patient relationship in the twenty-first century, which is supposed to be marked by transparency? Is it more wrong than it might otherwise be because we also worry about the long-term consequences of the medications being prescribed so freely? And if we think the answer to any or all these questions is yes, what are the alternatives?

Psychiatry has at least one possible alternative, but it would require an act of great professional and ethical courage. It could decide to return to a less hierarchical understanding of its place in the mental health and medical systems; one that would not necessarily or even probably be a return to Freudian orthodoxies, but which would acknowledge that mental suffering is a larger category than mental illness, and that even disorders with a likely or possible biological basis are not *just* medical, because the experiences of all human beings, ill or otherwise, are shaped by their cultural, social, and familial circumstances. Psychiatry could thereby become the medical arm of a fluid and cooperative ecosystem of mental health experts: psychologists, counselors, nurses, social workers, social service providers, and patient-run organizations. Much routine care for the "worried well" and much support for the seriously mentally ill is already outsourced to these other professionals. Nevertheless, the fiction persists that all this work, regardless of the kind of patient, is carried out in the service of the same medical mission. Psychiatrists create all the diagnoses and jealously guard their prescribing rights. A general consensus remains, implicitly, that the knowledge and practices of all the nonmedically trained workers are by definition subordinate to those of the medically trained ones.

What if an effort were made instead to flatten current hierarchies, lift all boats, and encourage regular cross-association gatherings? What if there was also systematic engagement with the many primary care physicians who currently write so many prescriptions, especially for patients with milder forms of distress? If this happened, medication might still play a role in supporting some of the patients not believed to actually have a disease; but its pros and cons could be disaggregated from the need to medicalize and could be discussed more honestly. After all, many women want pain medication during childbirth, but this does not mean being in labor is a disease. Prescribing drugs would thus no longer be the main way psychiatry specifically defended its status as a real branch of medicine, and the field would be freed to find ways to rest its authority and status on more authentic foundations. The solution would not be perfect, and it would demand a lot of brave alliance-building and fence-mending, but it could be a workable one.

Psychiatry could then gain immediate credibility by grappling with the failure of its past policies toward the seriously mentally ill—and especially with the shameful ways deinstitutionalization in the 1960s and '70s led to homelessness, incarceration, and premature death for many. Given its very mixed record with pursuing a narrowly medication-based approach to the care of this population, one of the first things psychiatry could do would be to step back from its current biological habits of mind and ask what might help most, even if all the answers do not necessarily feel medical. There is good social science research, for example, showing that many people with serious mental disorders often benefit far more from being given their own apartment and/or access to supportive communities than from being given a script for a new or stronger antipsychotic. In 2016 Shekhar Saxena, the director of the World Health Organization's mental health unit, was asked where he'd prefer to be if he were diagnosed with schizophrenia. He said he'd choose a city like Addis Ababa in Ethiopia or Colombo in Sri Lanka, rather than New York or London. The reason was that in the former, he had the potential to find a niche for himself as a productive if eccentric member of a community. In the latter, he was far more apt to end up stigmatized and on the margins of society. The field must seek the best solutions where they are to be found, regardless of who claims ownership of them.[4]

Even as it became more modest in focus, the kind of psychiatry I am advocating would be decidedly more ambitious—more expansive—in the way it would pursue research into the biomedical basis of mental illnesses. Important efforts are already under way to evaluate the conceptual, theoretical and methodological limitations of the biochemical, brain imaging, and genetic work of previous decades.[5] The field's stock-taking and call for a new beginning could, however, go further. It could look beyond current frameworks and toolkits, perhaps by actively recruiting scientists from outside the field (e.g., from microbiome science or neuroimmunology) with perspectives and tools that might productively destabilize entrenched habits (in ways analogous to what happened in the 1940s and '50s, when physicists entered the then-nascent field of molecular biology).

This new biological psychiatry I am envisioning could also aim to overcome its persistent reductionist habits and commit to an ongoing dialogue with the scholarly world of the social sciences and even the humanities. The goal of such a dialogue would be an intellectually rigorous one: to ensure that, even as it retains its focus on biological processes and disease, it seeks to understand ways that human brain functioning, disordered or not, is sensitive to culture and context (as the recent crisis over the placebo effect in psychopharmacology, among other things, has likely shown).

Finally, this psychiatry I am envisioning could commit to practicing a patient-oriented research ethic. There are good historical reasons why trust in psychiatry is brittle these days, but that could begin to change if patient groups, ethicists, and families were invited to help ensure that future questions and methods are aligned with the values and goals of those in whose name its work is being carried out.

As the new psychiatry does all these things, it will need to resist self-serving declarations of imminent breakthroughs and revolutions. In contrast with much that has gone before, it will need to make a virtue of modesty, continually acknowledging just how complex are the scientific challenges that it faces.

The scale of this complexity is not something about which psychiatry needs to feel in any way embarrassed. After all, current brain science still has little understanding of the biological foundations of many—indeed, most—*everyday* mental activities. This being the case, how could current psychiatry possibly expect to have a mature understanding of how such activities become disordered—and may possibly be reordered? In the early years of neurophysiology, Sir Charles Scott Sherrington predicted that when all was said and done, the effort to understand how different brain systems related to mental activity would likely "resolve into components for which at present we have no names."[6] If we think Sherrington was right, we may well anticipate that the psychiatry of the future will have little use for diagnostic categories like "schizophrenia," "bipolar disorder," and "depression." The fact that we don't know what terms it will use instead is just one measure of how far we still are from the promised land of real medical understanding of real mental illness.

NOTES

Introduction: Our Biological Enthusiasms

1. "The Psychological Society," May 31, 1978, *Firing Line* broadcast records, Program S0324, Hoover Institution Archives, https://digitalcollections.hoover.org/objects/6503.
2. Lois Timnick, "Look into the '80s: Psychiatry's Focus Turns to Biology," *Los Angeles Times*, July 21, 1980.
3. Donald F. Klein and Paul H. Wender, "The Promise of Biological Psychiatry," *Psychology Today* 15 (1981): 25.
4. Victor Cohn, "Charting 'the Soul's Frail Dwelling-House': Brain Waves: Scientists Stalk the Lodging of the Mind," *Washington Post*, September 5, 1982.
5. Jon Franklin, "The Mind Fixers," *Baltimore Sun*, July 23–31, 1984.
6. Nancy C. Andreasen, *The Broken Brain: The Biological Revolution in Psychiatry* (New York: Harper & Row, 1984).
7. Samuel B. Guze, "Biological Psychiatry: Is There Any Other Kind?" *Psychological Medicine* 19, no. 2 (May 1989): 322.
8. In *Broken Brain*, Nancy Andreasen was one of the first to frame the story of the so-called biological revolution of the 1980s as a pitched battle for the soul of psychiatry between followers of Freud and followers of Kraepelin. She was also one of the first to suggest that in triumphing over Freud in particular, the biologists were claiming a heritage bequeathed to them by a tribe of nineteenth-century scientific brethren. See Andreasen, *Broken Brain*, p. 14.
9. Harry Collins, "Actors' and Analysts' Categories in the Social Analysis of Science," *Clashes of Knowledge* (New York: Springer, 2008), pp. 101–10.
10. Thomas Insel, "Transforming Diagnosis," *NIMH Director's BlogPosts from*

2013 (blog), April 29, 2013, www.nimh.nih.gov/about/directors/thomas
-insel/blog/2013/transforming-diagnosis.shtml.

11. Steven E. Hyman, "Psychiatric Drug Development: Diagnosing a Crisis,"
Cerebrum: Dana Forum on Brain Science (April 2013); Steven E. Hyman, "The
Diagnosis of Mental Disorders: The Problem of Reification," *Annual Review
of Clinical Psychology* 6 (annurev.clinpsy.3.022806.091532 1146): 12.1–
12.25; Steven E. Hyman, "Revolution Stalled," *Science Translational Medicine*
4, no. 155 (October 10, 2012): 155cm11–155cm11; and Insel, "Transforming
Diagnosis."

Chapter 1: Betting on Anatomy

1. Nancy C. Andreasen, *The Broken Brain: The Biological Revolution in Psychiatry*
(New York: Harper & Row, 1984), pp. 14, 29.
2. Richard Noll, *The Encyclopedia of Schizophrenia and Other Psychotic Disorders*
(Infobase Publishing, 2009), p. xix; Michael R. Trimble and Mark George, *Biological Psychiatry* (New York: John Wiley & Sons, 2010), p. 3.
3. For an argument that more people should be learning from nineteenth- and early
twentieth-century clinicians, see Edward Shorter, *What Psychiatry Left Out of the
DSM-5: Historical Mental Disorders Today* (London: Routledge, 2015).
4. The rise of the therapeutic asylum has probably been subject to more analyses than any other chapter in the history of psychiatry. Most of the scrutiny
has focused on the goals and effects of these new institutions. Were they really
benevolent efforts motivated (even if perhaps not always fully successful) to
assist the mentally ill in their recovery? Or were they actually places that had
perfected a range of disciplinary routines designed to manage a major social
problem, while refashioning the mentally ill into compliance and social confor-
mity? For some of the classic skeptical discussions on this question, see Michel
Foucault, *Déraison et folie: Histoire de la folie à l'âge classique* (Paris: Librairie
Plon, 1961); David J. Rothman, *The Discovery of the Asylum: Social Order and
Disorder in the New Republic* (Boston: Little, Brown, 1971); Andrew T. Scull,
*Museums of Madness: The Social Organization of Insanity in Nineteenth-Century
England* (New York: Viking, 1979); Klaus Doerner, *Madmen and the Bourgeoi-
sie : A Social History of Insanity and Psychiatry* (London: Blackwell, 1984); and
Andrew T. Scull, *Social Order / Mental Disorder: Anglo-American Psychiatry in
Historical Perspective* (Berkeley: University of California Press, 1989). For a
more meliorist perspective, see Gerald N. Grob, *Mental Institutions in America:
Social Policy to 1875* (New Brunswick, NJ: Transaction Publishers, 2008).
5. John Conolly, *The Treatment of the Insane Without Mechanical Restraints* (London: Smith, Elder & Co., 1856), p. 154.
6. William Joseph Corbet, "On the Increase of Insanity," *American Journal of
Insanity* 50 (1893): 224–38.
7. Scull, *Social Order / Mental Disorder*, pp. 245–47.
8. For more, see E. Hare, "Was Insanity on the Increase? The Fifty-Sixth Maudsley Lecture," *British Journal of Psychiatry* 142, no. 5 (1983): 439ff.
9. Henry Maudsley, *The Physiology and Pathology of the Mind* (New York: D.
Appleton, 1867), p. 201.

10. Daniel Pick, *Faces of Degeneration: A European Disorder, c.1848–1918* (New York: Cambridge University Press, 1993).

11. E. Ray Lankester, *Degeneration: A Chapter in Darwinism* (London: Macmillan and Co., 1880). See Peter Bowler, "Holding Your Head Up High: Degeneration and Orthogenesis in Theories of Human Evolution," in *History, Humanity and Evolution: Essays for John C. Greene*, ed. James Richard Moore (Cambridge: Cambridge University Press, 1989), pp. 329–53.

12. Quoted in Gary Greenberg, *Manufacturing Depression: The Secret History of a Modern Disease* (New York: Simon & Schuster, 2010), p. 72. For more on Kraepelin's commitment to theories of degeneration, see Eric J. Engstrom, "'On the Question of Degeneration' by Emil Kraepelin (1908)," *History of Psychiatry* 18, no. 3 (September 1, 2007): 389–98.

13. "The Assassin's Trial," *Lewiston Evening Journal*, January 13, 1882. See also Henry H. Alexander, James Abram Garfield, and Edward Denison Easton, *Report of the Proceedings in the Case of* The United States vs. Charles J. Guiteau… (Washington, DC: U.S. Government Printing Office, 1882), p. 2303. The classic analysis of this case is Charles E. Rosenberg, *The Trial of the Assassin Guiteau: Psychiatry and the Law in the Gilded Age* (Chicago: University of Chicago Press, 1995).

14. For a thoughtful discussion of the whole Lombrosian tradition, see Jeff Ferrell et al., *Cultural Criminology Unleashed* (London: Routledge, 2004), p. 72.

15. See College of Physicians of Philadelphia, *The College of Physicians of Philadelphia* (Charleston, SC: Arcadia, 2012), p. 74.

16. Paul Broca, "Remarques sur le siège de la faculté du langage articulé, suivies d'une observation d'aphémie (perte de la parole)," *Bulletins de la Société Anatomique* 36 (1861): 330–57; Broca, "Du siège de la faculté du langage articulé," *Bulletins de la Société d'Anthropologie* 6 (1865): 377–93; Anne Harrington, *Medicine, Mind and the Double Brain* (Princeton, NJ: Princeton University Press, 1987).

17. Anne Harrington, "Beyond Phrenology: Localization Theory in the Modern Era," in *The Enchanted Loom: Chapters in the History of Neuroscience*, ed. P. Corsi (New York: Oxford University Press, 1991).

18. Wilhelm Griesinger, *Mental Pathology and Therapeutics*, trans. C. Lockhart Robertson and James Rutherford, rev. ed. (London: New Sydenham Society, 1867), p. 1. The original German edition was *Die Pathologie und Therapie der psychischen Krankheiten, für Ärzte und Studierende* (Stuttgart: Adolph Krabbe, 1845), online at http://www.deutschestextarchiv.de/book/view/griesinger psychische_1845?p=1.

19. While this was definitely the rhetoric, some scholarship has begun to show that it exaggerated the actual situation, pointing out evidence of interest in neuroanatomical work within psychiatry in the first half of the nineteenth century (perhaps especially in the German-speaking countries), long before the neurologists mounted their challenge. Michael Kutzer, "Der pathologisch-anatomische Befund und seine Auswertung in der deutschen Psychiatrie der ersten Hälfte des 19. Jahrhunderts," *Medizinhistorisches Journal* 26, nos. 3–4 (January 1, 1991): 214–35.

20. E. C. Spitzka, "Reform in the Scientific Study of Psychiatry," *Journal of Nervous and Mental Disease* 5 (1878): 201–28.

21. E. C. Spitzka, "Merits and Motives of the Movement for Asylum Reform," *Journal of Nervous and Mental Disease* 5 (1878): 694–714.

22. Brian Burrell, *Postcards from the Brain Museum: The Improbable Search for Meaning in the Matter of Famous Minds* (New York: Broadway Books, 2005).

23. Theodor Meynert, "Über die Nothwendigkeit und Tragweite einer anatomischen Richtung in der Psychiatrie," *Wiener medizinische Wochenschrift* 18 (May 3, 1868): 573–76, quoted in Scott Phelps, *Blind to Their Blindness*, Ph.D. diss., Harvard University, 2014.

24. Quoted in Peter Berner, *Psychiatry in Vienna* (Vienna: Brandstätter, 1983), p. 11.

25. George Makari, *Revolution in Mind: The Creation of Psychoanalysis* (New York: HarperCollins, 2008), p. 182.

26. Katja Guenther, *Localization and Its Discontents: A Genealogy of Psychoanalysis and the Neuro Disciplines* (Chicago: University of Chicago Press, 2015), pp. 55–57.

27. Irving Stone, *The Passions of the Mind: A Novel of Sigmund Freud* (New York: Doubleday, 1971).

28. Sigmund Freud, *Standard Edition of the Complete Psychological Works of Sigmund Freud*, ed. James Strachey and Anna Freud (London: Hogarth Press, 1893), p. 3:11–23.

29. Eric J. Engstrom, *Clinical Psychiatry in Imperial Germany: A History of Psychiatric Practice* (Ithaca, NY: Cornell University Press, 2003), pp. 61–62.

30. Kalyan B. Bhattacharyya, *Eminent Neuroscientists Their Lives and Works* (India: Academic Publishers, 2011), p. 96.

31. Quoted in Kalyan B. Bhattacharyya, "Johann Bernhard Aloys von Gudden and the Mad King of Bavaria," *Annals of Indian Academy of Neurology* 20, no. 4 (2017): 348–51

32. "Bavaria's 'Mad King' Ludwig May Not Have Been So Mad After All," *Telegraph*, February 6, 2014.

33. Quoted in C. Barry Chabot, *Freud on Schreber: Psychoanalytic Theory and the Critical Act* (Amherst: University of Massachusetts Press, 1982), p. 15.

34. As Flechsig wrote in 1882: "Collecting data from corpses offers in general the most direct way to advance knowledge of the lawful dependent relationship between mental disorders and brain anomalies." The original German here reads: "So bietet ueberhaupt die Erhebung des Leichenbefundes den direkteste Weg, um zur Erkenntnis gesetzmaessiger Abhaenigkeitsverhaeltnisse zwischen Geistesstoerungen und Hirnanomalien vorzudringen." See Paul Emil Flechsig, *Die körperlichen Grundlagen der Geistesstörungen: Vortrag gehalten beim Antritt des Lehramtes an der Universität Leipzig* (Leipzig: Verlag von Veit & Comp., 1882), p. 11.

35. Martin Stingelin, "Die Seele als Funktion des Körpers," in *Diskursanalysen 2: Institution Universität* (Wiesbaden: VS Verlag für Sozialwissenschaften, 1990), pp. 101–15; and Eric L. Santner, *My Own Private Germany: Daniel Paul Schreber's Secret History of Modernity* (Princeton, NJ: Princeton University Press, 1997), p. 71.

36. For more on this, see Sarah Ferber and Sally Wilde, eds., *The Body Divided: Human Beings and Human "Material" in Modern Medical History* (Farnham, UK: Ashgate Publishing, Ltd., 2013).

37. One might make a partial exception for the unusual histological changes in the brain found in a case of early-onset dementia, and first reported in the early twentieth century by an assistant of Emil Kraepelin, Alois Alzheimer. In the 1910 edition of his textbook in psychiatry, Kraepelin had proposed calling this newly discovered dementia "Alzheimer's disease." For fifty years or more, however, the disease was supposed to be very rare, and few clinicians took an interest in it. See Hanns Hippius and Gabriele Neundörfer, "The Discovery of Alzheimer's Disease," *Dialogues in Clinical Neuroscience* 5, no. 1 (March 2003): 101–8.

38. John Gach, "Biological Psychiatry in the Nineteenth and Twentieth Century," in *History of Psychiatry and Medical Psychology*, ed. Edwin R. Wallace IV and John Gach (New York: Springer, 2008).

39. Although Jaspers would become famous for his "brain mythology" critique, it actually seems to have been Jasper's mentor at Heidelberg, the neurohistologist Franz Nissl, who first coined the term. See Katja Guenther, "Recasting Neuropsychiatry: Freud's 'Critical Introduction' and the Convergence of French and German Brain Science," *Psychoanalysis and History* 14, no. 2 (July 1, 2012): 210.

40. Jaspers quoted in Katja Guenther, *Localization and Its Discontents: A Genealogy of Psychoanalysis and the Neuro Disciplines* (Chicago: University of Chicago Press, 2015), p. 13.

41. Quoted in Bernard Bolech, *Gehirn, Geist und Gesellschaft: Orte des Subjekts in den Wiener Humanwissenschaften um 1900*, Ph.D. diss., University of Vienna, 2014. Translation mine.

42. Quoted in Scott Phelps, *Blind to Their Blindness*, Ph.D. diss., Harvard University, 2014.

43. Thomas G. Dalzell, *Freud's Schreber Between Psychiatry and Psychoanalysis: On Subjective Disposition to Psychosis* (London: Routledge, 2011), pp. 132–35.

44. Eric J. Engstrom and Matthias M. Weber, "The Directions of Psychiatric Research by Emil Kraepelin 1887," *History of Psychiatry* 16, no. 3 (2005): 345–64; and Eric. J. Engstrom, "On Attitude Toward Philosophy and Psychology in German Psychiatry, 1867–1917," in *Philosophical Issues in Psychiatry III: The Nature and Sources of Historical Change*, ed. K. S. Kendler and J. Parnas (Oxford, UK: Oxford University Press, 2015), pp. 140–64.

45. Paul Hoff, "The Kraepelinian Tradition," *Dialogues in Clinical Neuroscience* 17, no. 1 (2015): 31.

46. Kraepelin quoted in Hannah S. Decker, "How Kraepelinian Was Kraepelin? How Kraepelinian Are the Neo-Kraepelinians?—From Emil Kraepelin to DSM-III," *History of Psychiatry* 18, no. 71, pt. 3 (2007): 337–60.

47. German E. Berrios, Rogello Luque, and Jose M. Villagran, "Schizophrenia: A Conceptual History," *International Journal of Psychology and Psychological Therapy* 3 (2003): 111–40.

48. That said, the materials on which he based his conclusions were not all complete, his follow-through was often scanty, and he did not always follow his own injunctions to stick to description and avoid speculation about cause. See Decker, "How Kraepelinian Was Kraepelin?" p. 341.

49. In the course of doing this work, Kraepelin also ended up affirming the existence of several other "natural entities" in psychiatry (paranoia, involutional

melancholy), but these would be more controversial and less influential. It was his distinction between manic-depression and dementia praecox that would have the greatest impact. For more on the fate of these other diagnostic categories, see Kenneth S. Kendler, "Kraepelin and the Diagnostic Concept of Paranoia," *Comprehensive Psychiatry* 29, no. 1 (January 1, 1988): 4–11; Richard P. Brown et al., "Involutional Melancholia Revisited," *American Journal of Psychiatry* 141, no. 1 (1984): 24–28.

50. Ulrich Palm and Hans-Jürgen Möller, "Reception of Kraepelin's Ideas 1900– 1960," *Psychiatry and Clinical Neurosciences* 65, no. 4 (June 1, 2011): 318–25; and David Healy et al., "Historical Overview: Kraepelin's Impact on Psychiatry," *European Archives of Psychiatry and Clinical Neuroscience* 258, no. 2 (June 1, 2008): 18.

51. Christopher G. Goetz, Michel Bonduelle, and Toby Gelfand, *Charcot: Constructing Neurology* (New York: Oxford University Press, 1995).

52. Georges Didi-Huberman, *Invention of Hysteria: Charcot and the Photographic Iconography of the Salpêtrière* (Cambridge, MA: MIT Press, 2004).

53. Didi-Huberman, *Invention of Hysteria*, pp. 115–16.

54. Quoted in Didi-Huberman, *Invention of Hysteria*, p. 32.

55. A bit of background: Until the mid-nineteenth century, the term *hypnosis* did not exist, but there was considerable interest in a therapeutic practice called animal magnetism or mesmerism, after the Austrian physician Anton Mesmer who pioneered it in the late eighteenth century. Mesmer had taught that the human body contained an invisible physical force called animal magnetism; when one's animal magnetism became depleted and/or blocked, one fell ill. To get well, one must be treated by a special kind of healer called a magnetizer, someone possessed of a strong supply of animal magnetism that he could "transfer" to his patent. The magnetizer typically gazed into the patient's eyes, blew on her face, and made long stroking gestures across her body, without actually touching it. (The eyes, breath, and hands were all key portals for animal magnetism.) In the early years, patients would typically respond to such ministrations by collapsing into convulsions. Later, they more commonly sank into a strange sleeplike state where they nevertheless were highly receptive to the voice and wishes of the magnetizer. Many also became impervious to pain, or reported remarkable healings. And a few magnetizers experimented with carrying out surgical procedures on patients while they were in a "magnetic" sleeplike state.

By the early nineteenth century, though, mainstream medicine had widely denounced animal magnetism as both fraudulent and immoral (because women in a trance were said to be susceptible to being seduced). Then in the late 1870s—inspired both by his colleague Charles Richet and by some experiences he had himself with therapies involving metals and magnets—Charcot decided that the consensus was wrong and that hypnosis deserved a place in medicine as a research tool. Because he didn't believe there was any such thing as animal magnetism, to describe the practice he adopted a term that had been coined in England a decade or two earlier: *hypnosis*. What made hypnosis worth taking seriously, he announced, was not its capacity to take away pain or heal people, but its capacity to create symptoms of hysteria on command in susceptible patients. For more, see Alison Winter, *Mesmerized: Powers of Mind in Victorian Britain* (Chicago: University of Chicago Press, 2000); C. Richet, "Du somnambulisme provoqué," *Journal de l'anatomie et de la physiologie normales et pathologiques de l'homme et des animaux* 2 (1875): 348–77; and Anne Harrington, "Metals and Magnets in Medicine—Hysteria, Hypnosis and Medical Culture in Fin-de-siècle Paris," *Psychological Medicine* 18 (1988): 21–38.

56. See, for example, Hippolyte Bernheim, "Hypnotisme et suggestion: Doctrine de la Salpêtrière et doctrine de Nancy," *Le Temps* (supplément) (January 29, 1891): 1–2.

57. Jean-Martin Charcot, "A Tuesday Lesson: Hysteroepilepsy" (1888), translated and reprinted in Greg Eghigian, ed., *From Madness to Mental Health: Psychiatric Disorder and Its Treatment in Western Civilization* (New Brunswick, NJ: Rutgers University Press, 2009), p. 198.

58. Sigmund Freud, *Letters of Sigmund Freud, 1873–1939*, ed. Ernst L. Freud (London: Hogarth Press, 1970), p. 196.

59. Sigmund Freud, "Some Points for a Comparative Study of Organic and Hysterical Motor Paralyses" (1893), in *The Standard Edition Complete Psychological Work of Sigmund Freud*, vol. 1, *Pre-psychoanalytic Papers and Unpublished Drafts* (London: Hogarth Press, 1966), pp. 160–72.

60. Pierre Janet, *L'état mental des hystériques* (Paris: F. Alcan, 1892).

61. On this development, see Mark S. Micale, "Charcot and les névroses traumatiques: Scientific and Historical Reflections 1," *Journal of the History of the Neurosciences* 4, no. 2 (1995): 101–19. See also J.-M. Charcot, preface to Janet, *L'état mental des hystériques*.

62. Sigmund Freud and Josef Breuer, *Studies in Hysteria* (New York: Penguin, 1895), pp. 160–61.

63. Sigmund Freud, "The Aetiology of Hysteria," trans. James Strachey (1896), reproduced in Jeffrey Masson, *The Assault on Truth: Freud's Suppression of the Seduction Theory* (New York: Pocket Books, 1998), appendix.

64. As he put it, "If hysterical subjects trace back their symptoms to traumas that are fictitious, then the new fact which emerges is precisely that they create such scenes in fantasy." Freud, "On the History of the Psycho-Analytic Movement" (1914), quoted in Masson, *Assault on Truth*, p. 17.

65. Sigmund Freud, *The History of the Psychoanalytic Movement* (New York: Nervous and Mental Disease Pub. Co., 1917).

66. The following section is adapted from my previous book *The Cure Within: A History of Mind-Body Medicine* (New York: Norton, 2008). I am grateful to W. W. Norton for allowing me to reuse this material in a limited capacity.

67. Quoted in Great Britain and Anthony Richards, *Report of the War Office Committee of Enquiry into "Shell-Shock" (Cmd. 1734): Featuring a New Historical Essay on Shell Shock* (1922; reprinted London: Imperial War Museum, 2004), pp. 48, 50–51.

68. Wilfred Owen, "Mental Cases" (1918), in *The Collected Poems of Wilfred Owen*, ed. C. Day Lewis (New York: New Directions, 1965), p. 69.

69. Michael Hagner, "Cultivating the Cortex in German Neuroanatomy," *Science in Context* 14, no. 4 (December 2001): 541–63.

70. Quoted in Juliet D. Hurn, *The History of General Paralysis of the Insane in Britain,*

1830 to 1950, Ph.D. diss., University of London, 1998, p. 6, http://discovery.ucl
.ac.uk/1349281/. For a vivid compilation of descriptions from the literature, see
James George Kiernan, "Paretic Dementia: Is It a Psychosis, a Neuro-Psychosis
or a Complication of the Psychosis?" *Alienist and Neurologist* 6, no. 2 (April 1,
1885): 219–24.

71. G. H. Savage, "General Paralysis," in *A Dictionary of Psychological Medicine*, ed.
D. Hack Tuke (London: J & A Churchill, 1892), pp. 1:519–44, esp. 535.

72. For more on the history of syphilis and its treatments, see Allan M. Brandt,
*No Magic Bullet: A Social History of Venereal Disease in the United States Since
1880* (New York: Oxford University Press, 1987); Roger Davidson and Lesley
A. Hall, *Sex, Sin and Suffering: Venereal Disease and European Society Since 1870*
(New York: Routledge, 2003).

73. Harry Oosterhuis, *Stepchildren of Nature: Krafft-Ebing, Psychiatry, and the Making of Sexual Identity* (Chicago: University of Chicago Press, 2000), p. 91.

74. Hideyo Noguchi and Joseph W. Moore, "A Demonstration of Treponema Pallidum in the Brain in Cases of General Paralysis," *Journal of Experimental Medicine* 17, no. 2 (1913): 232.

Chapter 2: Biology in Disarray

1. Lisa Appignanesi and John Forrester, *Freud's Women* (New York: Basic
Books, 1992).

2. David Schuster, *Neurasthenic Nation: The Medicalization of Modernity in the
United States, 1869–1920*, Ph.D. diss., University of California at Santa Barbara, 2006. See also David G. Schuster, *Neurasthenic Nation: America's Search
for Health, Happiness, and Comfort, 1869–1920* (New Brunswick, NJ: Rutgers
University Press, 2011).

3. George M. Beard, "The Influence of Mind in the Causation and Cure of Disease: The Potency of Definite Expectation," *Medical Record: A Weekly Journal
of Medicine and Surgery* 11 (1876): 461–62. I was alerted to this source by Eric
Caplan, *Mind Games: American Culture and the Birth of Psychotherapy* (Berkeley: University of California Press, 1998), pp. 93–94.

4. Hammond commentary in Beard, "Influence of Mind in Causation and Cure,"
p. 462.

5. Eric Michael Caplan, "Trains, Brains, and Sprains: Railway Spine and the Origins of Psychoneuroses," *Bulletin of the History of Medicine* 69 (1995), 387–419.

6. Anne Harrington, *The Cure Within: A History of Mind-Body Medicine* (New
York: Norton, 2008); and Eugene Taylor, *Shadow Culture: Psychology and Spirituality in America* (Washington, DC: Counterpoint, 1999).

7. Sonu Shamdasani, "'Psychotherapy': The Invention of a Word," *History of the
Human Sciences* 18, no. 1 (February 1, 2005): 1–22.

8. Quoted in Edward M. Brown, "Neurology's Influence on American Psychiatry,
1865–1915," in *History of Psychiatry and Medical Psychology*, ed. Edwin R. Wallace IV and John Gach (New York: Springer, 2010), p. 528.

9. Henri Ellenberger, "Pierre Janet and His American Friends" (1973), in George
E. Gifford, Jr., ed., *Psychoanalysis, Psychotherapy and the New England Medical
Scene, 1894–1944* (New York: Science History Publications, 1977), pp. 63–72.

10. Julien Bogousslavsky and Thierry Moulin, "Birth of Modern Psychiatry and the Death of Alienism: The Legacy of Jean-Martin Charcot," in *Frontiers of Neurology and Neuroscience*, ed. J. Bogousslavsky (Basel: Karger, 2010), pp. 29:1–8.

11. Some have suggested that at the time, Jung was actually better known and more of a draw than Freud. See Eugene Taylor, "Jung Before Freud, Not Freud before Jung: The Reception of Jung's Work in American Psychoanalytic Circles Between 1904 and 1909," *Journal of Analytical Psychology* 43, no. 1 (January 1, 1998): 97–114.

12. Ernest Jones, *The Life and Work of Sigmund Freud*, vol. 1, *1856–1900: The Formative Years and the Great Discoveries* (London: Hogarth Press, 1953), pp. 59–60.

13. Sigmund Freud, "The Origin and Development of Psychoanalysis," *American Journal of Psychology* 21 (April, 1910): 181–218. This issue of the journal (available free online through JSTOR) also includes an essay by Carl Gustav Jung on "the association method," (pp. 219–69) and two articles on Freud's dream theory, one by Ernest Jones (pp. 283–308) and one by Sandor Ferenczi (pp. 309–28).

14. Russell George Vasile, *James Jackson Putnam: From Neurology to Psychoanalysis: A Study of the Reception and Promulgation of Freudian Psychoanalytic Theory in America, 1895–1918* (Oceanside, NY: Dabor Science Publications, 1977).

15. Brown, "Neurology's Influence on American Psychiatry." See also James J. Putnam, "Personal Experience with Freud's Psychoanalytic Method," *Journal of Nervous and Mental Disease* 37, no. 11 (1910): 657–74; Fred H. Matthews, "The Americanization of Sigmund Freud: Adaptations of Psychoanalysis Before 1917," *Journal of American Studies* 1, no. 1 (1967): 39–62.

16. Freud, "Origin and Development of Psychoanalysis. See also Ricard Skues, "Clark Revisited: Reappraising Freud in America," in *After Freud Left: A Century of Psychoanalysis in America*, ed. John Burnham (Chicago: University of Chicago Press, 2012), p. 76.

17. Nathan Hale, examining media coverage of Freud and psychoanalysis between 1910 and 1918, found a steadily expanding and largely positive trajectory: eleven largely positive articles about Freud up through 1914, and about thirty-one articles, including at least one in a women's magazine, between 1915 and 1918. See Nathan G. Hale, *Freud and the Americans: The Beginnings of Psychoanalysis in the United States, 1876–1917* (Oxford, UK: Oxford University Press, 1995), p. 397.

18. Charles Burr, "A Criticism of Psychoanalysis," in *Proceedings of the American Medico Psychological Association at the Seventieth Annual Meeting Held in Baltimore, Md.* (Baltimore: Lord Baltimore Press, 1914), pp. 70: 303–17, 318–324. See also J. Victor Haberman, "A Criticism of Psychoanalysis," *Journal of Abnormal Psychology* 9, no. 4 (1914): 265–80. For an attempt to summarize and point out the weakness of all the criticisms, see John F. W. Meagher, "Psychoanalysis and Its Critics," *Psychoanalytic Review* 9 (January 1, 1922): 324–36.

19. Matthew Gambino, "'These Strangers Within Our Gates': Race, Psychiatry and Mental Illness Among Black Americans at St Elizabeths Hospital in Washington, DC, 1900–40," *History of Psychiatry* 19, no. 4 (December 1, 2008): 387–408. Much more work needs to be done on the ways Jim Crow–era assumptions about African-American racial inferiority shaped the projects and assumptions of early American psychoanalysts.

20. Susan Lamb, *Pathologist of the Mind: Adolf Meyer and the Origins of American Psychiatry* (Baltimore: Johns Hopkins University Press, 2014), p. 214. For more on Meyer's complicated relationship with psychoanalysis, see Ruth Leys, "Meyer's Dealings with Jones: A Chapter in the History of the American Response to Psychoanalysis," *Journal of the History of the Behavioral Sciences* 17 (1981): 445–65; and Nathan G. Hale, Jr., *The Rise and Crisis of Psychoanalysis in the United States: Freud and the Americans, 1917–1985* (New York: Oxford University Press, 1995), pp. 168–72.

21. Adolf Meyer, "The Dynamic Interpretation of Dementia Praecox," *American Journal of Psychology* 21, no. 3 (July 1910): 385–403, esp. 398.

22. Elmer E. Southard, "Cross-Sections of Mental Hygiene 1844, 1869, 1894," *American Journal of Psychiatry* 76, no. 2 (October 1, 1919): 91–111, esp. 107.

23. S. Weir Mitchell, "Address Before the Fiftieth Annual Meeting of the American Medico-Psychological Association, Held in Philadelphia, May 16th, 1894," *Journal of Nervous and Mental Disease* 19, no. 7 (1894): 413–37.

24. See Kenneth J. Weiss, "Asylum Reform and the Great Comeuppance of 1894— Or Was It?" *Journal of Nervous and Mental Disease* 199, no. 9 (September 2011): 631–38.

25. "John B. Chapin, M.D., LL.D. (1829–1918), Advocate for the Chronic Insane of New York, and the Removal of All Insane Persons from the County Almshouses," *American Journal of Insanity* 74 (1918): 689–705.

26. Walter Channing, "Some Remarks on the Address Delivered to the American Medico-Psychological Association, by S. Weir Mitchell, M.D., May 16, 1894," *American Journal of Psychiatry* 51, no. 2 (October 1, 1894): 171–81.

27. See, for example, Adolf Meyer, "Presidential Address: Thirty–Five Years of Psychiatry in the United States and Our Present Outlook" (1928), cited in Weiss, "Asylum Reform," p. 636.

28. Quoted in Lamb, *Pathologist of the Mind*, p. 42. See also Adolf Meyer, "Aims and Plans of the Pathological Institute for the New York State Hospitals," in *The Collected Papers of Adolf Meyer*, ed. Eunice E. Winters, 4 vols. (Baltimore: Johns Hopkins University Press, 1950–52), p. 2:93, quoted in Andrew Scull and Jay Schulkin, "Psychobiology, Psychiatry, and Psychoanalysis: The Intersecting Careers of Adolf Meyer, Phyllis Greenacre, and Curt Richter," *Medical History* 53, no. 1 (January 2009): 5.

29. Adolf Meyer, "The Role of Mental Factors in Psychiatry" (1908), quoted in Eric Caplan, *Mind Games: American Culture and the Birth of Psychotherapy* (Berkeley: University of California Press, 1998), p. 113. See also Michael Rutter, "Meyerian Psychobiology, Personality Development, and the Role of Life Experiences," *American Journal of Psychiatry* 143, no. 9 (1986): 1077–108.

30. Richard Noll, *American Madness: The Rise and Fall of Dementia Praecox* (Cambridge, MA: Harvard University Press, 2011).

31. Ruth Leys, "Types of One: Adolf Meyer's Life Chart and the Representation of Individuality," *Representations*, no. 34 (1991): 1–28.

32. For a fuller discussion of Meyer's work at the New York Pathological Institute, see Lamb, *Pathologist of the Mind*, pp. 55–58.

33. When Meyer left, the New York Pathological Institute appointed a third director, the neurologist August Hoch. A devotee of psychoanalysis, Hoch promptly

spent three months in the spring of 1909 in Switzerland working with Freud's (then) closest ally, Carl Gustav Jung. And he went on to serve a term (in 1913) as president of the newly established American Psychoanalytic Association. The dismantling of the institute as a German-style center for neuroanatomical research was complete. See Joseph Schwartz, *Cassandra's Daughter: A History of Psychoanalysis* (London: Karnac Books, 2003), p. 147.

34. Janet Farrar Worthington, "When Psychiatry Was Very Young," *Hopkins Medicine* (Winter 2008).

35. Roy Abraham Kallivayalil, "The Burghölzli Hospital: Its History and Legacy," *Indian Journal of Psychiatry* 58, no. 2 (2016): 226–28.

36. George Makari, *Revolution in Mind: The Creation of Psychoanalysis* (New York: HarperCollins, 2008), p. 182.

37. Makari, *Revolution in Mind*, p. 183.

38. Carl Gustav Jung, "The Content of the Psychoses," *Collected Papers on Analytical Psychology*, ed. Constance Long, 2nd ed. (New York: Moffat, Yard & Co., 1917), p. 322. Originally published as "The Psychology of Dementia Praecox," translated by Brill and Peterson, *Monograph Series of the Journal of Nervous and Mental Diseases* (New York, 1910).

39. Makari, *Revolution in Mind*, p. 184.

40. Eugen Bleuler, review of *Interpretations of Dreams*, 1904, quoted in Ernst Falzeder, *Psychoanalytic Filiations: Mapping the Psychoanalytic Movement* (London: Karnac Books, 2015), p. 179.

41. Freud to Wilhelm Fliess, April 26,1904, quoted in Jeffrey Masson, *The Assault on Truth: Freud's Suppression of the Seduction Theory* (New York: Pocket Books, 1998), p. 461.

42. For an excellent discussion of this, see Makari, *Revolution in Mind*, pp. 187–93.

43. John Read and Jacqui Dillon, *Models of Madness: Psychological, Social and Biological Approaches to Psychosis* (London: Routledge, 2013), p. 35.

44. Andrew Moskowitz and Gerhard Heim, "Eugen Bleuler's 'Dementia Praecox or the Group of Schizophrenias' (1911): A Centenary Appreciation and Reconsideration," *Schizophrenia Bulletin* 37, no. 3 (May 1, 2011): 471–79.

45. Ernst Falzeder, "The Story of an Ambivalent Relationship: Sigmund Freud and Eugen Bleuler," *Journal of Analytical Psychology* 52, no. 3 (2007): 343–68.

46. Richard Noll, "The American Reaction to Dementia Praecox, 1900," *History of Psychiatry* 15, no. 1 (March 1, 2004): 127–28.

47. E. E. Southard, "The Mind Twist and Brain Spot Hypotheses in Psychopathology and Neuropathology," *Psychological Bulletin* 11, no. 4 (April 1914): 117–30, esp. 120.

48. In Europe, there was also interest in the idea that schizophrenia might be caused by "intoxication" or brain poisoning, but the focus was more on the possibility it was caused by some kind of metabolic imbalance. Late in life, Emil Kraepelin became an advocate of this theory, as did Eugen Bleuler. Kraepelin also believed that the most likely source of these metabolic problems was an inherited defect of the sex organs. In the 1920s he injected some dementia praecox patients with various glandular extracts to see if it would improve their condition. See Richard Noll, "Kraepelin's 'Lost Biological Psychiatry'? Autointoxication, Organotherapy and Surgery for Dementia Praecox," *History of Psychiatry* 18,

no. 3 (2007): 301–20. In 1925—a year before his death—Kraepelin met with Alan Gregg from the Rockefeller Foundation. As Gregg recorded the visit, "I questioned K. offhand on any shift that may have taken place in his interests in psychiatry in the last ten years, and he replied that the development of serology had greatly changed his attitude.... He stated that it had been very difficult for him to write the last edition of his book, in view of the great progress made in that field. He mentioned nothing besides serology; he is openly intolerant of Freud and Jung." Quoted in Richard Noll, "Whole Body Madness," *Psychiatric Times* 29, no. 12 (2012): 13–14. For more, see Richard Noll, "Historical Review: Autointoxication and Focal Infection Theories of Dementia Praecox," *World Journal of Biological Psychiatry* 5, no. 2 (January 2004): 66–72.

49. See Henry A. Cotton, "The Etiology and Treatment of the So-Called Functional Psychoses: Summary of Results Based on the Experience of Four Years," *American Journal of Psychiatry* 79 (1922): 157–210. The authoritative study of Cotton's work is Andrew T. Scull, *Madhouse: A Tragic Tale of Megalomania and Modern Medicine* (New Haven, CT: Yale University Press, 2005).

50. Andrew Scull and Jay Schulkin, "Psychobiology, Psychiatry, and Psychoanalysis: The Intersecting Careers of Adolf Meyer, Phyllis Greenacre, and Curt Richter," *Medical History* 53, no. 1 (January 2009): 5–36.

51. Richard Noll, "Infectious Insanities, Surgical Solutions: Bayard Taylor Holmes, Dementia Praecox, and Laboratory Science in Early Twentieth-Century America," pt. 1, *History of Psychology* 17 (June 1, 2006): 183–204.

52. Bayard Holmes and Julius Retinger, "The Relation of Cecal Stasis to Dementia Precox," *Lancet-Clinic* 116 (August 12, 1916): 145–50; Richard Noll, "The Blood of the Insane," *History of Psychiatry* 17, no. 4 (2006): 395–418; M. Sullivan-Fowler, "Doubtful Theories, Drastic Therapies: Autointoxication and Faddism in the Late Nineteenth and Early Twentieth Centuries," *Journal of the History of Medicine and Allied Sciences* 50 (1995): 364–90; and Richard Noll, "Infectious Insanities, Surgical Solutions: Bayard Taylor Holmes, Dementia Praecox and Laboratory Science in Early Twentieth-Century America" pt. 2, *History of Psychiatry* 17, no. 3 (2006): 299–311.

53. Jonathan Davidson, "Bayard Holmes (1852–1924) and Henry Cotton (1869–1933): Surgeon-Psychiatrists and Their Tragic Quest to Cure Schizophrenia," *Journal of Medical Biography* 24, no. 4 (December 2014), pp. 550–59; and Noll, "Infectious Insanities, Surgical Solutions," pt. 2.

54. This school was originally called the New Jersey Home for the Education and Care of Feebleminded Children (1888). In 1893 the name was changed to the New Jersey Training School. By the time Goddard was appointed in 1906, it seems to have gone by several names: the Training School at Vineland, the Vineland Training School for Backward and Feeble-minded Children, and the Vineland Training School for Feeble-Minded Girls and Boys.

55. For the lively scholarship on all this, see Stephen Jay Gould, *The Mismeasure of Man* (1981; reprinted New York: Norton, 1996); Steven A. Gelb, "Myths, Morons, Psychologists: The Kallikak Family Revisited," *Review of Education/Pedagogy/Cultural Studies* 11, no. 4 (1985): 255–59; Raymond E. Fancher, "Henry Goddard and the Kallikak Family Photographs: 'Conscious Skulduggery' or 'Whig History'?" *American Psychologist* 42, no. 6 (1987): 585; and

NOTES TO PAGES 50-55 ⬤ 289

Martin A. Elks, "Visual Indictment: A Contextual Analysis of the Kallikak Family Photographs," *Mental Retardation* 43, no. 4 (2005): 268–80.

56. Henry H. Goddard, *The Kallikak Family: A Study in the Heredity of Feeble-Mindedness* (New York: Macmillan, 1912). Goddard actually later came to see the conclusions he drew in this book as flawed. For more, see Leila Zenderland, *Measuring Minds: Henry Herbert Goddard and the Origins of American Intelligence Testing* (New York: Cambridge University Press, 2001).

57. Garland Allen, "The Eugenics Record Office at Cold Spring Harbor, 1910–1940: An Essay on Institutional History," *Osiris* 2 (1986): 225–64.

58. Meyer's leadership role here is reported by Davenport himself in C. B. Davenport, "Report of Committee on Eugenics," *Journal of Heredity* 1, no. 2 (April 1, 1910): 126–29, esp. 126.

59. Ian Robert Dowbiggin, *Keeping America Sane: Psychiatry and Eugenics in the United States and Canada, 1880–1940* (Ithaca, NY: Cornell University Press, 1997), p. 113.

60. See Adolf Meyer, "Organization of Eugenics Investigations," *Eugenical News* 2 (1917): 66–69; and James W. Trent, *Inventing the Feeble Mind: A History of Mental Retardation in the United States* (Berkeley: University of California Press, 1995), p. 195.

61. Allen M. Hornblum, Judith L. Newman, and Gregory J. Dober, *Against Their Will: The Secret History of Medical Experimentation on Children in Cold War America* (New York: St. Martin's Press, 2013), pp. 35–36. For a succinct overview of Meyer's activities on the eugenics front, see Ruth Clifford Engs, *The Progressive Era's Health Reform Movement: A Historical Dictionary* (Santa Barbara, CA: Greenwood Publishing Group, 2003), p. 214.

62. Dowbiggin, *Keeping America Sane*, p. 114.

63. Marion Marle Woodson, *Behind the Door of Delusion by "Inmate Ward 8"* (New York: Macmillan, 1932).

64. The Racial Integrity Act was not overturned until 1967; the Sterilization Act was not formally repealed until 1979.

65. "The Supreme Court and the Sterilization of Carrie Buck," *Facing History and Ourselves*, n.d., www.facinghistory.org/resource-library/supreme-court-and -sterilization-carrie-buck.

66. Paul A. Lombardo, *Three Generations, No Imbeciles: Eugenics, the Supreme Court, and Buck v. Bell* (Baltimore: Johns Hopkins University Press, 2008), p. 127.

67. *Buck v. Bell*, 274 US 200 (Supreme Court 1927).

68. Mark P. Mostert, "Useless Eaters: Disability as Genocidal Marker in Nazi Germany," *Journal of Special Education* 36, no. 3 (2002): 157–70.

69. Foster Kennedy, "The Problem of Social Control of the Congenital Defective," *American Journal of Psychiatry* 99, no. 1 (July 1, 1942): 13–16.

70. Leo Kanner, "Exoneration of the Feebleminded," *American Journal of Psychiatry* 99, no. 1 (July 1942): 17–22, esp. 20.

71. Kanner, "Exoneration of the Feebleminded," p. 21.

72. "Comment: Euthanasia," *American Journal of Psychiatry* 99, no. 1 (July 1942): 140–43, esp. 143. For a full summary and discussion of this 1942 exchange, see Jay Joseph, "The 1942 'Euthanasia' Debate in the American Journal of Psychiatry," *History of Psychiatry* 16, no. 2 (June 1, 2005): 171–79.

73. Joel T. Braslow, "In the Name of Therapeutics: The Practice of Sterilization in a California State Hospital," *Journal of the History of Medicine and Allied Sciences* 51, no. 1 (1996): 29–52.

74. L. D. Hubbard, "Hydrotherapy in the Mental Hospital," *American Journal of Nursing* 27, no. 8 (1927): 642.

75. Russell Barnes (1903–1987), former psychiatric aid Jacksonville (Illinois) State Hospital, interview by Rodger Streitmatter, 1972, Mental Health Care Project, Norris L. Brooken Library, Archives/Special Collections, University of Illinois, Springfield.

76. Robert Foster Kennedy, "Preface," in Manfred Sakel, *The Pharmacological Shock Treatment of Schizophrenia*, trans. Joseph Wortis, rev. ed. (New York: Nervous and Mental Disease Pub. Co., 1938).

77. Julius Wagner-Jauregg, "The Treatment of General Paresis by Inoculation of Malaria," *Journal of Nervous and Mental Disease* 55, no. 5 (May 1922): 369–75. Did the treatment really work? Maybe sometimes. Even today no one is quite sure how, but one theory is that the high fever induced by the malaria may have triggered an intense immune response in some patients that also helped them fight the bacterial infection. See Gretchen Vogel, "Malaria as Lifesaving Therapy," *Science* 342, no. 6159 (November 8, 2013): 686.

78. Quoted in Edward M. Brown, "Why Wagner-Jauregg Won the Nobel Prize for Discovering Malaria Therapy for General Paresis of the Insane," *History of Psychiatry* 11 (2000): 371–82.

79. Quoted in Joel T. Braslow, *Mental Ills and Bodily Cures: Psychiatric Treatment in the First Half of the Twentieth Century* (Berkeley: University of California Press, 1997), p. 82.

80. Quoted in Joel Braslow, "The Influence of a Biological Therapy on Physicians' Narratives and Interrogations: The Case of General Paralysis of the Insane and Malaria Fever Therapy, 1910–1950," *Bulletin of the History of Medicine* 70, no. 4 (1996): 577–608. Braslow was the first to make the point about the effect of malaria fever treatment on clinicians' attitudes toward their GPI patients. Paul de Kruif was an American microbiologist and science popularizer of Dutch descent, best known for his 1926 heroic history of microbiology, *Microbe Hunters*.

81. For more information, see Matthew Gambino, "Fevered Decisions: Race, Ethics, and Clinical Vulnerability in the Malarial Treatment of Neurosyphilis, 1922–1953," *Hastings Center Report* 45, no. 4 (2015): 39–50.

82. George Jahn, "Investigator: Orphans Injected with Malaria Bug," Associated Press, May 4, 2014.

83. Clare Chapman, "Austrians Stunned by Nobel Prize-Winner's Nazi Ideology," *Scotland on Sunday*, January 25, 2004.

84. Edward Shorter and David Healy, *Shock Therapy: A History of Electroconvulsive Treatment in Mental Illness* (New Brunswick, NJ: Rutgers University Press, 2007), p. 11.

85. Shorter and Healy, *Shock Therapy*, p. 11.

86. Sakel also later claimed to have first become aware of insulin's therapeutic potential while directing a clinic for addicts; he then claimed to have carefully tested the treatment on animals; and he finally claimed to have subsequently developed the optimal method for using it on schizophrenic patients. Sakel's

self-serving narratives have been widely disseminated, but historians Edward Shorter and David Healy have corrected the record. See Shorter and Healy, *Shock Therapy,* pp. 14–15.

87. Kingsley Jones, "Insulin Coma Therapy in Schizophrenia," *Journal of the Royal Society of Medicine* 93, no. 3 (2000): 147–49.

88. Joseph Wortis, "Fragments of a Freudian Analysis," *American Journal of Orthopsychiatry* 10, no. 4 (October 1940): 843–49.

89. "Shock Therapy for the Insane Called a Success: Commission Asks Insulin Treatment Be Available in All State Hospitals," *New York Herald Tribune,* August 27, 1944; John J. O'Neill, "Insane Now Get Chance to Live Life Over Again: Insulin Shock Rolls Back Time. . . . ," *New York Herald Tribune,* May 15, 1937; "Dementia Praecox Curbed by Insulin: Psychiatrists Report Shock Produced by Drug Has Aided Many Insane," *New York Times,* January 13, 1937; "Insulin Rocks the Foundations of Reason and Yet Seems to Restore Sanity in Many Cases," *Los Angeles Times,* March 24, 1940; and "Thousands of 'Living Dead' May Live Again Through 'Insulin Shock,'" *Austin American,* October 10, 1937.

90. Joseph Wortis, "45. Early Experiences with Sakel's Hypoglycemic Insulin Treatment of the Psychoses in America," *American Journal of Psychiatry* 94, no. 6S (1938): 307–8. In fact, we do see some early criticism of the treatment, particularly from psychoanalytically oriented clinicians. One 1940 review of a book Sakel had written about the treatment suggested that interest in insulin coma therapy was rapidly waning, as clinicians discovered its grave limitations. The author then smugly told his colleagues that the real interest of Sakel's book was as "a manifestation of the age-long reaction formation against anxiety, a reaction which insists that everything is physical and everything else is mortal sin." G. Z., review of *The Pharmacological Shock Treatment of Schizophrenia* by Manfred Sakel, *Psychoanalytic Quarterly* 9 (1940): 419–20.

91. Benjamin Malzberg, "Outcome of Insulin Treatment of One Thousand Patients with Dementia Praecox," *Psychiatric Quarterly* 12, no. 3 (1938): 528–53.

92. Quoted in Eric Cunningham Dax, "Modern Mental Treatment 1947," p. 13, www.wakefieldasylum.co.uk/management-and-treatment/modern-mental-treatment-1947/.

93. Deborah Blythe Doroshow, "Performing a Cure for Schizophrenia: Insulin Coma Therapy on the Wards," *Journal of the History of Medicine and Allied Sciences* 62, no. 2 (April 1, 2007): 213–43.

94. Harold Bourne, "Insulin Coma in Decline," *American Journal of Psychiatry* 114, no. 11 (May 1, 1958): 1015–17; and Harold Bourne, "The Insulin Myth," *Lancet* 2 (1953): 964–68.

95. J. Nyirö and A. Jablonsky, "Einige Daten zur Prognose der Epilepsie, mit besonderer Rucksicht auf die Konstitution," *Psychiatrische Neurologische Wochenschrift* 31 (1929): 547–49.

96. Max Fink, "Meduna and the Origins of Convulsive Therapy," *American Journal of Psychiatry* 141, no. 9 (September 1984): 1034–41, doi.org/10.1176/ajp.141.9.1034.

97. Fink, "Meduna and Origins of Convulsive Therapy."

98. Louis H. Cohen, "The Early Effects of Metrazol Therapy in Chronic Psychotic

Over-Activity," *American Journal of Psychiatry* 95, no. 2 (September 1, 1938): 327–33, esp. 327.

99. Hunter Gillies and E. F. J. Dunlop, "Convulsion Therapy in Schizophrenia," *Lancet* 231, no. 5990 (June 18, 1938): 1418.

100. Quoted in Robert Whitaker, *Mad in America: Bad Science, Bad Medicine, and the Enduring Mistreatment of the Mentally Ill* (Cambridge MA: Perseus, 2002).

101. Alessandro Aruta, "Shocking Waves at the Museum: The Bini-Cerletti Electro-Shock Apparatus," *Medical History* 55, no. 3 (July 2011): 407–12.

102. Ugo Cerletti, "Electroshock Therapy," in *The Great Physiodynamic Therapies in Psychiatry*, ed. Arthur M. Sackler et al. (New York: Hoeber-Harper, 1956), pp. 91–120, esp. 92.

103. Ferdinando Accornero, "An Eyewitness Account of the Discovery of Electro-shock," *Convulsive Therapy* 4, no. 1 (1988): 44.

104. Accornero, "Eyewitness Account of Discovery."

105. Quoted in Elliot Valenstein, *Great and Desperate Cures: The Rise and Decline of Psychosurgery and Other Radical Treatments for Mental Illness* (New York: Perseus, 1987), p. 51. The variation between the accounts is significant. The Italian historian Roberta Passione has suggested that they are best read as quasi-novels rather than used as documentary reports of what really happened during that first critical experiment. It seems to be untrue, for example, that Cerletti actually made any momentous declaration at the end of the first experiment. Other reports omit the fact that the researchers put this patient through at least three failed attempts before finally achieving the convulsive state they wanted. See Roberta Passione, *Il Romanzo dell'elettroshock* (Reggio Emilia: Aliberti, 2007).

106. There was some evidence that it was helpful for patients suffering specifically from the abnormal movement disorder known as catatonia, widely supposed to be a symptom or subtype of schizophrenia.

107. This account is taken from "Brain Surgery Feat Arouses Sharp Debate: Dr. Walter Freeman's Report Creates Stir at Medical Convention," *Baltimore Sun*, November 21, 1936.

108. "Brain Surgery Feat Arouses Sharp Debate."

109. Jack D. Pressman, *Last Resort: Psychosurgery and the Limits of Medicine* (New York: Cambridge University Press, 2002).

110. See Walter Freeman and James W. Watts, "Prefrontal Lobotomy in the Treatment of Mental Disorders," *Southern Medical Journal* 30, no. 1 (1937): 23–31.

111. Hugh Levinson, "The Strange and Curious History of Lobotomy," *BBC News Magazine*, November 8, 2011, www.bbc.com/news/magazine-15629160.

112. For more, see Gretchen J. Diefenbach et al., "Portrayal of Lobotomy in the Popular Press: 1935–1960," *Journal of the History of the Neurosciences* 8, no. 1 (April 1, 1999): 60–69.

113. Here is a fuller list of newspaper reports: "Abnormal Worry Is Reported Relieved by Brain Operation: Southern Medical Group Hears George Washington Physicians Describe Success of Nerve Surgery in Aiding Sufferers from Anxiety," *Washington Post*, November 21, 1936; John J. O. Neill, "In the Realm of Science: Experiments Indicate Forebrain Is Civilizing Center of Man's Body: Judgment Seat Is Man's Guide to Decisions Area Appears to Assume Role of Court of Rea-

son for Other Parts of Brain," *New York Herald Tribune*, August 27, 1939; "Brain Surgery Urged as Aid in Mental Illness: Fulton of Yale Would Limit Operations to Specific Parts Affecting Emotions," *New York Herald Tribune*, January 14, 1951; "'Hopelessly' Insane Are Released with Action Part of Brain Out," *New York Herald Tribune*, January 8, 1947; "Brain Surgery Spares Cancer Patients Pain," *Austin Statesman*, April 19, 1947; "Right Up in Front: Human Personality's Brain Seat Discovered," *Los Angeles Times*, September 9, 1949; "Worry Stopped by Operation on Brain Lobe: Southern Medical Group Hears of New Surgery for Mental Conditions. Ideas Stay, 'Drive' Goes," *New York Herald Tribune*, November 21, 1936, p. 10; Stephen J. McDonouch, "Sever 'Worry Nerves' of Brain, Restore Insane to Normal," *Toronto Globe and Mail*, June 13, 1941; Thomas R. Henry, "Using Soul Surgery to Combat Worry, Fear," *Baltimore Sun*, June 23, 1940; James Hague, "Doctors Tell Lobotomy's Aftermath," *Washington Post*, November 7, 1951; and William L. Laurence, "Surgery Used on the Soul-Sick Relief of Obsessions Is Reported: New Brain Technique Is Said to Have Aided 65% of the Mentally Ill Persons on Whom It Was Tried as Last Resort, but Some Leading Neurologists Are Highly Skeptical of It," *New York Times*, June 7, 1937.

114. Waldemar Kaempffert, "Turning the Mind Inside Out," *Saturday Evening Post*, May 24, 1941, pp. 18–19, 69, 71–72, 74, esp. 18.

115. Kaempffert, "Turning the Mind Inside Out," p. 74.

116. "Swiss and Portuguese Doctors Split 1949 Nobel Medical Prize," *New York Herald Tribune*, October 28, 1949.

117. Doris Kearns Goodwin, *The Fitzgeralds and the Kennedys* (New York: Macmillan, 1991), p. 643.

118. Walter Freeman and James W. Watts, "Prefrontal Lobotomy," *American Journal of Psychiatry* 101, no. 6 (May 1, 1945): 739–48.

119. In a 2005 documentary, *My Lobotomy*, Sallie Ionesco (who was then eighty-eight years old) and her daughter, Angelene Forester, recalled their memories of the procedure:

SALLIE ELLEN IONESCO: He was just a great man. That's all I can say.
FORESTER: Do you remember what his face looked like mama?
IONESCO: I don't remember.
FORESTER: Do you remember his office?
IONESCO: I don't remember that either. I don't remember nothing else, and I'm very tired.
FORESTER: Do you want to go lie down? I remember sitting on his lap and his beard was pointed and it was very soft. As a child you kind of see into people's souls and he was good—at least then. I don't know what happened after that. I wish he hadn't gotten quite so out of hand.

My Lobotomy, co-produced by Howard Dully, Priya Kochhar, and Dave Isay (November, 2005), transcript, at https://exchange.prx.org/pieces/7480/transcripts/7480.

120. For reports heralding this developments, see "Asylum Frees 'Hopeless' Insane with Action Part of Brain Out," *New York Herald Tribune*, January 8, 1947.

121. "Prefrontal Lobotomy: The Problem of Schizophrenia," *American Journal of Psychiatry* 101.6 (1945): 739–48, esp. 748.

122. Glenn Frankel, "D.C. Neurosurgeon Pioneered 'Operation Icepick' Technique," *Washington Post*, April 7, 1980.

123. Glenn Frankel, "Psychosurgery's Effects Still Linger," *Washington Post*, April 6, 1980.

124. Katherine A. Kean, "Spencer State Hospital," *Times Record/Roane County Reporter*, July 6, 1989, West Virginia Archives and History, www.wvculture .org/history/government/spencer03.html.

Chapter 3: A Fragile Freudian Triumph

1. Norman Dain, *Clifford W. Beers: Advocate for the Insane* (Pittsburgh: University of Pittsburgh Press, 1980).

2. Christina Cogdell, *Eugenic Design: Streamlining America in the 1930s* (Philadelphia: University of Pennsylvania Press, 2010), p. 157.

3. For an introduction to the contested and quarrelsome literature on the Progressive Era, see Adam Quinn, "Reforming History: Contemporary Scholarship on the Progressive Era," Society for Historians of the Gilded Age and Progressive Era (H-SHGAPE), H-Net (forum), May 9, 2017, https://networks.h-net .org/node/20317/discussions/179222/reforming-history-contemporary -scholarship-progressive-era, and Quinn's generous bibliography. For more on the complex roles of both race and racism in the suffrage movement, see Brent Staples, "How the Suffrage Movement Betrayed Black Women," *New York Times*, July 28, 2018, https://www.nytimes.com/2018/07/28/opinion/sunday/ suffrage-movement-racism-black-women.html; and Rosalyn Terborg-Penn, *African American Women in the Struggle for the Vote, 1850–1920* (Bloomington: Indiana University Press, 1998).

4. C. Macfie Campbell, "The Mental Health of the Community and the Work of the Psychiatric Dispensary," *Mental Hygiene* 1 (1917): 572–84, esp. 572.

5. Johannes Coenraad Pols, *Managing the Mind: The Culture of American Mental Hygiene, 1910–1950*, Ph.D. diss., University of Pennsylvania, 1997, p. 103.

6. "Childhood: The Golden Period for Mental Hygiene," *Mental Hygiene* 4 (April 1920): 266–67.

7. The best analysis is Sol Cohen, "The Mental Hygiene Movement, the Development of Personality and the School: The Medicalization of American Education," *History of Education Quarterly* 23, no. 2 (Summer 1983) (1983): 123–49.

8. Harry Nathaniel Rivlin, *Educating for Adjustment. The Classroom Applications of Mental Hygiene* (Oxford, UK: Appleton-Century, 1936); Lawrence Augustus Averill, *Mental Hygiene for the Classroom Teacher* (Oxford, UK: Pitman, 1939).

9. F. McKinney, "An Outline of a Series of Lectures on Mental Hygiene for College Freshmen," *Journal of Abnormal and Social Psychology* 29, no. 3 (1934): 276–86.

10. See Campbell, "Mental Health of the Community," p. 572. In 1914 Campbell offered a more measured assessment: C. Macfie Campbell, "The Role of the Psychiatric Dispensary: A Review of the First Year's Work of the Dispensary of the Phipps Psychiatric Clinic," *American Journal of Psychiatry* 71, no. 3 (January 1, 1915): 439–57. For more on the Phipps Clinic, see S. D. Lamb, *Pathologist of the Mind: Adolf Meyer and the Origins of American Psychiatry* (Baltimore: Johns Hopkins University Press, 2014).

11. Southard even collaborated with a social worker, Mary C. Jarrett, on what became a monumental study of the social origins of mental disorder. See Elmer E. Southard and Mary C. Jarrett, *The Kingdom of Evils: Psychiatric Social Work Presented in One Hundred Case Histories, Together with a Classification of Social Divisions of Evil* (New York: Macmillan, 1922). For a comprehensive history of the Boston Psychopathic Hospital and its impact, see Elizabeth Lunbeck, *The Psychiatric Persuasion: Knowledge, Gender, and Power in Modern America* (Princeton, NJ: Princeton University Press, 1995).

12. "Psychopathic Clinic at Sing Sing Clinic," *Bulletin of the Rockefeller Foundation*, 1916, p. 15.

13. For more on how these outpatient clinics worked, see E. S. Rademacher, "A Day in a Mental Hygiene Clinic," *Yale Journal of Biology and Medicine* 2 no. 6 (1930): 443–50.

14. George S. Stevenson and Geddes Smith, *Child Guidance Clinics: A Quarter Century of Development* (New York: Commonwealth Fund, 1934), reviewed in *Psychoanalytic Review* 22, no. 4 (1935): 479–80.

15. Kathleen W. Jones, *Taming the Troublesome Child: American Families, Child Guidance, and the Limits of Psychiatric Authority* (Cambridge, MA: Harvard University Press, 1999).

16. On this concept, see the important essay by Jacquelyn Dowd Hall, "The Long Civil Rights Movement and the Political Uses of the Past," *Journal of American History* 91, no. 4 (2005): 1233–63.

17. Gerald Markowitz and David Rosner, *Children, Race, and Power: Kenneth and Mamie Clark's Northside Center* (New York: Routledge, 2013). See also Ed Edwin, "Interview of Dr. Mamie Clark, May 25, 1976," *Social and Cultural History: Letters and Diaries Online*, Alexander Street Press, https://asp6new alexanderstreet.com/ladd/ladd.help.aspx?dorpID=1000605705.

18. S. I. Hayakawa, "Second Thoughts," *Chicago Defender*, January 11, 1947, national ed., p. 15. For more on the *Chicago Defender*'s critical role as an activist paper during the Jim Crow era in the United States, see Ethan Michaeli, *The Defender: How the Legendary Black Newspaper Changed America* (Boston: Houghton Mifflin Harcourt, 2016).

19. On Northside, see Markowitz and Rosner. On the Lafargue Clinic, see Gabriel N. Mendes, *Under the Strain of Color: Harlem's Lafargue Clinic and the Promise of an Antiracist Psychiatry* (Ithaca, NY: Cornell University Press, 2015). See also Dennis Doyle, *Psychiatry and Racial Liberalism in Harlem, 1936–1968* (Rochester, NY: University of Rochester Press, 2016).

20. Many were less influenced by Freud's writings directly than by new psychoanalytic theories associated with ego psychology and object relations theory. One particularly influential text for this community was the British psychoanalyst J. M. Flugel's *The Psychoanalytic Study of the Family* (London: Hogarth Press, 1921). See Kathleen Jones, "'Mother Made Me Do It': Mother-Blaming and the Women of Child Guidance," in *"Bad" Mothers: The Politics of Blame in Twentieth-Century America*, ed. Molly Ladd-Taylor and Lauri Umansky (New York: NYU Press, 1998), pp. 99–124, esp. 101. For more on the history of the child guidance movement, see Kathleen W. Jones, *Taming the Troublesome Child: American Families, Child Guidance, and the Limits of Psychiatric Authority* (Cambridge, MA: Harvard University Press, 1999).

21. Frankwood E. Williams and International Congress for Mental Hygiene, eds., *Proceedings of the First International Congress on Mental Hygiene, Held at Washington, D.C., U.S.A., May 5th to 10th, 1930* (New York: American Foundation for Mental Hygiene,1932).
22. Quoted in Edward J. K. Gitre, "The Great Escape: World War II, Neo-Freudianism, and the Origins of U.S. Psychocultural Analysis," *Journal of the History of the Behavioral Sciences* 47, no. 1 (2011): 18–43.
23. For a thoughtful discussion, see Stephen A. Mitchell and Adrienne Harris, "What's American About American Psychoanalysis?" *Psychoanalytic Dialogues* 14, no. 2 (2004): 165–91.
24. Gregory Zilboorg, *A History of Medical Psychology* (New York: Norton, 1941), pp. 486–87.
25. Hans Pols and Stephanie Oak, "War and Military Mental Health," *American Journal of Public Health* 97, no. 12 (December 2007): 2132–42.
26. Ellen Herman, *The Romance of American Psychology: Political Culture in the Age of Experts* (Berkeley: University of California Press, 1995).
27. Nathan G. Hale, Jr., *The Rise and Crisis of Psychoanalysis in the United States: Freud and the Americans, 1917–1985* (New York: Oxford University Press, 1995), pp. 191, 200.
28. Roy R. Grinker and John P. Spiegel, *War Neuroses* (Philadelphia: Blakiston, 1945), p. 82, quoted in Hans Pols and Stephanie Oak, "War and Military Mental Health," *American Journal of Public Health* 97, no. 12 (December 2007): 2132–42.
29. Michael Kernan, "1981 Review of 'Let There Be Light': War Casualty," *Washington Post*, May 24, 2012.
30. For another perspective on why the film might have been banned, see Richard Ledes, "'Let There Be Light': John Huston's Film and the Concept of Trauma in the United States After WWII," paper delivered to the Après-Coup Psychoanalytic Association, 1998, 1–24.
31. Pols and Oak, "War and Military Mental Health."
32. Andrew Scull, "The Mental Health Sector and the Social Sciences in Post–World War II USA," pts. 1 and 2, *History of Psychiatry* 22, no. 1 (2011): 3–19, and no. 3 (2011): 268–84.
33. Ben Shephard, *A War of Nerves: Soldiers and Psychiatrists in the Twentieth Century* (Cambridge, MA: Harvard University Press, 2001), p. 32; see also Scull, "Mental Health Sector and Social Sciences," pt. 1.
34. "The American Psychiatric Association: Proceedings of the One Hundred and Fourth Annual Meeting. Hotel Statler, Washington, D.C., May 17–20, 1948," *American Journal of Psychiatry* 105, no. 11 (May 1, 1949): 851–68, esp. 851. For a further discussion, see Rebecca Jo Plant, "William Menninger and American Psychoanalysis, 1946–48," *History of Psychiatry* 16, no. 2 (June 1, 2005): 181–202.
35. José Bertolote, "The Roots of the Concept of Mental Health," *World Psychiatry* 7, no. 2 (June 2008): 113–16.
36. Lawrence Davidson, "The Strange Disappearance of Adolf Meyer," *Orthomolecular Psychiatry* 9, no. 2 (1980): 135–43.
37. Albert Deutsch, *The Story of GAP. Relating to the Origins, Goals, and Activities of a Unique Medical Organization . . .* (New York: Group for the Advancement of Psychiatry, 1959), p. 4.

38. "Shock Therapy," Report No. 1, Group for the Advancement of Psychiatry, September 15, 1947, http://gap-dev.s3.amazonaws.com/documents/assets/000/000/150/original/reports_shock_therapy9151.pdf?1429591297.

39. "Research on Prefrontal Lobotomy," Report No. 6, Group for the Advancement of Psychiatry, June 1948, http://gap-dev.s3.amazonaws.com/documents/assets/000/000/155/original/reports_researchon_prefronta.pdf?1429591321.

40. Gerald N. Grob, *The Mad Among Us: A History of the Care of America's Mentally Ill* (New York: Free Press, 1994).

41. Clyde H. Ward, "Psychiatric Training in University Centers," *American Journal of Psychiatry* 3 (1954): 123–31, esp. 123.

42. Hale, *Rise and Crisis of Psychoanalysis*, pp. 211–12.

43. See, for example, Robert E. L. Faris and H. Warren Dunham, *Mental Disorders in Urban Areas: An Ecological Study of Schizophrenia and Other Psychoses* (Chicago: University of Chicago Press, 1939); H. Warren Dunham, "Current Status of Ecological Research in Mental Disorders," *Social Forces* 25 (March 1947): 321–26; August B. Hollingshead and Frederick C. Redlich, *Social Class and Mental Illness: A Community Study* (New York: Wiley, 1958); and Leo Srole et al., *Mental Health in the Metropolis: The Midtown Manhattan Study* (New York: McGraw-Hill, 1962). For a nice summary of this moment, see Matthew Smith, "The Art of Medicine. An Ounce of Prevention," *Lancet* 386 (August 1, 2015): 424–25.

44. Gene Martin Lyons, *The Uneasy Partnership* (New York: Russell Sage Foundation, 1969), p. 276.

45. Portions of this section are adapted from Anne Harrington, "Mother Love and Mental Illness: An Emotional History," *Osiris* 31, no. 1 (2016): 94–115.

46. Helene Deutsch, *The Psychology of Women: A Psychoanalytic Interpretation*, vol. 2, *Motherhood* (New York: Grune and Stratton, 1945), p. 20, and Karen Horney, "Maternal Conflicts" (1933), reprinted in Horney, *Feminine Psychology*, ed. Harold Kelman (New York: Norton, 1967), pp. 175–81.

47. Deutsch, *Psychology of Women*, p. v.

48. Janet Sayers, *Mothers of Psychoanalysis: Helene Deutsch, Karen Horney, Anna Freud, Melanie Klein*, rev. ed. (New York: Norton, 1993).

49. Quoted in Mari Jo Buhle, *Feminism and Its Discontents: A Century of Struggle with Psychoanalysis* (Cambridge, MA: Harvard University Press, 2009), p. 135.

50. Inge Pretorius, "The Hampstead War Nurseries and the Origins of the Anna Freud Centre," August 12, 2010, www.annafreud.org/war_nurseries.htm.

51. Rene A. Spitz, "The Role of Ecological Factors in Emotional Development in Infancy," Child Development 20, no. 3 (September 1, 1949): 145–55.

52. John Bowlby, *Maternal Care and Mental Health* (Geneva: World Health Organization, 1951).

53. David M. Levy, *Maternal Overprotection* (New York: Columbia University Press, 1943).

54. C. H. Rogerson, "The Psychological Factors in Asthma-Prurigo," *QJM: An International Journal of Medicine* 6, no. 4 (October 1, 1937): 367–94.

55. Martha Lewenberg, "IV. Marital Disharmony as a Factor in the Etiology of Maternal Over-protection," *Smith College Studies in Social Work* 2, no. 3 (1932): 224–36.

56. "Mother's Perplexing Problems: How Does One Stop Being Over-Protective?" *Boston Globe*, December 8, 1940.

57. Edward Adam Strecker, *Their Mothers' Sons: The Psychiatrist Examines an American Problem...* (Philadelphia: Lippincott, 1946).

58. John L. Zimmerman, review of *Their Mothers' Sons*, in *Military Affairs* 11, no. 3 (Autumn 1947): 191–92.

59. Amram Scheinfeld, "Are American Moms a Menace?" *Ladies' Home Journal* (November, 1945), reprinted in *Women's Magazines, 1940–1960: Gender Roles and the Popular Press*, ed. Nancy Walker (Boston: Bedford/St. Martin's, 1998), pp. 108–14.

60. Rebecca Jo Plant, *Mom: The Transformation of Motherhood in Modern America* (Chicago: University of Chicago Press, 2010).

61. Abram Kardiner and Lionel Ovesey, *The Mark of Oppression* (New York: Norton, 1951).

62. Jack Dworin and Oakley Wyant, "Authoritarian Patterns in the Mothers of Schizophrenics," *Journal of Clinical Psychology* 13, no. 4 (October 1957): 332–38.

63. Quoted in Ann-Louise S. Silver, *Psychoanalysis and Psychosis* (New York: International Universities Press, 1989), p. 28.

64. Tellingly, Freud had actually cautioned against drawing that conclusion. Psychotic patients were too disconnected from reality, he said, to be able to establish a viable therapeutic relationship with a clinician. See Sigmund Freud, "On Narcissism" (1914), in Peter Fonagy, Ethel Spector Person, and Joseph Sandler, eds., *Freud's "On Narcissism": An Introduction* (London: Karnac Books, 2012).

65. Marguerite Sechehaye, *Symbolic Realization: A New Method of Psychotherapy Applied to a Case of Schizophrenia* (New York: International Universities Press, 1951), p. 51; and Marguerite Sechehaye, *Autobiography of a Schizophrenic Girl* (New York: Grune and Stratton, 1951), where the patient describes this incident with the apples from her own perspective. Sechehaye is quoted in Annie G. Rogers, "Marguerite Sechehaye and Renee: A Feminist Reading of Two Accounts of a Treatment," *International Journal of Qualitative Studies in Education* 5, no. 3 (1992): 245–51.

66. Edith Weigert, "In Memoriam, Frieda Fromm-Reichmann, 1889–1957," *Psychiatry* 21 (February 1958): 91–95, esp. 94.

67. Quoted in Edward Shorter, *The Health Century* (New York: Doubleday, 1987), p. 304.

68. Henri Laborit and P. Huguenard, "L'hibernation artificielle par moyens pharmacodynamiques et physiques," *La Presse médicale* 59, no. 64 (October 13, 1951): 1326–29.

69. Thomas A. Ban, "Fifty Years Chlorpromazine: A Historical Perspective," *Neuropsychiatric Disease and Treatment* 3, no. 4 (August 2007): 495–500.

70. J. Delay, P. Deniker, and J. M. Harl, "Traitement des états d'excitation et d'agitation par une méthode médicamenteuse dérivée de l'hibernothérapie," *Annales médico-psychologiques, revue psychiatrique* 110 (July 1952): 267–73.

71. A. Caldwell, "History of Psychopharmacology," in *Principles of Psychopharmacology*, ed. William Gilbert Clark, J. Del Giudice, and Gary C. Aden (New York: Academic Press, 1978), p. 30.

72. Elliot Valenstein has written that even before Laborit's work, some workers for Rhône-Poulenc had independently observed that chlorpromazine had a variety of physiological properties with possible relevance for psychiatry, including the

abilities to provide relief from depression and anxiety and to mute the emotional salience of hallucinations and delusional thoughts. Most of these early observations, Valenstein noted, were buried in the internal reports of the company. Elliot S. Valenstein, *Blaming the Brain: The Truth About Drugs and Mental Health* (New York: Free Press, 1998), p. 22.

73. Heinz E. Lehmann, interview by William E. Bunney, Jr., in *Recollections of the History of Psychopharmacology through Interviews Conducted by William E. Bunney, Jr.* (Risskov, Denmark: International Network for the History of Neuropsychopharmacology, 1994).

74. Heinz E. Lehmann and Gorman E. Hanrahan, "Chlorpromazine: New Inhibiting Agent for Psychomotor Excitement and Manic States," *AMA Archives of Neurology and Psychiatry* 71, no. 2 (1954): 227–37.

75. Nathan Kline, "Discussion of Pharmacologic Treatment of Schizophrenics," in *Psychopharmacology Frontiers: Proceedings of the Psychopharmacology Symposium*, ed. Nathan S. Kline (Boston: Little, Brown, 1959), p. 426.

76. See for example Mortimer Ostow and Nathan S. Kline, "The Psychic Action of Reserpine and Chlorpromazine," in *Psychopharmacology Frontiers*, ed. Kline, pp. 45–58.

77. Thorazine advertisement, *Mental Hospitals* 7, no. 8 (1956): 2.

78. *The Year in Review: Annual Report Smith, Kline & French Laboratories, 1961* (Philadelphia: Smith, Kline & French Laboratories, 1962).

79. F. M. Berger, "The Mode of Action of Myanesin," *British Journal of Pharmacology* 2, no. 4 (1947): 241–50.

80. Frank Berger, interview by Thomas Ban, April 6, 1999, in *Recollections of the History of Neuropharmacology Through Interviews Conducted by Thomas A. Ban*, ed. Peter R. Martin (Córdoba, Argentina: International Network for the History of Neuropsychopharmacology 2014), p. 80.

81. Jonathan Michel Metzl, *Prozac on the Couch: Prescribing Gender in the Era of Wonder Drugs* (Durham, NC: Duke University Press, 2003), p. 73.

82. Andrea Tone, *The Age of Anxiety: A History of America's Turbulent Affair with Tranquilizers* (New York: Basic Books, 2008).

83. "Happiness by Prescription," *Time*, March 11, 1957, p. 59.

84. "Domestic Tranquility," *New Republic*, June 24, 1957, pp. 5–6, esp. 5.

85. For more on this argument, see Jonathan M. Metzl, "'Mother's Little Helper': The Crisis of Psychoanalysis and the Miltown Resolution," *Gender and History* 15, no. 2 (2003): 240–67.

Chapter 4: Crisis and Revolt

1. Ellen Herman, *The Romance of American Psychology: Political Culture in the Age of Experts* (Berkeley: University of California Press, 1995), pp. 113–18.

2. Albert J. Glass, "Military Psychiatry and Changing Systems of Mental Health Care," *Journal of Psychiatric Research* 8 (1971): 499–512.

3. J. T. English, "Early Models of Community Mental Health Programs: The Vision of Robert Felix and the Example of Alan Kraft," *Psychiatric Quarterly* 62, no. 3 (1991): 257–65.

4. Quoted in D. L. Cutler and C. Huffine, "Heroes in Community Psychiatry: Gerald Caplan," *Community Mental Health Journal* 40, no. 3 (June 2004): 193.

5. Markam Bryant, "The Thirteen Thousand," *Antioch Review* 7, no. 1 (1947): 83–98.
6. Albert Q. Maisel, "Bedlam 1946: Most US Mental Hospitals Are a Shame and a Disgrace," *Life* 20, no. 18 (1946): 102–18.
7. Bryant, "Thirteen Thousand."
8. Albert Deutsch, *The Shame of the States* (New York: Harcourt, Brace, 1948).
9. John K. Wing, "Institutionalism in Mental Hospitals," *British Journal of Clinical Psychology* 1, no. 1 (1962): 38–51; John K. Wing and George W. Brown, *Institutionalism and Schizophrenia* (Cambridge, UK: Cambridge University Press, 1970).
10. Addison M. Duval and Douglas Goldman, "The New Drugs (Chlorpromazine & Reserpine): Administrative Aspects," *Mental Hospitals* (February 1956), reprinted in *Psychiatric Services* 51, no. 3 (March 1, 2000): 327–31. In a sign of the changing times brought about by deinstitutionalization, by 1966 the journal *Mental Hospitals* had changed its name to *Hospital and Community Psychiatry*.
11. This view is widespread in the literature, in part because the psychiatric leadership promoted it for many decades. For a recent example, see Henry A Nasrallah, "A Saga of Psychiatric Serendipities," *Current Psychiatry* 12, no. 9 (September 1, 2013): 7.
12. Joni Lee Pow et al., "Deinstitutionalization of American Public Hospitals for the Mentally Ill Before and After the Introduction of Antipsychotic Medications," *Harvard Review of Psychiatry* 23, no. 3 (June 2015): 176–87.
13. For a typical example of testimony to this effect, see E. Fuller Torrey, *American Psychosis: How the Federal Government Destroyed the Mental Illness Treatment System* (New York: Oxford University Press, 2013), p. 33.
14. "Excerpts from the Report of the Joint Commission on Mental Illness and Health," *Journal of Psychosocial Nursing and Mental Health Services* 1, no. 4 (July 1, 1963): 336–45.
15. John F. Kennedy, "Message from the President of the United States Relative to Mental Illness and Mental Retardation," *American Journal of Psychiatry* 120, no. 8 (1964): 729–37; and John F. Kennedy, "Mental Illness and Mental Retardation: Message from the President of the United States Relative to Mental Illness and Mental Retardation," *American Psychologist* 18, no. 6 (1963): 280.
16. Act of October 31, 1963 ("Mental Retardation Facilities and Community Health Centers Construction Act of 1963"), Public Law 88-164, 77 STAT 282, General Records of the United States Government, 1778–2006: Enrolled Acts and Resolutions of Congress, 1789–2011, National Archives and Records Administration, Office of the Federal Register, https://catalog.archives.gov/id/299883.
17. "Kennedy's Vision for Mental Health Never Realized," *Epoch Times*, 2013.
18. David A. Rochefort, "Origins of the 'Third Psychiatric Revolution': The Community Mental Health Centers Act of 1963," *Journal of Health Politics Policy and Law* 9, no. 1 (April 1, 1984): 1–30.
19. Paul R. Friedman, "The Mentally Handicapped Citizen and Institutional Labor," *Harvard Law Review* (1974): 567–87.
20. *Deinstitutionalization, Mental Illness, and Medications*, Hearing before the Committee on Finance, U.S. Senate, 103rd Congress, 2nd sess, May 10, 1994; H. Richard Lamb and Leona L. Bachrach, "Some Perspectives on Deinstitutionalization," *Psychiatric Services* 52, no. 8 (August 1, 2001): 1039–45; Gerald N. Grob, "Historical Origins of Deinstitutionalization," *New Directions for Men-*

tal Health Services 17 (1983): 15–29; and Ann Braden Johnson, *Out of Bedlam: The Truth About Deinstitutionalization* (New York: Basic Books, 1992).

21. The historian Gerald Grob called particular attention to this point in a review of Edward Shorter's 1997 *A History of Psychiatry: From the Era of the Asylum to the Age of Prozac,* in *Bulletin of the History of Medicine* 72, no 1 (Spring 1998): 153–55.

22. F. J. Ayd, Jr., "A Survey of Drug-Induced Extrapyramidal Reactions," *JAMA* 175 (1961): 1054–60.

23. Oryx Cohen, *Psychiatric Survivor Oral Histories: Implications for Contemporary Mental Health Policy* (Amherst: Center for Public Policy and Administration, University of Massachusetts, 2001), p. 29.

24. Bongos, Bass & Bob, "The Thorazine Shuffle" (2009), www.youtube.com/wat ch?v=1E6ywsBBSj0&feature=youtube_gdata_player.

25. For more, see Anne E. Parsons, *From Asylum to Prison: Deinstitutionalization and the Rise of Mass Incarceration After 1945* (Chapel Hill: University of North Carolina Press, 2018). A further important though as yet unpublished contribution is Antonia Hylton, "Carceral Continuities: Tracing Black Bodies from the Asylum to the Penal State," undergraduate senior thesis, March 2015, Harvard College Libraries, accession 2017.556, box 1.

26. See the acknowledgement in Thomas J. Scheff, "The Societal Reaction to Deviance: Ascriptive Elements in the Psychiatric Screening of Mental Patients in a Midwestern State," *Social Problems* 11, no. 4 (Spring 1964), pp. 401–13, esp. 401n.

27. Thomas J. Scheff, *Being Mentally Ill: A Sociological Theory* (New Brunswick, NJ: Transaction Publishers, 1970).

28. Erving Goffman, *Asylums: Essays on the Social Situation of Mental Patients and Other Inmates* (1960; reprinted London: Routledge, 2017). The historian Matthew Gambino has recently suggested that the situation for patients at St. Elizabeths in these years was not as dire and oppressive as Goffman had so famously suggested: "Group therapy, psychodrama, art and dance therapy, patient newspapers, and patient self-government—each of which debuted at the hospital in the 1940s and 1950s—provided novel opportunities for men and women to make themselves heard and to take their fate into their own hands. While these initiatives did not reach all of the patients at St. Elizabeths, surviving documentation suggests that those who participated found their involvement rewarding and empowering," Matthew Gambino, "Erving Goffman's Asylums and Institutional Culture in the Mid-Twentieth-Century United States," *Harvard Review of Psychiatry* 21, no. 1 (February 2013): 52–57.

29. Michel Foucault, *Madness and Civilization: A History of Insanity in the Age of Reason* (London: Tavistock, 1961).

30. Ronald D. Laing, *The Divided Self: A Study of Sanity and Madness* (London: Penguin, 1960), p. 39.

31. Ronald D. Laing and Aaron Esterson, *Sanity, Madness and the Family* (1964; reprinted London: Taylor & Francis, 2016).

32. Ronald D. Laing, *The Politics of Experience and the Bird of Paradise* (London: Penguin, 1967).

33. Laing, *Politics of Experience*, p. 65.

34. Laing, *Politics of Experience*, p. 129.

35. Thomas S. Szasz, *The Myth of Mental Illness: Foundations of a Theory of Personal Conduct*, rev. ed. (New York: Harper & Row, 1974).

36. Thomas S. Szasz, *Psychiatric Justice* (Syracuse, NY: Syracuse University Press, 1965).

37. Thomas S. Szasz, *Law, Liberty, and Psychiatry: An Inquiry Into the Social Uses of Mental Health Practices* (Syracuse, NY: Syracuse University Press, 1963), p. 223.

38. Henry Davidson, "The New War on Psychiatry" (response to a paper by Thomas Szasz), *American Journal of Psychiatry* 121, no. 6 (December 1964): 528–34. For Szasz's take on this event, see Thomas Szasz, "Reply to Slovenko," in *Szasz Under Fire: A Psychiatric Abolitionist Faces His Critics*, ed. Jeffrey A. Schaler (Chicago: Open Court, 2015), pp. 159–178, esp. 174–78.

39. Many years later, one of Szasz's psychiatric colleagues expressed regret that Szasz felt the need to go rogue: "Organized psychiatry has shabbily treated Szasz. Few psychiatrists even tried to deal with the serious issues he raised by responding with calm and reflective dialogue. Rather, he was attacked in the worst kind of ad hominem ways and subjected to scorn and ridicule. I have always felt that if organized psychiatry had responded to his first critical book, *The Myth of Mental Illness*, with a truly intellectual dialogue, that perhaps Szasz would have been more temperate in his later writings." Seymour L. Halleck, review of Thomas Szasz, *A Lexicon of Lunacy: Metaphoric Malady, Moral Responsibility, and Psychiatry*, in *Academic Psychiatry* 17, no. 3 (1993): 165–67.

40. Judi Chamberlin, *On Our Own: Patient-Controlled Alternatives to the Mental Health System* (New York: Hawthorn Books, 1978).

41. Sherry Hirsch, ed., *Madness Network News Reader* (San Francisco: Glide, 1974), p. 75.

42. Quoted in Maggie Scarf, "Normality Is a Square Circle or a Four-Sided Triangle," *New York Times*, October 3, 1971.

43. Bruce J. Ennis, *Prisoners of Psychiatry: Mental Patients, Psychiatrists, and the Law* (New York: Harcourt Brace Jovanovich, 1972).

44. For more on this history, see Ralph Slovenko, *Psychiatry in Law / Law in Psychiatry*, 2nd ed. (New York: Routledge, 2009).

45. "Photograph of Tom Cruise and Thomas Szasz, circa 2004," *Szasz Blog*, July 1, 2005, http://theszaszblog.blogspot.com/2005/07/photograph-of-thomas-szasz-and-tom.html. For more on the Szasz-Scientology alliance, see Donald A. Westbrook, "'The Enemy of My Enemy Is My Friend': Thomas Szasz, the Citizens Commission on Human Rights, and Scientology's Anti-Psychiatric Theology," *Nova Religio: The Journal of Alternative and Emergent Religions* 20, no. 4 (2017): 37–61.

46. D. L. Rosenhan, "On Being Sane in Insane Places," *Science*, new ser., 179, no. 4070 (January 19, 1973): 250–58, esp. 252.

47. Rosenhan, "On Being Sane," p. 258.

48. Samuel B. Guze, interview by Marion Hunt, 1994, Washington University School of Medicine Oral History Project, Becker Medical Library, http://becker exhibits.wustl.edu/oral/interviews/guze1994.html.

49. Quoted in Candace O'Connor, "Rethinking Psychiatry: 'Troublemakers' in the Department of Psychiatry Later Were Hailed for Having Reshaped the Profession," *Outlook Magazine*, Washington University in St. Louis School of Medicine, February 2011, https://outlook.wustl.edu/2011/feb/psychiatry/.

50. Samuel Guze, interview by Marion Hunt, 1994, Washington University School of Medicine Oral History Project, transcript, http://beckerexhibits.wustl.edu/oral/interviews/guze1994.html.

51. For the larger story, see Gerald N. Grob, "Origins of DSM-I: A Study in Appearance and Reality," *American Journal of Psychiatry* 148, no. 4 (1991): 421.

52. *Diagnostic and Statistical Manual: Mental Disorders (DSM-I)* (Washington, DC: American Psychiatric Associaton Mental Hospital Service, 1952).

53. Quoted in M. Wilson, "DSM-III and the Transformation of American Psychiatry: A History," *American Journal of Psychiatry* 150 (1993): 399–410, esp. 406.

54. P. Ash, "The Reliability of Psychiatric Diagnosis," *Journal of Abnormal and Social Psychology* 44 (1949): 272–77; A. Beck, "Reliability of Psychiatric Diagnoses: I: A Critique of Systematic Studies," *American Journal of Psychiatry* 119 (1962): 210–16.

55. Gerald L. Klerman, "The Evolution of a Scientific Nosology," in *Schizophrenia: Science and Practice*, ed. J. C. Shershow (Cambridge, MA: Harvard University Press, 1978), pp. 99–121, esp. 104.

56. John P. Feighner et al, "Diagnostic Criteria for Use in Psychiatric Research," *Archives of General Psychiatry* 26, no. 1 (1972): 57–63.

57. For more on the history of this paper, see Roger K. Blashfield, "Feighner et al., Invisible Colleges, and the Matthew Effect," *Schizophrenia Bulletin* 8, no. 1 (1982): 1–6.

58. Ronald Bayer, *Homosexuality and American Psychiatry: The Politics of Diagnosis* (Princeton, NJ: Princeton University Press, 1981).

59. She later learned that some government officials derisively referred to her project as the "Fairy Project." See Katharine S. Milar, "The Myth Buster," *Monitor on Psychology* 42, no. 2 (February 2011), www.apa.org/monitor/2011/02/myth-buster.aspx.

60. Evelyn Hooker, "The Adjustment of the Male Overt Homosexual," *Journal of Projective Techniques* 21, no. 1 (1957): 18–31. Hooker's story is recounted in detail by gay studies scholar Henry Minton in *Departing from Deviance: A History of Homosexual Rights and Emancipatory Science in America* (Chicago: University of Chicago Press, 2002), pp. 219–64.

61. Ronald Bayer, *Homosexuality and American Psychiatry: The Politics of Diagnosis* (Princeton, NJ: Princeton University Press, 1981), p. 103.

62. Quoted in *American Psychiatry and Homosexuality: An Oral History*, ed. J. Drescher and J. P. Merlino (Binghamton, NY: Haworth Press, 2007).

63. Quoted in Bayer, *Homosexuality and American Psychiatry*, p. 127.

64. "The A.P.A. Ruling on Homosexuality," *New York Times*, December 23, 1973, italics added.

65. Michael Strand, "Where Do Classifications Come from? The DSM-III, the Transformation of American Psychiatry, and the Problem of Origins in the Sociology of Knowledge," *Theory and Society* 40, no. 3 (2011): 273–313.

66. Robert L. Spitzer, "On Pseudoscience in Science, Logic in Remission, and Psychiatric Diagnosis: A Critique of Rosenhan's 'On Being Sane in Insane Places,'" *Journal of Abnormal Psychology* 84, no. 5 (1975): 442–522. See also Robert L. Spitzer, "More on Pseudoscience in Science and the Case for Psychiatric Diagnosis: A Critique of D. L. Rosenhan's 'On Being Sane in Insane Places' and 'The

Contextual Nature of Psychiatric Diagnosis,'" *Archives of General Psychiatry* 33, no. 4 (April 1, 1976): 459–70.

67. Quoted in Hannah S. Decker, *The Making of DSM-III: A Diagnostic Manual's Conquest of American Psychiatry* (New York: Oxford University Press, 2013), p. 103.

68. Spitzer, "More on Pseudoscience in Science," p. 467.

69. Quoted in M. Wilson, "DSM-III and the Transformation of American Psychiatry: A History," *American Journal of Psychiatry* 150, no. 3 (1993): 399.

70. Quoted in Rick Mayes and Allan V. Horwitz, "DSM-III and the Revolution in the Classification of Mental Illness," *Journal of the History of the Behavioral Sciences* 41 (2005): 249–67.

71. See especially the excellent Decker, *Making of DSM-III*.

72. Richard Friedman, "Diagnostic and Statistical Manual of Mental Disorders, Third Edition (DSM-III), Prepared by the Committee on Nomenclature and Statistics of the American Psychiatric Association Task Force. Draft Edition, 1977," *Modern Psychoanalysis* 2, no. 2 (1977): 270–73, esp. 270.

73. Gerald L. Klerman, George E. Vaillant, Robert L. Spitzer, and Robert Michels, "A Debate on DSM-III," *American Journal of Psychiatry* 141, no. 4 (1984): 539–53.

74. Shorter, *History of Psychiatry*, p. 302.

Chapter 5: Schizophrenia

1. For a pessimistic appraisal of biological research on schizophrenia in this period, see Wray Herbert, "Schizophrenia: From Adolescent Insanity to Dopamine Disease," *Science News* 121, no. 11 (March 13, 1982): 173–75. For an example of work from this time, see the once-widely reviewed (but now forgotten) 1945 Salmon Memorial Lecture by a former student of Walter Bradford Cannon, Roy G. Hoskins, published in book form as *The Biology of Schizophrenia* (New York: Norton, 1946). Reviews of *The Biology of Schizophrenia* include Clifford Allen, reviewer, in *Nature* 159, no. 4048 (1947): 725; W. O. Jahrreiss, reviewer, in *Quarterly Review of Biology* 21, no. 4 (1946): 415–16; Riley H. Guthrie, reviewer, in *American Journal of Psychiatry* 104, no. 6 (1947): 428–28; Ernest Groves, reviewer, in *Social Forces* 25, no. 1 (January 1, 1946): 101; Sol W. Ginsburg, reviewer, in *American Journal of Orthopsychiatry* 17, no. 2 (1947): 362–63; and Anton T. Boisen, reviewer, in *Journal of Religion* 27, no. 4 (1947): 298–99.

2. Kieran McNally, *A Critical History of Schizophrenia* (New York: Palgrave Macmillan, 2016), p. 5.

3. Quoted in Kieran McNally, *A Critical History of Schizophrenia* (London: Palgrave Macmillan, 2016), p. 53.

4. Ralph Waldo Gerard, "The Academic Lecture: The Biological Roots of Psychiatry I," *American Journal of Psychiatry* 112 (1955): 81–90, esp. 81.

5. Donald Jackson, "Psychiatrists' Conceptions of the Schizophrenogenic Parent," *AMA Archives of Neurology and Psychiatry* 79 (April 1958): 448–59.

6. For a review of family systems theory in relation to schizophrenia, see John G. Howells and Waguih R. Guirguis, *The Family and Schizophrenia* (New York:

International Universities Press, 1985). For an important overview of the history, see Deborah Weinstein, *The Pathological Family: Postwar America and the Rise of Family Therapy* (Ithaca, NY: Cornell Univeristy Press, 2013).

7. C. Christian Beels, "Notes for a Cultural History of Family Therapy," *Family Process* 41, no. 1 (March 2002): 67–82.
8. Beels, "Notes for Cultural History of Family Therapy."
9. Gregory Bateson, Don D. Jackson, Jay Haley, and John Weakland, "Toward a Theory of Schizophrenia," *Behavioral Science* 1, no. 4 (1956): 251–64.
10. Bateson, Jackson, Haley, and Weakland, "Toward a Theory of Schizophrenia."
11. Jerry Osterweil, "Discussion," *Family Process* 1 (1962): 141–45.
12. Jay Haley quoted in Paul H. Glasser and Lois N. Glasser, *Families in Crisis* (New York: Harper & Row, 1970), p. 188.
13. Milton Silverman and Margaret Silverman, "Psychiatry Inside the Family Circle," *Saturday Evening Post*, July 28, 1962, pp. 46–51.
14. Lester Grinspoon, P. H. Courtney, and H. M. Bergen, "The Usefulness of a Structured Parents' Group in Rehabilitation," in *Mental Patients in Transition: Steps in Hospital-Community Rehabilitation,* ed. M. Greenblatt, D. J. Levinson, and G. L. Klerman (Springfield, IL: Charles C. Thomas, 1961), p. 245.
15. Quoted in T. M. Luhrmann, "Down and Out in Chicago," *Raritan* 29, no. 3 (January 1, 2010): 140–66.
16. Lenore Korkes, *The Impact of Mentally Ill Children upon Their Families*, Ph.D. diss., New York University, 1956.
17. August B. Hollingshead and Fredrick C. Redlich, *Social Class and Mental Illness: A Community Study* (New York: Wiley,1958).
18. Louise Wilson, *This Stranger My Son: A Mother's Moving, Harrowing Story to Save Her Deeply Disturbed Child* (New York: New American Library, 1969), quoted in Torrey Edwin Fuller, *Surviving Schizophrenia: A Family Manual* (New York: Harper & Row, 1983), pp. 156, 157.
19. Betty Friedan, *The Feminine Mystique* (1963; reprinted New York: Norton, 2010), p. 276.
20. Phyllis Chesler, *Women and Madness* (New York: Doubleday, 1972), p. 95.
21. Paulin B. Bart, "Sexism and Social Science: From the Gilded Cage to the Iron Cage, or the Perils of Pauline," *Journal of Marriage and Family* 33 (1971): 734–45.
22. Thomas H. Maugh, II, "Obituary: Albert Hofmann, 102; Swiss Chemist Discovered LSD," *Los Angeles Times*, April 30, 2008, p. 102.
23. Albert Hofmann and Jonathan Ott, *LSD. My Problem Child* (Oxford, UK: Oxford University Press, 2013), p. 20.
24. Michael Horowitz, "Interview with Albert Hofmann," *High Times* 11 (1976), reprinted at *The Vaults of Erowid*, https://erowid.org/culture/characters/hofmann_albert/hofmann_albert_interview1.shtml.
25. Kurt Beringer, *Der Meskalinrausch: Seine Geschichte und Erscheinungsweise* (Berlin: J. Springer, 1927); and G. Tayler Stockings, "A Clinical Study of the Mescaline Psychosis, with Special Reference to the Mechanism of the Genesis of Schizophrenic and Other Psychotic States," *British Journal of Psychiatry* 86, no. 360 (1940): 29–47.
26. His Swiss colleague went one step further and called the drug a "psychosis

agent." A. M Becker, "Zur Psychopathologie der Lysergsäurediäthylamid-wirkung," *Wiener Zeitschrift für Nervenheilkunde* 2, no. 4 (1949): 402–40.

27. W. A. Stoll, "Lysergsäure-Diäthylamid, Ein Phantastikum aus der Mutter-korngruppe," *Schweizer Archiv für Neurologie und Psychiatrie* 60, no. 1 (1947): 279–323.

28. Gion Condrau, "Klinische Erfahrungen an Geisteskranken mit Lysergsaeure-diaethylamid," *Acta Psychiatrica Scandinavica* 24, no. 1 (1949): 9–32; and Hud-son Hoagland, "A Review of Biochemical Changes Induced in Vivo by Lysergic Acid Diethylamide and Similar Drugs," *Annals of the New York Academy of Sciences* 66, no. 3 (1957): 445–58.

29. Max Rinkel, "Experimentally Induced Psychoses in Man," in *Neuropharmacology: Transactions of the Second Conference, May 25, 26, and 27, 1955, Princeton, N.J.*, ed. Harold A. Abramson (New York: Josiah Macy, Jr., Foundation, 1956), p. 235.

30. Like Werner Stoll's original report, the pamphlet that Sandoz distributed with these drug samples emphasized above all LSD's ability to create brief schizophrenia-like conditions but also pointed to possible therapeutic benefits of the drug for the analyst. Hofmann and Ott, *LSD*.

31. For his first publication on this matter, see Max Rinkel et al., "Experimental Schizophrenia-like Symptoms," *American Journal of Psychiatry* 108, no. 8 (February 1, 1952): 572–78.

32. Quoted in Andy Roberts, *Albion Dreaming: A Popular History of LSD in Britain*, rev. ed. (Singapore: Marshall Cavendish International Asia Pte, 2008), p. 20.

33. Max Rinkel at Harvard was the epicenter of the East Coast work; Sidney Cohen at UCLA spearheaded the West Coast effort. See Steven J. Novak, "LSD Before Leary: Sidney Cohen's Critique of 1950s Psychedelic Drug Research," *Isis* 88, no. 1 (1997): 87–110.

34. On the Saskatchewan group and its pioneering work on LSD and alcoholism, see Erika Dyck, *Psychedelic Psychiatry: LSD from Clinic to Campus* (Baltimore: Johns Hopkins University Press, 2008). For Lauretta Bender, see Lauretta Bender, Lothar Goldschmidt, and D. V. Siva Sankar, "Treatment of Autistic Schizophrenic Children with LSD-25 and UML-492," *Recent Advances in Biological Psychiatry* 4 (1962): 170–77; and Lauretta Bender, Lothar Goldschmidt, and D. V. Siva Sankar, "LSD-25 Helps Schizophrenic Children," *American Druggist* 146, no. 13 (December 24, 1962): 33. On the use of LSD to catalyze breakthroughs in psychotherapy, including Ronald Sandison's early work, see Harold Alexander Abramson, *The Use of LSD in Psychotherapy: Transactions* (New York: Josiah Macy, Jr., Foundation, 1960).

35. See Erika Dyck, *Psychedelic Psychiatry: LSD from Clinic to Campus* (Baltimore: Johns Hopkins University Press, 2008); Martin A. Lee and Bruce Shlain, *Acid Dreams: The Complete Social History of LSD : The CIA, the Sixties, and Beyond* (New York: Grove Press, 1992).

36. "Examined Life: What a Trip," *Stanford Magazine* (January–February 2002).

37. Humphry Osmond, "On Being Mad," *Saskatchewan Psychiatric Services Journal* 1, no.2 (September 1952).

38. H. Osmond and J. Smythies, "Schizophrenia: A New Approach," *Journal of Mental Science* 98, no. 411 (April 1, 1952): 309–15.

39. Elliot S. Valenstein, *Blaming the Brain: The Truth About Drugs and Mental Health* (New York: Free Press, 1998), p. 75.

40. Julius Axelrod, "An Unexpected Life in Research," *Annual Review of Pharmacology and Toxicology* 28, no. 1 (1988): 95.

41. Stephen Szara, Julius Axelrod, and Seymour Perlin. "Is Adrenochrome Present in the Blood?" *American Journal of Psychiatry* 115 (1958): 162.

42. For a fuller discussion, see John A. Mills, "Hallucinogens as Hard Science: The Adrenochrome Hypothesis for the Biogenesis of Schizophrenia," *History of Psychology* 13, no. 2 (May 2010): 178–95, esp. 186–88.

43. Huxley quoted in Steven J. Novak, "LSD Before Leary: Sidney Cohen's Critique of 1950s Psychedelic Drug Research," *Isis* 88, no. 1 (1997): 95.

44. Humphry Osmond, "A Review of the Clinical Effects of Psychotomimetic Agents," *Annals of the New York Academy of Sciences* 66, no. 3 (March 1, 1957): 428.

45. For a fuller discussion, see Eugene Alonzo Smith III, *Within the Counterculture: The Creation, Transmission, and Commercialization of Cultural Alternatives During the 1960s*, Ph.D. diss., Carnegie Mellon University, 2001. The long-aborted film of the Merry Pranksters' journey across America has recently been rescued through the magic of digital technology and can now be purchased online at Key-Z Productions, a small mail-order company in Oregon whose mission is to "enlighten people of their psychedelic past and to enable them to learn about the people who brought them to the present." See http://www.key-z.com/video.html.

46. John S. Hughes, "Labeling and Treating Black Mental Illness in Alabama, 1861–1910," *Journal of Southern History* 58, no. 3 (1992): 452.

47. "Pellagra in Man and Black Tongue in Dogs Found to Be Due to Similar Cause," *Annals of Internal Medicine* 2, no. 4 (October 1, 1928): 388–89.

48. Alan Kraut, *Goldberger's War: The Life and Work of a Public Health Crusader* (New York: Hill & Wang, 2003)

49. Conrad Elvehjem, Robert J. Madden, F. M. Strong, and D. W. Woolley. "The Isolation and Identification of the Anti-Black Tongue Factor," *Journal of Biological Chemistry* 123 (1938): 137–49.

50. John A. Mills, "Hallucinogens as Hard Science: The Adrenochrome Hypothesis for the Biogenesis of Schizophrenia," *History of Psychology* 13, no. 2 (May 2010): 178–95.

51. Abram Hoffer et al., "Treatment of Schizophrenia with Nicotinic Acid and Nicotinamide," *Journal of Clinical and Experimental Psychopathology* 18, no. 2 (1957): 131–57.

52. Humphry Osmond and Abram Hoffer, "Massive Niacin Treatment in Schizophrenia: Review of a Nine-Year Study," *Lancet* 279, no. 7224 (1962): 316–20.

53. A. Saul, "An interview with Abram Hoffer," *Journal of Orthomolecular Medicine* 24, nos. 3–4 (2009): 122–29, esp. 123–24.

54. Linus Pauling, "Orthomolecular Psychiatry," *Science* 160, no. 3825 (1968): 265–71.

55. APA Council on Research and Development and APA Task Force on Vitamin Therapy in Psychiatry, *Megavitamin and Orthomolecular Therapy in Psychiatry* (Washington, DC: American Psychiatric Association, 1973), p. 7.

56. Elliot S. Valenstein, *The War of the Soups and the Sparks: The Discovery of Neurotransmitters and the Dispute over How Nerves Communicate* (New York: Columbia University Press, 2005), p. 158. See also Lester H. Margolis, "Pharmacotherapy in Psychiatry: A Review," *Annals of the New York Academy of Sciences* 66, no. 3 (March 1, 1957): 698–718.

57. Theodore L. Sourkes, "Acetylcholine—From Vagusstoff to Cerebral Neurotransmitter," *Journal of the History of the Neurosciences* 18, no. 1 (January 2009): 47–58.

58. D. W. Woolley and F. N. Shaw, "Evidence for the Participation of Serotonin in Mental Processes," *Annals of the New York Academy of Sciences* 66, no. 3 (March 1, 1957): 649–67.

59. John H. Gaddum, "Antagonism Between Lysergic Acid Diethylamide and 5-Hydroxytryptamine," *Journal of Physiology* 121, no. 1 (1953): 1–15.

60. B. M. Twarog and I. H. Page, "Serotonin Content of Some Mammalian Tissues and Urine and a Method for Its Determination," *American Journal of Physiology* 175 (1953): 157–61.

61. D. W. Woolley and E. Shaw, "A Biochemical and Pharmacological Suggestion About Certain Mental Disorders," *Proceedings of the National Academy of Sciences* 40, no. 4 (1954): 228–31. There is a modest dispute in the literature as to whether Woolley or John Gaddum first proposed this idea. For more on Gaddum's role, see A. R. Green, "Gaddum and LSD: The Birth and Growth of Experimental and Clinical Neuropharmacology Research on 5-HT in the UK," *British Journal of Pharmacology* 154 (2008): 1583–99.

62. E. Rothlin, "Lysergic Acid Diethylamide and Related Substances," *Annals of the New York Academy of Sciences* 66, no. 3 (March 1, 1957): 674.

63. Seymour Kety, "The Implications of Psychopharmacology in the Etiology and Treatment of Mental Illness," *Annals of the New York Academy of Sciences* 66, no. 3 (March 1, 1957): 840.

64. Jal Vakil Rustom, "A Clinical Trial of Rauwolfia Serpentina in Essential Hypertension," *British Heart Journal* 2 (1949): 350–55. In England, the cardiologist Robert Wilkins did further studies on the drug as a hypertensive medication, using tablets manufactured by a company in Bombay. See Ivan Oransky, "Robert W Wilkins [Obituary]," *Lancet* 362 (July 26, 2003): 335. The postcolonial interactions and power dynamics in play between the varied Anglo-American and Indian scientific and commercial stakeholders in the early history of reserpine warrants further study.

65. J. M. Mueller, E. Schlittler, and H. J. Bein, "Reserpin, der sedative Wirkstoff aus *Rauwolfia serpentina* Benth," *Experientia* 8, no. 9 (September 1952): 338.

66. Alfred Pletscher, Parkhurst A. Shore, and Bernard B. Brodie, "Serotonin Release as a Possible Mechanism of Reserpine Action," *Science*, new ser., 122, no. 3165 (August 26, 1955): 374–75.

67. Dilworth Wayne Woolley, *The Biochemical Bases of Psychoses; or, The Serotonin Hypothesis about Mental Diseases* (New York: Wiley, 1962), italics added.

68. Arvid Carlsson, interview by William Bunney, Jr., December 12, 1998, in *Recollections of the History of Neuropsychopharmacology through Interviews Conducted by William E. Bunney, Jr.*, ed. Peter R. Martin (Cordoba, Argentina: International Network for the History of Neuropsychopharmacology, 1994), pp. 28–37.

69. Arvid Carlsson, Margit Lindqvist, and T. O. R. Magnusson, "3, 4-Dihydroxy-phenylalanine and 5-Hydroxytryptophan as Reserpine Antagonists," *Nature* 180 (November 30, 1957): 1200.

70. Arvid Carlsson, interview by William E. Bunney, Jr., in *Recollections of the History of Neuropsychopharmacology through Interviews Conducted by William E. Bunney, Jr.* (Risskov, Denmark: International Network for the History of Neuropsychopharmacology, 1994), pp. 28–37.

71. There is a small but significant priority dispute behind this discovery. Three months before Carlsson's group published, a largely unsung female researcher from England, Kathleen Montagu, had published her findings of the same compounds in rat brains. See K. A. Montagu, "Catechol Compounds in Rat Tissues and in Brains of Different Animals," *Nature* 180, no. 4579 (1957): 244–45. Partly because Carlsson was more prominent, partly because he was a man, and partly because he went further than Montagu in identifying the clinical significance of dopamine, he is generally identified as the discoverer of this neurotransmitter.

72. Oleh Hornykiewicz, "From Dopamine to Parkinson's Disease: A Personal Research Record," in *The Neurosciences: Paths of Discovery II*, ed. F. Samson and G. Adelman (Boston: Birkhäuser, 1992), pp. 125–46.

73. Carlsson, Lindqvist, and Magnusson, "3,4 Dihydroxyphenylalanine."

74. Hornykiewicz, "From Dopamine to Parkinson's Disease."

75. Harold M. Schmeck, Jr., "A Drug for Parkinson's Disease Gets Cautious F.D.A. Approval," *New York Times*, June 5, 1970.

76. The full technical story is told by Solomon H. Snyder, "What Dopamine Does in the Brain," *Proceedings of the National Academy of Sciences* 108, no. 47 (November 22, 2011): 18869–71.

77. J. van Rossum, "The Significance of Dopamine-Receptor Blockade for the Action of Neuroleptic Drugs," in *Neuro-Psycho-Pharmacology: Proceedings of the Fifth International Congress of the Collegium Internationale Neuro-Psycho-Pharmacologicum*, ed. H. Brill et al. (Amsterdam: Excerpta Medica Foundation, 1967), pp. 321–99. For a long time, the laboratory evidence did not allow a definitive conclusion, since it turned out that the drugs blocked not just dopamine but also other neurotransmitters like norepinephrine and serotonin. See Arvid Carlsson and Margit Lindqvist, "Effect of Chlorpromazine or Haloperidol on Formation of 3-Methoxytyramine and Normetanephrine in Mouse Brain," *Basic and Clinical Pharmacology and Toxicology* 20, no. 2 (1963): 140–44; and Bertha K. Madras, "History of the Discovery of the Antipsychotic Dopamine D2 Receptor: A Basis for the Dopamine Hypothesis of Schizophrenia," *Journal of the History of the Neurosciences* 22, no. 1 (January 2013): 62–78.

78. P. Seeman and T. Lee, "Antipsychotic Drugs: Direct Correlation between Clinical Potency and Presynaptic Action on Dopamine Neurons," *Science* 188, no. 4194 (1975): 1217–19.

79. Nicolas Rasmussen, *On Speed: From Benzedrine to Adderall* (New York: NYU Press, 2009).

80. "Harry Hipster Gibson—Who Put The Benzedrine in Mrs. Murphys Ovaltine" (1944), posted by warholsoup100, April 24, 2011, www.youtube.com/watch?v=l2WJqnK3gAY.

81. John C. Kramer, M.D, "Introduction to Amphetamine Abuse," *Journal of Psychedelic Drugs* 2, no. 2 (April 1, 1969): 6–7.
82. Jonathan Black, "The 'Speed' That Kills Or Worse," *New York Times*, June 21, 1970.
83. E. H. Ellinwood and Abraham Sudilovsky, "Chronic Amphetamine Intoxication: Behavioral Model of Psychoses," in *Psychopathology and Psychopharmacology*, ed. J. Cole, A. Freedman, and A. Friedhoff (Baltimore: Johns Hopkins University Press, 1973), pp. 51–70; Philip Henry Connell, *Amphetamine Psychosis* (London: Institute of Psychiatry, 1958).
84. As clinicians became disenchanted with the old LSD model of schizophrenia, some pointed out that while diagnosed schizophrenics typically heard voices, persons who took LSD typically had visual hallucinations and only rarely heard voices. The effort to insist that these two experiences were interchangeable had—according to the new consensus—always been misguided. Barry G. Young, "A Phenomenological Comparison of LSD and Schizophrenic States," *British Journal of Psychiatry* 124, no. 578 (1974): 64–74.
85. Jonathan M. Metzl, "Living in Mental Health: Guns, Race, and the History of Schizophrenic Violence," in *Living and Dying in the Contemporary World: A Compendium*, ed. Veena Das and Clara Han (Berkeley: University of California Press, 2015), pp. 205–31, esp. 209. Metzl originally developed this argument in his *The Protest Psychosis: How Schizophrenia Became a Black Disease* (New York: Beacon Press, 2010).
86. Thus in the early 1960s, the FBI hung *Armed and Dangerous* posters throughout the southern states warning citizens to beware of Robert Williams, head of the Monroe, North Carolina, chapter of the NAACP and author of the 1962 book *Negroes with Guns*, which advocated gun rights for African Americans seeking to protect themselves against the Ku Klux Klan. The posters pulled no punches: "Williams allegedly has possession of a large quantity of firearms, including a .45 caliber pistol. . . . He has previously been diagnosed as schizophrenic and has advocated and threatened violence." Jonathan Metzl, "The Art of Medicine: Why Are the Mentally Ill Still Bearing Arms?" *Lancet* 377 (June 25, 2011): 2172–73, esp. 2173. See also Jonathan M. Metzl, "Living in Mental Health: Guns, Race, and the History of Schizophrenic Violence," in *Living and Dying in the Contemporary World: A Compendium*, ed. Veena Das and Clara Han (Berkeley: University of California Press, 2015), pp. 205–31, esp. 209; and Metzl, *Protest Psychosis*.

The FBI didn't quite dare to slap a label of "schizophrenia" onto Martin Luther King, Jr., though it did blackmail and threaten him. Nevertheless, King was as aware as anyone of the ways the government recruited psychiatry and psychology to use its diagnostic labels to silence dissent and support the status quo. In September 1967, at the annual convention of the American Psychological Association in Washington, he challenged the attendees to reflect on the political implications of their entire vision of mental disorder. He called attention particularly to a word they still used "more than other word in psychology": *maladjusted*. He had no problem with the word in principle but wanted to make perfectly clear "that there are some things in our society, some things in our world, to which we should never be adjusted." No one should ever "adjust themselves" to racial and religious bigotry, or to economic policies that deprived the poor of necessities so the rich could enjoy more luxuries, or to "the madness of militarism and the self-defeating effects of physical violence." On the contrary: when confronted with all these things, what was needed was not "adjustment" but resistance. "It may well be," he concluded, "that our world is in dire need of a new organization, The International Association for the Advancement of Creative Maladjustment." See Martin L. King, Jr., "The Role of the Behavioral Scientist in the Civil Rights Movement," *American Psychologist* 23, no. 3 (1968): 180.

87. D. S. Bell, "Comparison of Amphetamine Psychosis and Schizophrenia," *British Journal of Psychiatry* 111, no. 477 (August 1, 1965): 701–7, doi.org/10.1192/bjp.111.477.701.

88. A. Randrup and I. Munkvad, "Stereotyped Activities Produced by Amphetamine in Several Animal Species and Man," *Psychopharmacology* 11, no. 4 (1967): 300–10.

89. "Molecular and clinical studies suggest that both the schizophrenia-like symptoms of amphetamine psychosis and the specific ability of phenothiazines to relieve the symptoms of schizophrenia and amphetamine psychosis may be the result of interactions with dopamine systems in the brain." Solomon H. Snyder, "Amphetamine Psychosis: A 'Model' Schizophrenia Mediated by Catecholamines," *American Journal of Psychiatry* 130, no. 1 (January 1, 1973): 61–67.

90. F. K. Goodwin, "Behavioral Effects of L-Dopa in Man," *Psychiatric Complications of Medical Drugs*, ed. R. I. Shader (New York: Raven Press 1972), pp. 149–74.

91. Oliver Sacks, *Awakenings* (1972; reprinted New York: Vintage, 1999), p. 210.

92. Snyder, "Amphetamine Psychosis."

93. Seymour Kety, "It's Not All in Your Head," *Saturday Review*, February 21, 1976, pp. 28–32, esp. 28.

94. P. J. Caplan and Ian Hall McCorquodale, "Mother-Blaming in Major Clinical Journals," *American Journal of Orthopsychiatry* 55, no. 3 (July 1985): 345–53.

95. George E. Gardner, "Childhood Schizophrenia: Round Table, 1953: Discussion," *American Journal of Orthopsychiatry* 24, no. 3 (1954): 517.

96. Leo Kanner, "Autistic Disturbances of Affective Contact," *Nervous Child* 2 (1943): 217–50.

97. Quoted in Shelby Louise Hyvonen, *Evolution of a Parent Revolution: Exploring Parent Memoirs of Children with Autism Spectrum Disorders*, Psy.D. thesis, Wright Institute, 2004, pp. 14–15.

98. Bruno Bettelheim, *The Empty Fortress: Infantile Autism and the Birth of the Self* (New York: Free Press, 1967), p. 125.

99. Bruno Bettelheim, *Truants from Life: The Rehabilitation of Emotionally Disturbed Children* (Glencoe, IL: Free Press, 1955).

100. Cited in Hyvonen, *Evolution of Parent Revolution*, p. 47.

101. *Refrigerator Mothers*, directed by David E. Simpson, Kartemquin Films, 2002.

102. John Joseph Donvan and Caren Brenda Zucker, *In a Different Key: The Story of Autism* (New York: Crown, 2017), p. 121.

103. Donvan and Zucker, *In a Different Key*, p. 93. Adam Feinstein records Kanner's

words at that meeting as being slightly different and a touch more dramatic: "Parents, I acquit you!." See Adam Feinstein, *A History of Autism: Conversations with the Pioneers* (New York: John Wiley, 2010), p. 99.

104. M. Rutter, "Childhood Schizophrenia Reconsidered," *Journal of Autism and Childhood Schizophrenia* 2, no. 4 (1972): 315–37.

105. As Richard Lewontin, Steven Rose, and Leon Kamin tartly wrote in their 1984 book, *Not in Our Genes*, "The lineage of the effort to find genetic predispositions runs back through the eugenic thinking of the 1930s and 1920s, with its belief in genes for criminal degeneracy, sexual profligacy, alcoholism, and every other type of activity disapproved of by bourgeois society. It is deeply embedded in today's determinist ideology. Only thus can we account for the extraordinary repetitive perseverance and uncritical nature of research into the genetics of schizophrenia." Richard C. Lewontin, Steven Rose, and Leon J. Kamin, *Not in Our Genes: Biology, Ideology, and Human Nature* (New York: Pantheon, 1984), p. 207.

106. Franz J. Kallmann, "The Genetic Theory of Schizophrenia: An Analysis of 691 Schizophrenic Twin Index Families," *American Journal of Psychiatry* 103 (1946): 309–22.

107. For Kallmann's complex Nazi past, see Elliot S. Gershon, "The Historical Context of Franz Kallmann and Psychiatric Genetics," *Archiv für Psychiatrie und Nervenkrankheiten* 229, no. 4 (December 1, 1981): 273–76, esp. 273; and E. Fuller Torrey and Robert H. Yolken, "Psychiatric Genocide: Nazi Attempts to Eradicate Schizophrenia," *Schizophrenia Bulletin* 36, no. 1 (January 1, 2010): 26–32.

108. H. Stierlin and David Rosenthal, eds., *The Genain Quadruplets: A Study of Heredity and Environment in Schizophrenia* (New York: Basic Books, 1963).

109. Leonard Heston, "Psychiatric Disorders in Foster-Home-Reared Children of Schizophrenic Mothers," *British Journal of Psychiatry* 112 (1966): 819–25.

110. Seymour S. Kety, "Biochemical Theories of Schizophrenia," *Science* 129, no. 3362 (1959): 1528–32.

111. "Seymour S. Kety," in *The History of Neuroscience in Autobiography*, ed. Larry Squire (Washington, DC: Society for Neuroscience, 1996), 1:382–413.

112. Bent Sigurd Hansen, "Something Rotten in the State of Denmark: Eugenics and the Ascent of the Welfare State," in *Eugenics and the Welfare State: Sterilization Policy in Denmark, Sweden, Norway and Finland*, ed. Gunnar Broberg and Nils Roll-Hansen (Ann Arbor: Michigan State University Press, 2007), pp. 9–76.

113. Seymour S. Kety et al., "The Types and Prevalence of Mental Illness in the Biological and Adoptive Families of Adopted Schizophrenics," *Journal of Psychiatric Research* 6, supp. 1 (November 1968): 345–62.

114. David Rosenthal and Seymour S. Kety, eds., *The Transmission of Schizophrenia; Proceedings of the Second Research Conference of the Foundations' Fund for Research in Psychiatry, Dorado, Puerto Rico, 26 June to 1 July 1967* (New York: Pergamon Press, 1968).

115. Kety et al., "Types and Prevalence of Mental Illness."

116. Carlos E. Sluzki, "Lyman C. Wynne and Transformation of the Field of Family-and-Schizophrenia," *Family Process* 46, no. 2 (June 2007): 143–49.

117. Rosenthal and Kety, *Transmission of Schizophrenia*.

118. Theodore Lidz, "Reply to Kety et al.," *Schizophrenia Bulletin* (1977): 522–26;

Theodore Lidz, "Commentary on 'A Critical Review of Recent Adoption, Twin, and Family Studies of Schizophrenia: Behavioral Genetics Perspectives,'" *Schizophrenia Bulletin* 2, no. 3 (January 1, 1976): 402–12; and "A Reconsideration of the Kety and Associates Study of Genetic Factors in the Transmission of Schizophrenia," *American Journal of Psychiatry* 133, no. 10 (October 1, 1976): 1129–33.

119. Seymour Kety, "From Rationalization to Reason," *American Journal of Psychiatry* 131 (1974): 957–63, esp. 961.

120. P. Holzman, "Seymour S. Kety and the Genetics of Schizophrenia," *Neuropsychopharmacology* 25, no. 3 (September 2001): 299–304. See also Edward Dolnick, *Madness on the Couch: Blaming the Victim in the Heyday of Psychoanalysis* (New York: Simon & Schuster, 1998), p. 162.

121. Marjorie Wallace, *The Forgotten Illness* (London: Times Newspapers, 1987).

122. William Doll, "Family Coping with the Mentally Ill: An Unanticipated Problem of Deinstitutionalization," *Psychiatric Services* 27, no. 3 (1976): 183–85; Edward H. Thompson, Jr., and William Doll, "The Burden of Families Coping with the Mentally Ill: An Invisible Crisis," *Family Relations* 31, no. 3 (July 1982): 379–88.

123. Anomymous parent quoted in "U.S. Department of Health Bulletin on 'Schizophrenia" (1974), Archival Repository, *PAS/California Alliance for the Mentally Ill (CAMI)*, Los Angeles Department of Mental Health, http://histpubmh .semel.ucla.edu/archive/pascalifornia-alliance-mentally-ill-cami.

124. Quoted in Phyllis Vine, *Families in Pain: Children, Siblings, Spouses, and Parents of the Mentally Ill Speak Out* (New York: Pantheon, 1982), p. 225.

125. *When Medicine Got It Wrong* (film), directed by Kate Cadigan and Laura Murray, 2009, available from Documentary Educational Resources, www.der.org.

126. Roy W. Menninger and John Case Nemiah, eds., *American Psychiatry After World War II, 1944–1994* (New York: American Psychiatric Publications, 2008), p. 222.

127. Herbert Pardes, "NIMH During the Tenure of Director Herbert Pardes, M.D. (1978–1984): The President's Commission on Mental Health and the Reemergence of NIMH's Scientific Mission," *American Journal of Psychiatry* 155, no. 9 suppl. (1998). 14–19. For more on the politics behind Pardes's appointment, see American Psychopathological Association, *Recognition and Prevention of Major Mental and Substance Use Disorders* (New York: American Psychiatric Publications, 2007), p. 59.

128. Quoted in Athena McLean, "Contradictions in the Social Production of Clinical Knowledge: The Case of Schizophrenia," *Social Science and Medicine* 30, no. 9 (1990): 974.

129. Agnes B. Hatfield, "The Family Consumer Movement: A New Force in Service Delivery," *New Directions for Mental Health Services* 1984, no. 21 (March 1, 1984): 71–79.

130. "Editorials: Megavitamin and Orthomolecular Therapy of Schizophrenia," *Revue de l'Association des Psychiatres du Canada/Canadian Psychiatric Association Journal* 20, no. 2 (1975): 97–100, esp. 97. By way of contrast, a typical multivitamin pill today provides about 90 mg of vitamin C and 16 mg of vitamin B3.

131. *AMI Newsletter*, Alliance for the Mentally Ill of San Mateo County (formerly PAS), November 1982, in http://histpubmh.semel.ucla.edu/archive/pas california-alliance-mentally-ill-cami

132. *AMI Newsletter*, Alliance for the Mentally Ill of San Mateo County, November 1982.
133. Abram Hoffer and Humphry Osmond, *How to Live with Schizophrenia* (London: Johnson, 1966), p. 5
134. Edwin Fuller Torrey, *Surviving Schizophrenia: A Family Manual* (New York: Harper & Row, 1983).
135. Torrey, *Surviving Schizophrenia*, p. 2.
136. Torrey to NAMI, cited in Torrey, *Surviving Schizophrenia*, pp. 156, 157.
137. Michael Winerip, "Schizophrenia's Most Zealous Foe," *New York Times*, February 22, 1998.
138. Herbert Pardes, "Citizens: A New Ally for Research," *Psychiatric Services* 37, no. 12 (December 1, 1986): 1193.
139. Quoted in Athena McLean, "Contradictions in the Social Production of Clinical Knowledge: The Case of Schizophrenia," *Social Science and Medicine* 30, no. 9 (1990): 974, 976.
140. Richard R. J. Lewine, "Parents of Schizophrenic Individuals: What We Say Is What We See," *Schizophrenia Bulletin* 5, no. 3 (January 1, 1979): 434.
141. Carol M. Anderson, Gerard Hogarty, and Douglas J. Reiss, "The Psychoeducational Family Treatment of Schizophrenia," *New Directions for Mental Health Services* (1981): 79–94. See also Judith A. Cook, "Who 'Mothers' the Chronically Mentally Ill?" *Family Relations* 37 (1988): 42–49.
142. Thomas H. McGlashan, "The Chestnut Lodge Follow-up Study: II. Long-Term Outcome of Schizophrenia and the Affective Disorders," *Archives of General Psychiatry* 41, no. 6 (June 1, 1984): 586–601. In 2006 a colleague of McGlashan, Dr. Wayne Fenton of the NIMH, recalled marveling at McGlashan's nerve in standing up to the "giants of psychotherapy" and telling them there was "not a shred of evidence" that anything they were doing was effective. Quoted in Benedict Carey, "A Career That Has Mirrored Psychiatry's Twisting Path," *New York Times*, May 23, 2006.
143. "Madness," episode 7 of *The Brain*, WNET, New York: Kastel Enterprises, 1984.
144. Dan Weisburd, interview by Howard Padwa and Kevin Miller, July 29, 2010, *Oral Histories,* Los Angeles County Department of Mental Health, http://histpubmh.semel.ucla.edu/oral-histories/V-Z.
145. Alfie Kohn, "Getting a Grip on Schizophrenia," *Los Angeles Times,* June 25, 1990.
146. Rajiv Tandon, Matcheri Keshavan, and Henry Nasrallah, "Schizophrenia, 'Just the Facts': What We Know in 2008," pt. 1, *Schizophrenia Research* 100, no. 1 (March 2008): 4–19.
147. M. S. Keshavan, H. A. Nasrallah, and R. Tandon, "Schizophrenia, 'Just the Facts' 6. Moving Ahead with the Schizophrenia Concept: From the Elephant to the Mouse," *Schizophrenia Research* 127, nos. 1–3 (April 2011): 2–13, esp. 10.

Chapter 6: Depression

1. David Lowell Herzberg, *Happy Pills in America: From Miltown to Prozac* (Baltimore: Johns Hopkins University Press, 2009).
2. The work they studied was carried out by a research branch of the U.S. War

Department, by the Stirling County Study, and by the Midtown Manhattan Study. For more on this epidemiology and the central role of concerns with anxiety, see J. M. Murphy and A. H. Leighton, "Anxiety: Its Role in the History of Psychiatric Epidemiology," *Psychological Medicine* 39, no. 7 (July 2009): 1055–64. I am indebted for this reference to Allan V. Horwitz, "How an Age of Anxiety Became an Age of Depression," *Milbank Quarterly* 88, no. 1 (March 2010): 112–38.

3. *Diagnostic and Statistical Manual: Mental Disorders (DSM-I)* (Washington, DC: American Psychiatric Association Mental Hospital Service, 1952), p. 33.

4. Edward Shorter has called for a return to the distinction between neurotic depression (what he would call "nerves") and melancholy, claiming that the two are as distinct as "tuberculosis is from mumps." See Edward Shorter, *How Everyone Became Depressed: The Rise and Fall of the Nervous Breakdown* (New York: Oxford University Press, 2013).

5. *DSM-I*, p. 25

6. Lawrence Babb, *Sanity in Bedlam: A Study of Robert Burton's Anatomy of Melancholy* (Westport, CT: Greenwood Press, 1977).

7. Paul Schilder, "Notes on Psychogenic Depression and Melancholia," *Psychoanalytic Review* 20, no. 1 (1933): 10–18.

8. Gary G. Leonhardt, W. Ray Walker, and M. Evelyn McNeil, "Electroconvulsive Therapy: A Treatment Ahead of Its Time," *Resident and Staff Physician* 10, no. 35 (1989): 95–103. I am indebted to Shorter's *History of Psychiatry* for this reference.

9. Quoted in Joel Braslow, "History and Evidence-Based Medicine: Lessons from the History of Somatic Treatments from the 1900s to the 1950s," *Mental Health Services Research* 1, no. 4 (1999): 235–36.

10. Elliot Valenstein, *Great and Desperate Cures: The Rise and Decline of Psychosurgery and Other Radical Treatments for Mental Illness* (New York: Basic Books, 1986), pp. 50–51.

11. Jonathan Sadowsky, "Beyond the Metaphor of the Pendulum: Electroconvulsive Therapy, Psychoanalysis, and the Styles of American Psychiatry," *Journal of the History of Medicine and Allied Sciences* 61 (2005): 1–25; and Edgar Miller, "Psychological Theories of ECT: A Review," *British Journal of Psychiatry* 113 (1967): 201–311.

12. G. J. Wayne, "Some Unconscious Determinants in Physicians Motivating the Use of Particular Treatment Methods—With Special Reference to Electroconvulsive Treatment," *Psychoanalytic Review* 42, no. 1 (1955): 83–87.

13. "Two Health Plans Augment Benefits," *New York Times*, November 19, 1959, p. 1.

14. Alan Stone, interview by author, December 8, 2011.

15. "Not So Shocking," *Time*, September 8, 1947, pp. 42–47.

16. Quoted in Leonard Roy Frank, ed., *The Electroshock Quotationary*, June 2006, www.endofshock.com/102C_ECT.PDF.

17. David J. Impastato, "Prevention of Fatalities in Electroshock Therapy," *Diseases of the Nervous System*, July 1957, quoted in Frank, *Electroshock Quotationary*.

18. Abraham Myerson, *When Life Loses Its Zest* (Boston: Little, Brown, 1925); Nicolas Rasmussen, "Making the First Anti-Depressant: Amphetamine in American Medicine, 1929–1950," *Journal of the History of Medicine and Allied Sciences* 61, no. 3 (February 21, 2006): 288–323.

19. "Reports Finding Drug That Ends Urge to Suicide: Claims Discovery Also Cures Nervous Ills," *Chicago Tribune,* September 3, 1936, p. 26

20. "Tells of Drug Made to Act as Body Chemicals," *St. Louis Post-Dispatch,* May 6, 1936, p. 12.

21. "The Benzedrine 'Lift,'" *New York Herald Tribune,* December 30, 1938, p. 14. For other examples, see "New Drug Halts Suicide Mood, Eases Strain of Modern Tempo," *New York Herald Tribune,* September 3, 1936, p. 1; and Irving S. Cutter, "How to Keep Well: 'Blue Mondays' and Benzedrine," *Chicago Tribune,* June 21, 1937, p. 10.

22. Rasmussen, "Making the First Anti-Depressant."

23. Rasmussen, "Making the First Anti-Depressant"; Pierre Berton, "Benzy Craze," *Maclean's,* June 15, 1948.

24. "Wyeth Claims Drug to Relieve Anxieties and Mild Neuroses," *Wall Street Journal,* August 22, 1955, p. 1.

25. Ad for Dexamyl, *American Journal of Psychiatry* 112, no. 11 (May 1956).

26. Nicholas Weiss, "No One Listened to Imipramine," in *Altering American Consciousness: The History of Alcohol and Drug Use in the United States, 1800–2000,* ed. Caroline Jean Acker and Sarah W. Tracy (Amherst: University of Massachusetts Press, 2004), p. 332.

27. E. H. Robitzek, I. J. Selikoff, and G. G. Ornstein, "Chemotherapy of Human Tuberculosis with Hydrazine Derivatives of Isonicotinic Acid; Preliminary Report of Representative Cases," *Quarterly Bulletin of Sea View Hospital* 13, no. 1 (1952): 27–51.

28. Weiss, "No One Listened to Imipramine," p. 333. Also see Marco A. Ramos, "Drugs in Context: A Historical Perspective on Theories of Psychopharmaceutical Efficacy," *Journal of Nervous and Mental Disease* 201, no. 11 (2013): 926–33.

29. Quoted in Gary Greenberg, *Manufacturing Depression: The Secret History of a Modern Disease* (New York: Simon & Schuster, 2010), p. 187.

30. In an interview published in 2014, Ostow claimed to have immediately realized the photographs' potential meaning: "In 1956 or '57, my wife and I were having breakfast one morning, and I picked up the *New York Times,* and there was an article on the first page about some patients in a TB hospital who were given a new drug called isoniazid, and they seemed to become unusually cheerful. And I said to my wife, 'There will be the first antidepressant medication.'" Oliver Turnbull, "Mortimer Ostow," *Neuropsychoanalysis: An Interdisciplinary Journal for Psychoanalysis and the Neurosciences* 6, no. 2 (2014): 206–16, esp. 213.

31. N. S. Kline and T. B. Cooper, "Monoamine Oxidase Inhibitors as Antidepressants," in *Psychotropic Agents,* vol. 55 of *Handbook of Experimental Pharmacology* (New York: Springer, 1980), pp. 369–97. See also M. Chessin et al., "Modifications of Pharmacology of Reserpine by Iproniazid," in *Federation Proceedings* 15 (1956): 1334.

32. Harry P. Loomer, John C. Saunders, and Nathan S. Kline, "A Clinical and Pharmacodynamic Evaluation of Iproniazid as a Psychic Energizer," *Psychiatric Research Reports* 8 (1957): 129–41.

33. Some years after iproniazid had become an established treatment in psychiatry, one woman who was being treated for severe depression told her psychiatrist

NOTES TO PAGES 194–198

that she had experienced real happiness only once in her lifetime, during a religious conversion. After questioning her more closely, the psychiatrist learned that she had been in a sanitorium at the time and had been given iproniazid for her tuberculosis. "I couldn't quite bring myself to tell her," he said years later, "that her ecstatic experience might not have come from the Lord, but may have been instead a biochemical reaction to the medication." Maggie Scarf, "From Depression to Joy: New Insights into the Chemistry of Moods," *New York Times Magazine*, April 24, 1977, p. 33.

34. Quoted in Weiss, "No One Listened to Imipramine," pp. 334–35, originally recorded in *Journal of Clinical and Experimental Psychopathology and Quarterly Review of Psychiatry and Neurology* 18 (1957): 73.

35. "Three Hours Sleep per Night Enough?" *Newsweek*, July 7, 1960.

36. "Chefarzt Roland Kuhn: «Wir haben die Substanz nach und nach an 300 Fällen kennengelernt»," *St. Galler Tagblatt*, January 16, 2003, www .tagblatt.ch/ostschweiz/thurgau/kanton/Chefarzt-Roland-Kuhn-Wir -haben-die-Substanz-nach-und-nach-an-300-Faellen-kennengelernt; art123841,3267011; Edward Shorter, *A Historical Dictionary of Psychiatry* (New York: Oxford University Press, 2005), p. 141; and Walter Sneader, *Drug Discovery: A History* (Chichester, UK: John Wiley & Sons, 2005), p. 413.

37. David Healy, "The Antidepressant Drama," in *Treatment of Depression: Bridging the 21st Century*, ed. M. N.Weissman (Washington, DC: American Psychiatric Press, 2001), pp. 7–34.

38. The report was published in 1957 in the *Schweizerische Medizin Wochenschrift* and in English a year later: Roland Kuhn, "The Treatment of Depressive States with G 22355 (Imipramine Hydrochloride)," *American Journal of Psychiatry* 115, no. 5 (1958): 459–64.

39. Donald F. Klein, "Anxiety Reconceptualized," *Comprehensive Psychiatry* 21, no. 6 (1980): 411–27.

40. In 1970 Kuhn described the effects of imipramine as follows. "We have achieved a specific treatment of depressive states, not ideal but already going far in this direction. I emphasize 'specific' because the drug largely or completely restores what the illness has impaired—namely, the mental functions and capacity and what is of prime importance, the power to experience." Roland Kuhn, "The Imipramine Story," in *Discoveries in Biological Psychiatry*, ed. F. J. Ayd and B. Blackwell (Philadelphia: Lippincott, 1970), pp. 205–17, esp. 214.

41. Harold D. Watkins, "Probing the Mind: Scientists Speed New Drugs That May Help Treat the Mentally Ill," *Wall Street Journal*, March 5, 1959.

42. Frank Ayd, interview by Thomas A. Ban, July 19, 2001, Archives of the American College of Neuropsychopharmacology.

43. *Symposium in Blues,* Merck Sharp and Dohne promotion album, RCA Victor 1966, www.amazon.com/Symposium-Blues-Merck-Sharp-Promotion/ dp/B001IUWKX6/ref=sr_1_1?ie=UTF8&qid=1501743880&sr=8–1 &keywords=Symposium-Blues-Merck-Sharp-Promotion.

44. Maggie Scarf, "From Depression to Joy: New Insights Into the Chemistry of Moods," *New York Times Magazine*, April 24, 1977.

45. The 1977 Osheroff case against Chestnut Lodge is seen by some as a key moment in the triumph of biological psychiatry over psychoanalysis. For some of the

relevant literature, see first the classic defense of Osheroff's position: Gerald L. Klerman, "The Psychiatric Patient's Right to Effective Treatment: Implications of Osheroff v. Chestnut Lodge," *American Journal of Psychiatry* 147, no. 4 (1990): 409–18. Follow that with Alan A. Stone, "Law, Science, and Psychiatric Malpractice: A Response to Klerman's Indictment of Psychoanalytic Psychiatry," *American Journal of Psychiatry* 147, no. 4 (1990): 419–27. Additional interesting analyses from various perspectives can be found in John Gulton Malcolm, "Treatment Choices and Informed Consent in Psychiatry: Implications of the Osheroff Case for the Profession," *Journal of Psychiatry and Law* 14, nos. 1–2 (1986): 9–107; and Michael Robertson, "Power and Knowledge in Psychiatry and the Troubling Case of Dr. Osheroff," *Australasian Psychiatry* 13, no. 4 (2005): 343–50.

46. Merton Sandler interview, in David Healy, *The Psychopharmacologists: Interviews* (London: Altman, 1996), pp. 385–86.

47. Alfred Pletscher, Parkhurst A. Shore, and Bernard B. Brodie, "Serotonin Release as a Possible Mechanism of Reserpine Action," *Science*, new ser., 122, no. 3165 (August 26, 1955): 374–75.

48. Quoted in Elliot S. Valenstein, *Blaming the Brain: The Truth About Drugs and Mental Health* (New York: Free Press, 1998), p. 73.

49. For a more detailed but brief and accessible discussion of this work, see Solomon H. Snyder, "Turning off Neurotransmitters," *Cell* 125, no. 1 (April 7, 2006): 13–15. See also DeWitt Stetten, *NIH: An Account of Research in Its Laboratories and Clinics* (New York: Academic Press, 2014), pp. 40–41.

50. J. Axelrod, L. G. Whitby, and G. Hertting, "Effects of Psychotropic Drugs on the Uptake of H^3-Norepinephrine by Tissues," *Science* 133 (1961): 383–84.

51. Scarf, "From Depression to Joy."

52. Samuel H. Barondes, *Better than Prozac: Creating the Next Generation of Psychiatric Drugs* (New York: Oxford University Press, 2003).

53. J. J. Schildkraut, "The Catecholamine Hypothesis of Affective Disorders: A Review of Supporting Evidence," *American Journal of Psychiatry* 122, no. 5 (November 1965): 509–22.

54. Valenstein, *Blaming the Brain,* p. 78.

55. Thomas Fleming, "What's Happening in Psychiatry? Or, Where Are All the Analysts Hiding?" *Cosmopolitan,* March 1970, pp. 164–67, 182–83, esp. 167; "New Book Describes Journey through "Hell' of Depression," *Rushton Daily Leader* (Louisiana), February 28, 1975, p. 249; Scarf, "From Depression to Joy," p. 32.

56. "News About Blues: No Thanks on the Holiday? Check Your Chemicals," *Stars and Stripes,* November 22, 1977, italics added.

57. Cited in Thomas Szasz, "J'Accuse: How Dan White Got Away with Murder— And How American Psychiatry Helped Him Do It," *Inquiry* 20 (August 6, 1979): 17–21.

58. "A New Kind of Drug Abuse Epidemic," *Baltimore Sun,* February 5, 1975, p. 1; "Valium Abuse Remains High," *Hartford Courant,* May 23, 1977, p. 21; Norman Zinberg, "Abusers Imperil Valium," *Boston Globe,* August 29, 1976, p. 60; and "Pill-Popping can be Risky," *Boston Globe,* November 17, 1974, p. 1.

59. Mary Sykes Wylie, "Falling in Love again: A Brief History of Our Infatuation with Psychoactive Drugs," *Psychotherapy Networker* 38, no. 4 (July 2014).

60. For an insightful discussion, see Herzberg, *Happy Pills in America*.

61. Norman Sartorius, "Description and Classification of Depressive Disorders: Contributions for the Definition of the Therapy-Resistance and of Therapy-Resistant Depressions," *Pharmacopsychiatrie Neuro-Psychopharmacologie* 7, no. 2 (1974): 76–79.

62. Norman Sartorius and Thomas A. Ban, eds., *Assessment of Depression* (Berlin: Springer, 1985). For a thoughtful discussion of scales in depression studies, see Laura D. Hirshbein, "Science, Gender, and the Emergence of Depression in American Psychiatry, 1952–1980," *Journal of the History of Medicine and Allied Sciences* 61, no. 2 (January 5, 2006): 187–216.

63. See, for example, Aubrey Lewis, "'Endogenous' and 'Exogenous': A Useful Dichotomy?" *Psychological Medicine* 1, no. 3 (1971): 191–96.

64. For a slightly different pass through this history, see Edward Shorter, *How Everyone Became Depressed: The Rise and Fall of the Nervous Breakdown* (New York: Oxford University Press, 2013).

65. In this paragraph and the next, I am adapting text from my *The Cure Within* (New York: Norton, 1997). Some of my original references were L. Coleman, M.D., "Your Health: Stress Tolerance Differs," *Valley Independent* (Pittsburgh), May 21, 1973, p. 19; Alvin Toffler, *Future Shock* (New York: Random House, 1970); "The Hazards of Change," *Time*, March 1, 1971, p. 54; and Institute of Medicine, *Research on Stress and Human Health* (Washington, DC: National Academy Press, 1981), pp. 2–3.

66. "The Social Readjustment Rating Scale," *Psychosomatic Research* 11 (1967): 213–18.

67. Eugene S. Paykel et al., "Life Events and Depression: A Controlled Study," *Archives of General Psychiatry* 21, no. 6 (1969): 753–60.

68. Gerald Knox, "When the Blues Really Get You Down," *Better Homes and Gardens*, January 1974, pp. 12–18. For another popular discussion of the link between stress and depression, see David M. Alpern "All About Depression," *Cosmopolitan* August 1974, pp. 132–36.

69. Myrna M. Weissman and Gerald L. Klerman, "Sex Differences and the Epidemiology of Depression," *Archives of General Psychiatry* 34, no. 1 (January 1, 1977): 98–111.

70. Harold M. Schmeck, Jr., "Depression Is Called More Common in Women," *New York Times*, October 23, 1975.

71. Kathleen Brady, "Does Liberation Cause Depression?" *Harper's Bazaar*, February 1976, pp. 118–19. See also "Seems Work Stress Takes Toll on Liberated Women," *Jet*, March 1979, p. 44.

72. "Psychologist Cites Causes of Suicide Among Blacks," *Jet*, February 15, 1979, p. 44; and "Stresses and Strains on Black Women," *Ebony*, June 1974, pp. 33–40.

73. Richard S. Lazarus, James Deese, and Sonia F. Osler, "The Effects of Psychological Stress upon Performance," *Psychological Bulletin* 49, no. 4 (1952): 293.

74. Martin E. Seligman and Steven F. Maier, "Failure to Escape Traumatic Shock," *Journal of Experimental Psychology* 74, no. 1 (1967): 1.

75. Aaron T. Beck, *Cognitive Therapy of Depression* (New York: Guilford, 1979); Aaron T. Beck et al., "The Measurement of Pessimism: The Hopelessness

Scale," *Journal of Consulting and Clinical Psychology* 42, no. 6 (1974): 861; Steven D. Hollon and Aaron T. Beck, "Cognitive Therapy of Depression," in *Cognitive-Behavioral Interventions: Theory, Research, and Procedures*, ed. Philip C. Kendall and Steven D. Hollon (New York: Academic Press, 1979), 153–203; William R. Miller, Martin E. Seligman, and Harold M. Kurlander, "Learned Helplessness, Depression, and Anxiety," *Journal of Nervous and Mental Disease* 161, no. 5 (1975): 347–57; William R. Miller and Martin E. Seligman, "Depression and Learned Helplessness in Man," *Journal of Abnormal Psychology* 84, no. 3 (1975): 228; and David C. Klein, Ellen Fencil-Morse, and Martin E. Seligman, "Learned Helplessness, Depression, and the Attribution of Failure," *Journal of Personality and Social Psychology* 33, no. 5 (1976): 508.

76. Aaron Beck and Maria Kovacs, "A New, Fast Therapy for Depression," *Psychology Today*, January 1977, p. 94.

77. Augustus J. Rush et al., "Comparative Efficacy of Cognitive Therapy and Pharmacotherapy in the Treatment of Depressed Outpatients," *Cognitive Therapy and Research* 1, no. 1 (1977): 17–37.

78. George W. Ashcroft and D. F. Sharman, "5–Hydroxyindoles in Human Cerebrospinal Fluids," *Nature* 186 (1960): 1050–51. See also David Healy, *Let Them Eat Prozac: The Unhealthy Relationship Between the Pharmaceutical Industry and Depression* (New York: NYU Press, 2004), p. 11.

79. Alec Coppen et al., "Tryptophan in the Treatment of Depression," *Lancet* 290, no. 7527 (1967): 1178–80.

80. Alec Coppen, "The Biochemistry of Affective Disorders," *British Journal of Psychiatry* 113, no. 504 (November 1, 1967): 1237–64.

81. I am indebted for this narrative to Greenberg, *Manufacturing Depression*, pp. 167–69.

82. David T. Wong et al., "A Selective Inhibitor of Serotonin Uptake: Lilly 110140, 3-(p-Trifluoromethylphenoxy)-n-methyl-3-phenylpropylamine," *Life Sciences* 15, no. 3 (1974): 471–79, esp. 416.

83. Wong et al., "Selective Inhibitor of Serotonin Uptake," p. 416.

84. Carolyn Phillips, "Eli Lilly Facing a Shortage of New Products as Three Drugs Develop Serious Problems," *Wall Street Journal*, August 31, 1983, pp. 23, 44.

85. "Eli Lilly Drug Passes a Test," *New York Times*, September 12, 1987.

86. Martin H. Teicher, Carol Glod, and Jonathan O. Cole, "Emergence of Intense Suicidal Preoccupation During Fluoxetine Treatment," *American Journal of Psychiatry* 147, no. 2 (1990): 207; Erin Marcus, "Prozac: The Wonder Drug? The Maker of an Antidepressant Once Hailed as Safe Is Fighting Claims That the Drug Turned Patients Violent," *Washington Post*, September 9, 1990; and Natalie Angier, "Eli Lilly Facing Million-Dollar Suits on Its Antidepressant Drug Prozac," *New York Times*, August 16, 1990.

87. Peter D. Kramer, *Listening to Prozac* (New York: Penguin, 1994), pp. 9, 21.

88. Kramer, *Listening to Prozac*, p. 15.

89. Jean-Michel Bader, "Bestseller Not Drug Ad," *Lancet* 343, no. 8909 (May 28, 1994): 1353.

90. Greenberg, *Manufacturing Depression*, p. 269.

91. "Prozac Print Campaign," *Marketing Campaign Case Studies*, October 15, 2008,

http://marketing-case-studies.blogspot.com/2008/10/prozac-print-campaign.html; and Jean Grow, Jin Park, and Xiaoqi Han, "'Your Life Is Waiting!': Symbolic Meanings in Direct-to-Consumer Antidepressant Advertising," *Journal of Communication Inquiry* 30, no. 2 (2006): 163–88.

92. Quoted in Jim Folk and Marilyn Folk, "The Chemical Imbalance Theory: Officially Proven False!" June 26, 2018, www.anxietycentre.com/anxiety/chemical-imbalance.shtml.

93. Quoted in Jonathan M. Metzl, "Prozac and the Pharmacokinetics of Narrative Form," *Signs* 27, no. 2 (Winter 2002): 365–66.

94. "Study: Media Perpetuates Unsubstantiated Chemical Imbalance Theory of Depression," *Florida State University News* (March 3, 2008), http://news.fsu.edu/news/education-society/2008/03/03/study-media-perpetuates-unsubstantiated-chemical-imbalance-theory-depression/; Christopher M. France, Paul H. Lysaker, and Ryan P. Robinson, "The 'Chemical Imbalance' Explanation for Depression: Origins, Lay Endorsement, and Clinical Implications," *Professional Psychology: Research and Practice* 38, no. 4 (August 2007): 411–20; Anna Chur-Hansen and Deborah Zion, "'Let's Fix the Chemical Imbalance First, and Then We Can Work on the Problems Second': An Exploration of Ethical Implications of Prescribing an SSRI for 'Depression,'" *Monash Bioethics Review* 25, no. 1 (2006): 15–30; and Brett J. Deacon and Grayson L. Baird, "The Chemical Imbalance Explanation of Depression: Reducing Blame at What Cost?" *Journal of Social and Clinical Psychology* 28, no. 4 (April 2009): 415–35.

95. One of the most frightening claims for the risks of these drugs was that they increased the likelihood of suicidal behavior, particularly in children and adolescents. The psychiatrist (and historian of psychiatry) David Healy played a prominent role in calling attention to the evidence, which he claimed the psychopharmaceutical industry had been actively suppressing. Partly as a result of his whistle-blowing, the FDA conducted its own meta-analysis of 372 randomized clinical trials of antidepressants involving nearly 100,000 participants. They indeed found that the rate of suicidal thinking or suicidal behavior was 4 percent among patients assigned to receive an antidepressant, as compared with 2 percent among those assigned to receive placebo, but only when the patients were under eighteen. Following this finding, in October 2004, the FDA mandated that all antidepressant drugs on the market must now contain a new black-box warning (the most serious act it could take short of pulling a drug off the market), which called attention to the risk of suicidal thinking in children. The decision was controversial from the beginning, since untreated depression also puts one at (probably considerably greater) risk of suicide. See, for example, Richard A. Friedman, "Antidepressants' Black-Box Warning—10 Years Later," *New England Journal of Medicine* 371 (October 30, 2014): 1666–68. For more on David Healy's role, see Benedict Carey, "A Self-Effacing Scholar Is Psychiatry's Gadfly," *New York Times*, November 15, 2005.

96. Lauren Slater, *Blue Dreams: The Science and the Story of the Drugs That Changed Our Minds* (New York: Little, Brown, 2018).

Chapter 7: Manic-Depression

1. Richard Noll, *American Madness: The Rise and Fall of Dementia Praecox* (Cambridge, MA: Harvard University Press, 2011), p. 258.
2. J. J. Geoghegan, "Manic Depressive Psychosis and Electroshock," *Canadian Medical Association Journal* 55, no. 1 (1946): 54-55; Donald W. Hastings, "Circular Manic-Depressive Reaction Modified by 'Prophylactic Electroshock,'" *American Journal of Psychiatry* 118, no. 3 (1961): 258-60; G. H. Stevenson and A. McCausland, "Prefrontal Leucotomy for the Attempted Prevention of Recurring Manic-Depressive Illnesses," *American Journal of Psychiatry* 109, no. 9 (1953): 662-69; William W. Zeller et al., "Use of Chlorpromazine and Reserpine in the Treatment of Emotional Disorders," *Journal of the American Medical Association* 160, no. 3 (1956): 179-84; and M. Querol, F. Samanez, and M. Almeida, "Chlorpromazine in the Treatment of Schizophrenia and Manic-Depressive Psychoses," *Anales de la Facultad de Medicina* 40, no. 3 (1957): 729-46.
3. Max Byrd, *Visits to Bedlam: Madness and Literature in the Eighteenth Century* (Columbia: University of South Carolina Press, 1974); Jonathan Andrews et. al., *The History of Bethlem* (New York: Routledge, 1997).
4. E. Hare, "The Two Manias: A Study of the Evolution of the Modern Concept of Mania," *British Journal of Psychiatry* 138, no. 2 (1981): 91.
5. Christopher Baethge, Paola Salvatore, and Ross J. Baldessarini, "'On Cyclic Insanity' by Karl Ludwig Kahlbaum, MD: A Translation and Commentary," *Harvard Review of Psychiatry* 11, no. 2 (January 1, 2003): 78-90.
6. Quoted in David Healy, *The Antidepressant Era* (Cambridge, MA: Harvard University Press, 1997), p. 38.
7. As he wrote in 1920, "We have to live with the fact that the criteria applied by us are not sufficient to differentiate reliably in all cases between schizophrenia and manic-depressive insanity. And there are also many overlaps in this area." Quoted in Andreas Marneros and Jules Angst, eds., *Bipolar Disorders: 100 Years After Manic-Depressive Insanity* (New York: Springer Science and Business Media, 2007), p. 15. For the ongoing historical debate, see A. Jablensky, "The Conflict of the Nosologists: Views on Schizophrenia and Manic-Depressive Illness in the Early Part of the 20th Century," *Schizophrenia Research* 39 (1999): 95-100.
8. *Diagnostic and Statistical Manual: Mental Disorders (DSM-I)* (Washington, DC: American Psychiatric Association Mental Hospital Service, 1952), p. 25.
9. See Karl Abraham, "Notes on the Psycho-Analytical Investigation and Treatment of Manic-Depressive Insanity and Allied Conditions" (1911), in Abraham, *Selected Papers on Psychoanalysis* (New York: Basic Books, 1953). See also Sigmund Freud, "Mourning and Melancholia" (1917), in *Standard Edition of the Complete Psychological Works of Sigmund Freud*, ed. and trans. James Strachey (London: Hogarth Press, 1957), vol. 14.
10. Robert W. Gibson, "The Family Background and Early Life Experience of the Manic-Depressive Patient: A Comparison with the Schizophrenic Patient," *Psychiatry* 21, no. 1 (1958): 71-90, esp. 72.
11. Frieda Fromm-Reichmann et al., *An Intensive Study of Twelve Cases of Manic-Depressive Psychosis* (Washington, DC: Washington School of Psychiatry,

1953), pp. 74–75. See also Frieda Fromm-Reichmann, "Intensive Psychotherapy of Manic Depressives," *Confinia Neurologica* 9 (1949): 158–65.

12. Jack F. Cade, "John Frederick Joseph Cade: Family Memories on the Occasion of the 50th Anniversary of His Discovery of the Use of Lithium in Mania," *Australian and New Zealand Journal of Psychiatry* 33, no. 5 (October 1, 1999): 615–18.

13. John F. J. Cade, "Lithium Salts in the Treatment of Psychotic Excitement," *Medical Journal of Australia* 2 (1949): 349–52.

14. Cade, "Lithium Salts."

15. W. Felber, "[Lithium Prevention of Depression 100 Years Ago—An Ingenious Misconception]," *Fortschritte der Neurologie-Psychiatrie* 55, no. 5 (May 1987): 141–44.

16. For a thorough discussion, see Johan Schioldann, "From Guinea Pigs to Manic Patients: Cade's 'Story of Lithium,'" *Australian and New Zealand Journal of Psychiatry* 47, no. 5 (2013): 484–86; Johan Schioldann, *History of the Introduction of Lithium into Medicine and Psychiatry: Birth of Modern Psychopharmacology 1949* (Adelaide: Academic Press, 2009); and Johann Schioldann, "'On Periodical Depressions and Their Pathogenesis' by Carl Lange (1886)," *History of Psychiatry* 22, no. 85, pt. 1 (2011): 108–30.

17. James Greenblatt and Kayla Grossmann, *Lithium: The Untold Story of the Magic Mineral That Charges Cell Phones and Preserves Memory*, reviewed in *Townsend Letter*, October 2015, www.townsendletter.com/Oct2015/lithium 1015.html.

18. Quoted in Frederick Neil Johnson, *The History of Lithium Therapy* (Berlin: Springer, 1984), p. 48.

19. Lawrence W. Hanlon et al., "Lithium Chloride as a Substitute for Sodium Chloride in the Diet: Observations on Its Toxicity," *Journal of the American Medical Association* 139, no. 11 (March 12, 1949): 688–92; A. M. Waldron, "Lithium Intoxication," *Journal of the American Medical Association* 139, no. 11 (March 12, 1949): 733; and A. C. Corcoran, R. D. Taylor, and Irvine H. Page, "Lithium Poisoning from the Use of Salt Substitutes," *Journal of the American Medical Association* 139, no. 11 (March 12, 1949). 685–88.

20. Elliot S. Valenstein, *Blaming the Brain: The Truth about Drugs and Mental Health* (New York: Free Press, 1998), p. 43.

21. Charles Noack and Edward Trautner, "The Lithium Treatment of Maniacal Psychosis," *Medical Journal of Australia* 2, no. 7 (August 1951): 219–22. The argument for monitoring blood serum levels had been made first in response to concerns about the use of lithium compounds as a salt substitute. See J. H. Talbott, "Use of Lithium Salts as Substitutes for Sodium Chloride," *Archives of Internal Medicine* 85 (1950): 1–10.

22. Mogens Schou, "Lithium Perspectives," *Neuropsychobiology* 10, no. 1 (1983): 9.

23. Mogens Schou et al., "The Treatment of Manic Psychoses by the Administration of Lithium Salts," *Journal of Neurology, Neurosurgery, and Psychiatry* 17 (1954): 250–60.

24. Baastrup quoted in Johnson, *History of Lithium Therapy*, p. 71.

25. Poul Christian Baastrup, "The Use of Lithium in Manic-Depressive Psychosis," *Comprehensive Psychiatry* 5, no. 6 (1964): 396–408.

26. Edwin Diamond, "Lithium vs. Mental Illness," *New York Times*, January 12, 1969.

27. Poul Christian Baastrup and Mogens Schou, "Lithium as a Prophylactic Agent: Its Effect Against Recurrent Depressions and Manic-Depressive Psychosis," *Archives of General Psychiatry* 16 (1967): 162–72.

28. B. Blackwell and M. Shepherd, "Prophylactic Lithium: Another Therapeutic Myth? An Examination of the Evidence to Date," *Lancet* 1, no. 7549 (1968): 968–71.

29. Barry Blackwell, "Need for Careful Evaluation of Lithium," *American Journal of Psychiatry* 125, no. 8 (1969): 1131.

30. Paul Grof and Jules Angst, "The Lithium Controversy: Somewhat Different Hindsights, Reply to Barry Blackwell," *International Network for the History of Psychopharmacology*, November 1, 2014, http://inhn.org/controversies/barry -blackwell-the-lithium-controversy-a-historical-autopsy/comment-by-paul -grof-and-jules-angst.html.

31. Barry Blackwell, "Reply to Grof and Angst, Comment by Blackwell," *International Network for the History of Psychopharmacology*, February 5, 2015, http:// inhn.org/controversies/barry-blackwell-the-lithium-controversy-a-historical -autopsy/comment-by-paul-grof-and-jules-angst/reply-to-grof-and-angst -comment-by-blackwell.html.

32. Poul Christian Baastrup et al, "Prophylactic Lithium: Double Blind Discontinuation in Manic-Depressive and Recurrent-Depressive Disorders," *Lancet* 2, no. 7668 (August 15, 1970): 326–30.

33. Edwin Diamond, "Lithium vs Mental Illness," *New York Times*, January 12, 1969.

34. Diamond, "Lithium vs Mental Illness."

35. Stephen J. Sansweet, "Smith Kline & French Undertakes an Overhaul to Redirect Operations," *Wall Street Journal*, September 19, 1969.

36. Pfizer advertisement for Navane (thiothixene) together with an advertisment for Lithane (lithium carbonate), *American Journal of Psychiatry* 127 (August 1970).

37. Diamond, "Lithium vs Mental Illness."

38. "Dear Abby," *Austin American Statesman*, February 18, 1974, p. 37.

39. "How Drugs Are Used to Treat Mental Illness (The Better Way)," *Good Housekeeping*, March 1970, pp. 151–53.

40. Ruth Heyman, "Back from Manic-Depression," *Newsday*, June 9, 1974, p. 39.

41. "A.M.A. Speaker Says Manic Stage of Depression Aids Gifted," *New York Times*, June 25, 1973.

42. Heyman, "Back from Manic-Depression." p. 39. Similar stories can be found in Nathan Kline, *From Sad to Glad: Kline on Depression* (New York: Ballantine Books, 1987), e.g., p. 5.

43. Ronald R. Fieve, *Moodswing: The Third Revolution in Psychiatry* (New York: Morrow, 1975), p. 13.

44. Kline, *From Sad to Glad*, p. 86.

45. Very occasionally, journalists admitted this. See, for example, "How Drugs Are Used to Treat Mental Illness," *Good Housekeeping*, March 1970, p. 152.

46. Maggie Scarf, "From Depression to Joy: New Insights Into the Chemistry of Moods," *New York Times Magazine*, April 24, 1977.

47. Gina Kolata, "Manic-Depression: Is It Inherited?" *Science* 232, no. 4750 (1986): 575.
48. Thomas A. Ban, "Clinical Pharmacology and Leonhard's Classification of Endogenous Psychoses," *Psychopathology* 23, no. 4–6 (1990): 331–38.
49. Depression, he later clarified, came in two varieties: unipolar and bipolar—that is, cyclical depression, of the sort that Schou's brother suffered from, and that had responded to lithium.
50. C. A. Perris, "A Study of Bipolar (Manic-Depressive) and Unipolar Recurrent Psychotic Depression," *Acta Psychiatrica Scandinavica* 42, supp. 194. (1966): 9–14; J. Angst, "The Etiology and Nosology of Endogenous Depressive Psychoses," *Foreign Psychiatry* 2 (1966): 1–108.
51. Theodore Reich, Paula J. Clayton, and George Winokur, "Family History Studies: V. The Genetics of Mania," *American Journal of Psychiatry* 125, no. 10 (1969): 1358–69.
52. Hannah S. Decker, *The Making of DSM-III: A Diagnostic Manual's Conquest of American Psychiatry* (New York: Oxford University Press, 2013).
53. Quoted in Emily Martin, *Bipolar Expeditions: Mania and Depression in American Culture* (Princeton, NJ: Princeton University Press, 2009), p. 29.
54. Janice Egeland quoted in Patty Duke and Gloria Hochman, *Brilliant Madness: Living with Manic Depressive Illness* (New York: Random House, 2010), p. 87.
55. Jeanne Antol Krull, "Family Ties," *University of Miami Medicine Online*, 2004, http://www6.miami.edu/ummedicine-magazine/spring2004/fstory4.html.
56. Duke and Hochman, *Brilliant Madness*, p. 87.
57. Krull, "Family Ties."
58. Egeland and a colleague spelled out the arguments for seeing the Amish as a nearly perfect human laboratory for behavioral genetic research in Janice A. Egeland and Abram M. Hostetter, "Amish Study," pts. 1–3, *American Journal of Psychiatry* 401, no. 1 (1983): 56–61, 62–66, and 67–71.
59. For a critique of this assumption, see Jerry Floersch, Jeffrey Longhofer, and Kristine Latta, "Writing Amish Culture Into Genes: Biological Reductionism in a Study of Manic Depression," *Culture, Medicine and Psychiatry* 21, no. 2 (June 1, 1997): 137–59.
60. Ronald Kotulak, "Dark Heritage: Amish Study Shows Mental Illness Isn't All in the Mind," *Chicago Tribune*, May 10, 1988.
61. Janice A. Egeland et al., "Bipolar Affective Disorders Linked to DNA Markers on Chromosome 11," *Nature* 325, no. 6107 (1987): 786.
62. Steven Mark Paul, interview by Thomas Ban, December 12, 2001, in *Recollections of the History of Neuropharmacology Through Interviews Conducted by Thomas A. Ban*, ed. Peter R. Martin (Córdoba, Argentina: International Network for the History of Neuropsychopharmacology 2014), p. 912.
63. Richard Saltus, "Manic-Depression Caused by Gene, Study Indicates," *Boston Globe*, February 26, 1987, p. 1; Kotulak, "Dark Heritage."
64. John R. Kelsoe et al., "Re-Evaluation of the Linkage Relationship between Chromosome 11p Loci and the Gene for Bipolar Affective Disorder in the Old Order Amish," *Nature* 342, no. 6247 (1989): 238–43.
65. David Dunner, interview by Thomas Ban, December 13, 2001, in *An Oral History of Neuropsychopharmacology: The First Fifty Years, Peer Interviews*, vol. 7:

Special Areas. ed. Thomas A. Ban and Barry Blackwell (Brentwood, TN: American College of Neuropsychopharmacology, 2011), http://d.plnk.co/ACNP /50th/Transcripts/David%20Dunner%20by%20Thomas%20A.%20Ban.doc.

66. Fieve, *Moodswing*, p. 222. The theater producer Joshua Logan—Fieve's poster child for the brilliant manic-depressive patient—was convinced that his remarkable career on Broadway and in Hollywood owed a debt less to the medicine that made him well than to the disease that caused him such suffering. "Without my illness, active or dormant," Logan told journalists after he had "come out" about his illness, "I'm sure I would have lived only half of the life I've lived and that would be as unexciting as a safe and sane Fourth of July. I would have missed the sharpest, the rarest and, yes, the sweetest moments of my existence." "Joshua Logan, Stage and Screen Director, Dies at 79," *New York Times*, July 13, 1988.

67. Nancy Andreasen and Arthur Canter, "The Creative Writer: Psychiatric Symptoms and Family History," *Comprehensive Psychiatry* 15, no. 2 (1974): 131, 129.

68. Nancy Andreasen, "Creativity and Mental Illness: Prevalence Rates in Writers and Their First-Degree Relatives," *American Journal of Psychiatry* 144, no. 10 (October 1, 1987): 1288–92.

69. Kay Redfield Jamison, "Mood Disorders and Patterns of Creativity in British Writers and Artists," *Psychiatry*, 52, no. 2 (1989): 125–34.

70. Kay Redfield Jamison, *Touched with Fire : Manic-Depressive Illness and the Artistic Temperment* (New York: Free Press, 1993).

71. Frederick K. Goodwin and Kay Redfield Jamison, *Manic-Depressive Illness* (New York: Oxford University Press, 1990).

72. Kay Redfield Jamison, *An Unquiet Mind: A Memoir of Moods and Madness* (New York: Vintage, 1996).

73. Stephen Fried, "Creative Tension," *Washington Post Lifestyle Magazine*, April 16, 1995.

74. Quoted in Fried, "Creative Tension." Boorstin's actions here underscore the degree to which schizophrenia remained the most stigmatized mental disorder.

75. *The Diagnostic and Statistical Manual of Mental Disorders*, 3rd ed. (*DSM-III*) (Washington, DC: American Psychiatric Association, 1980), pp. 217–19.

76. David Dunner, interview by Thomas Ban, December 13, 2001, in *Recollections of the History of Neuropharmacology Through Interviews Conducted by Thomas A. Ban*, ed. Peter R. Martin (Córdoba, Argentina: International Network for the History of Neuropsychopharmacology, 2014).

77. Hagop S. Akiskal et al., "Cyclothymic Disorder: Validating Criteria for Inclusion in the Bipolar Affective Group," *American Journal of Psychiatry* 134 (1977): 1227–33.

78. See Hagop S. Akiskal, "The Bipolar Spectrum: New Concepts in Classification and Diagnosis," in *Psychiatry Update; The American Psychiatric Association Annual Review*, ed. Leonard Grinspoon (Washington, DC: American Psychiatric Press, 1983), pp. 2:271–92. See also S. Nassir Ghaemi, "Bipolar Spectrum: A Review of the Concept and a Vision for the Future," *Psychiatry Investigation* 10, no. 3 (September 2013): 218–24. I am indebted to Ghaemi for the Akiskal reference.

79. Hagop S. Akiskal and Olavo Pinto, "The Soft Bipolar Spectrum: Footnotes to Kraepelin on the Interface of Hypomania, Temperament and Depression,"

in *Bipolar Disorders: 100 Years after Manic-Depressive Insanity*, ed. Andreas Marneros and Jules Angst (New York: Springer Science and Business Media, 2007), pp. 37–62, esp. 54.

80. John McManamy, "Hagop Akiskal and the Mood Spectrum," *McMan's Depression and Bipolar Web*, May 16, 2011, http://www.mcmanweb.com/akiskal.html.

81. Goodwin and Jamison, *Manic-Depressive Illness*.

82. Goodwin and Jamison, *Manic-Depressive Illness*, pp. 4–5.

83. L. L. Judd and Hagop Akiskal, "The Prevalence and Disability of Bipolar Spectrum Disorders in the US Population: Re-Analysis of the ECA Database Taking Into Account Subthreshold Cases," *Journal of Affective Disorders* 73, nos. 1–2 (2003): 123–31.

84. Divalproex sodium, the main ingredient in Depakote, is converted into valproic acid in the stomach, which becomes the active ingredient in this medication. Valproic acid was also sold as an anticonvulsive medication under various brand names, the most common being Depakene.

85. David Healy, "The Latest Mania: Selling Bipolar Disorder," *PLOS Medicine* 3, no. 4 (April 11, 2006): e185.

86. Carmen Moreno et al., "National Trends in the Outpatient Diagnosis and Treatment of Bipolar Disorder in Youth," *Archives of General Psychiatry* 64, no. 9 (2007): 1032–39.

87. Sharna Olfman, *Bipolar Children: Cutting-Edge Controversy, Insights, and Research* (Santa Barbara, CA: Greenwood Publishing Group, 2007), pp. 4–5.

88. Dmitri F. Papolos and Janice Papolos, *The Bipolar Child: The Definitive and Reassuring Guide to Childhood's Most Misunderstood Disorder* (New York: Broadway Books, 1999).

89. "Heather," Amazon online review of *The Bipolar Child*, March 17, 2015, www.amazon.com/Bipolar-Child-Third-Definitive-Misunderstood-ebook/product-reviews/B000W969AY/ref=cm_cr_dp_d_show_all_btm?ie=UTF8 &reviewerType=all_reviews.

90. Healy, "Latest Mania," e185.

91. Shari Roan, "Parents Push for New Diagnosis of Volatile Children," *Chronicle-Telegram* (Elyria, OH), November 2, 2011, pp. 2, 7. See also Stuart L Kaplan, *Your Child Does Not Have Bipolar Disorder: How Bad Science and Good Public Relations Created the Diagnosis* (Santa Barbara, CA: Praeger, 2011).

Chapter 8: False Dawn

1. Ben Bursten, "Rallying 'Round the Medical Model," *Psychiatric Services* 32, no. 6 (June 1, 1981): 371.

2. Daniel Goleman, "Social Workers Vault into a Leading Role in Psychotherapy," *New York Times*, April 30, 1985.

3. W. Joseph Wyatt and Donna M. Midkiff, "Biological Psychiatry: A Practice in Search of a Science," *Behavior and Social Issues* 15, no. 2 (2006): 132.

4. For some contemporary perspectives on the turf wars, see Hillel Levin, "War Between the Shrinks." *New York Magazine*, May 21, 1979, pp. 52–54; and Melvin Berg, "Toward a Diagnostic Alliance Between Psychiatrist and Psychologist," *American Psychologist* 41, no. 1 (January 1986): 52–59. For a thoughtful

historical analysis, see Andrew Scull, "Contested Jurisdictions: Psychiatry, Psychoanalysis, and Clinical Psychology in the United States, 1940–2010," *Medical History* 55, no. 3 (July 2011): 401–6.

5. Goleman, "Social Workers Vault."

6. J. A. Beaulieu, *The Space Inside the Skull: Digital Representations, Brain Mapping and Cognitive Neuroscience in the Decade of the Brain*, Ph.D. diss., 2000, University of Amsterdam, https://dare.uva.nl/search?identifier=e9cc1834-d4fb-4071-a0ae-9e985a41bce5.

7. E. C. Johnstone et al., "Cerebral Ventricular Size and Cognitive Impairment in Chronic Schizophrenia," *Lancet* 2, no. 7992 (October 30, 1976): 924–26. See D. R. Weinberger et al., "Lateral Cerebral Ventricular Enlargement in Chronic Schizophrenia," *Archives of General Psychiatry* 36, no. 7 (July 1979): 735–39; and D. G. Owens et al., "Lateral Ventricular Size in Schizophrenia: Relationship to the Disease Process and Its Clinical Manifestations," *Psychological Medicine* 15, no. 1 (February 1985): 27–41.

8. Kay Redfield Jamison, *An Unquiet Mind: A Memoir of Moods and Madness* (New York: Vintage, 1996), p. 196.

9. Benedict Carey, "Can Brain Scans See Depression?" *New York Times*, October 18, 2005.

10. Tom Insel, "Understanding Mental Disorders as Circuit Disorders," National Institute of Mental Health, 2010.

11. Most of the woes of psychoanalysis in the 1990s had less directly to do with the growing prestige of biological psychiatry than with the rise of a new cohort of hostile critics. Some accused Freud personally of committing a wide range of ethical lapses, of lacking originality, and of failing his patients on a number of fronts. A separate cohort attacked the American Freudians for (among other things) systematically discrediting and silencing women who had experienced incest and other forms of traumatic sexual abuse.

   In 1993 the cover of *Time* featured a somber painting of a disappearing Freud (pieces taken out of his head like pieces from a jigsaw puzzle), accompanied by the pointed tagline "Is Freud Dead?" The accompanying cover story, "The Assault on Freud," mentioned drugs as just one reason for the decline in the fortunes of psychoanalysis and not clearly the most important. Paul Gray, "The Assault on Freud," *Time* (November 29, 1993), pp. 47–51.

   In 1998 the Library of Congress almost canceled an historical exhibition about Freud and psychoanalysis; it opened only after the exhibition designers made major changes to placate critics. A *New York Times* discussion of the drama made not a single mention of any role played by the rise of biological perspectives in psychiatry, though Margaret Talbot did observe that "managed care has been notoriously inhospitable to long-term psychotherapy and notoriously hospitable to the quicker, cheaper fixes of behavior mod and Prozac." Margaret Talbot, "The Museum Show Has an Ego Disorder," *New York Times*, October 11, 1998.

12. Marcia Angell, "The Truth About the Drug Companies," *New York Review of Books*, July 15, 2004.

13. Robert Whitaker and Lisa Cosgrove, *Psychiatry Under the Influence: Institutional Corruption, Social Injury, and Prescriptions for Reform* (New York: Palgrave Macmillan, 2015).

14. Ray Moynihan, "Key Opinion Leaders: Independent Experts or Drug Representatives in Disguise?" *BMJ* 336, no. 7658 (2008): 1402–3.

15. Quoted in Sera Davidow, "Dear NAMI: My Apologies. I've Been Unfair," *Mad in America* (blog), March 12, 2014, www.madinamerica.com/2014/03/dear-nami-apologies-ive-unfair/. The blogpost was published online but has been removed.

16. Gardiner Harris, "Drug Makers Are Advocacy Group's Biggest Donors," *New York Times*, October 21, 2009. See also Davidow, "Dear NAMI: My Apologies."

17. "Psychiatric Drug Discovery on the Couch," *Nature Reviews Drug Discovery* 6, no. 3 (March 1, 2007), doi.org/10.1038/nrd2268.

18. Pauline Anderson, "Direct-to-Consumer Ads Boost Psychiatric Drug Use," *Medscape Medical News* (September 19, 2016), www.medscape.com/viewarticle/868880.

19. Caroline Lappetito, "IMS Report 11.5% Dollar Growth in '03 US Prescription Sales" (February 17, 2004) *MS Health*, https://web.archive.org/web/20060322232805/http://www.imshealth.com/ims/portal/front/articleC/0,2777,6599_41382706_44771558,00.html.

20. Donald F. Klein, "Historical Aspects of Anxiety," *Dialogues in Clinical Neuroscience* 4, no. 3 (September 2002): 295–304.

21. Paul H. Wender and Donald F. Klein, "The Promise of Biological Psychiatry," *Psychology Today* 15 (February 1981), pp. 25–41 at 31.

22. R. L. Evans, "Alprazolam (Xanax, the Upjohn Company)," *Drug Intelligence and Clinical Pharmacy* 15, no. 9 (September 1981): 633–38; "Upjohn Drug Gets F.D.A. Approval," *New York Times*, November 3, 1981.

23. David Sheehan cited in Andrea Tone, *The Age of Anxiety: A History of America's Turbulent Affair with Tranquilizers* (New York: Basic Books, 2009), p. 281n18.

24. James C. Ballenger et al., "Alprazolam in Panic Disorder and Agoraphobia: Results from a Multicenter Trial: I. Efficacy in Short-Term Treatment," *Archives of General Psychiatry* 45, no. 5 (1988): 413–22; C. Ballenger, "Alprazolam in Panic Disorder and Agoraphobia," *Archives of General Psychiatry* 45 (1988): 413–22; and Gerald L. Klerman, "Overview of the Cross-National Collaborative Panic Study: I. Efficacy in Short-Term Treatment," *Archives of General Psychiatry* 45, no. 5 (1988): 407–12, esp. 408.

25. The researchers involved in this trial may have downplayed the evidence that the drug ceased to be more effective than placebo after about four weeks, while also tending to downplay the degree to which the drug, taken for any length of time, created dependency. See Robert Whitaker, "A Journalist's Dilemma," and "High Anxiety," *Consumer Reports Magazine*, January 1993.

26. L. Miller, "Listening to Xanax: How America Learned to Stop Worrying About Worrying and Pop Its Pills Instead," *New York Magazine*, March 26, 2012.

27. Miller, "Listening to Xanax."

28. Associated Press, "Xanax Is Ruining People's Lives," *New York Post* (blog), June 9, 2016.

29. Brendan I. Koerner, "Disorders Made to Order," *Mother Jones*, August 2002.

30. Bali Sunset, "Social Anxiety Disorder Campaign," *Marketing Campaign Case Studies* (blog), March 28, 2009, http://marketing-case-studies.blogspot.com/2009/03/social-anxiety-disorder-campaign.html.

31. Rebekah Bradley et al., "A Multidimensional Meta-Analysis of Psychotherapy for PTSD," *American Journal of Psychiatry* 162, no. 2 (2005): 214–27.
32. Koerner, "Disorders Made to Order."
33. Chandler Chicco Agency, "PTSD Alliance Offers Free Educational Resources," Newswise, August 16, 2002, www.newswise.com//articles/view/31140?print-article.
34. "FDA Approves Antidepressant for Generalized Anxiety Disorder," *Psychiatric News*, May 18, 2001, doi.org/10.1176/pn.36.10.0014b.
35. John Crilly, "The History of Clozapine and Its Emergence in the US Market: A Review and Analysis," *History of Psychiatry* 18, no. 1 (March 2007): 39–60.
36. Herbert Y. Meltzer, "The Role of Serotonin in Antipsychotic Drug Action," *Neuropsychopharmacology* 21, no. S1 (August 1, 1999): 1395370.
37. J. Kane et al., "Clozapine for the Treatment-Resistant Schizophrenic: A Double-Blind Comparison with Chlorpromazine," *Archives of General Psychiatry* 45, no. 9 (September 1988): 789–96.
38. Claudia Wallis and James Willwerth, "Awakenings: Schizophrenia: A New Drug Brings Patients Back to Life," *Time*, July 6, 1992.
39. Ken Duckworth, "Awakenings with the New Antipsychotics," *Psychiatric Times* 15, no. 5 (May 1, 1998): 65–66.
40. Quoted in Ben Wallace-Wells, "Bitter Pill," *Rolling Stone*, no. 1071 (2009): 56–63, 74–76.
41. Alex Berenson, "Disparity Emerges in Lilly Data on Schizophrenia Drug," *New York Times*, December 21, 2006; Alex Berenson, "Drug Files Show Maker Promoted Unapproved Use," *New York Times*, December 18, 2006; and Alex Berenson, "Eli Lilly Said to Play Down Risk of Top Pill," *New York Times*, December 17, 2006. All the leaked documents—even though a court ordered them to be returned to Eli Lilly—can still be found at https://web.archive.org/web/20081222083925/http://www.furiousseasons.com:80/zyprexadocs.html.
42. Alex Berenson, "Lilly Settles With 18,000 Over Zyprexa," *New York Times*, January 5, 2007.
43. Gardiner Harris and Alex Berenson, "Lilly Said to Be Near $1.4 Billion U.S. Settlement," *New York Times*, January 14, 2009.
44. Phoebe Sparrow Wagner, "Eli Lilly and the Dangers of a Drug" (letter to the editor), *New York Times*, December 20, 2006. Phoebe (previously Pamela) Wagner—a memoirist, poet and artist—generously gave permission for her 2006 letter to be quoted, but with the understanding that it also be made clear in a note that she would not write a letter like that today. Her current view, as she explained in an email, is that psychiatry and the drug companies have deceitfully promoted the idea that drugs ameliorate a "chemical imbalance" in the brain when they knew no such thing existed, and that drugs like Zyprexa are "not only useless, they are harmful."
45. The expression began to be widely used in the mid-1990s, as inferred from Google's Ngram Viewer: https://books.google.com/ngrams/graph?content=Big+Pharma&year_start=1800&year_end=2000&corpus=15&smoothing=3&share=&direct_url=t1%3B%2CBig%20Pharma%3B%2Cc0.
46. Marcia Angell, *The Truth About the Drug Companies: How They Deceive Us and What to Do About It* (New York: Random House, 2004). The quotations here

are from Marcia Angell, "The Truth About the Drug Companies," *New York Review of Books*, July 15, 2004.

47. Alison Bass, *Side Effects: A Prosecutor, a Whistleblower, and a Bestselling Antidepressant on Trial* (Chapel Hill, NC: Algonquin Books, 2008); Melody Petersen, *Our Daily Meds: How the Pharmaceutical Companies Transformed Themselves into Slick Marketing Machines and Hooked the Nation on Prescription Drugs* (New York: Farrar, Straus and Giroux, 2008); Christopher Lane, *Shyness: How Normal Behavior Became a Sickness* (New Haven, CT: Yale University Press, 2007); David Healy, *Let Them Eat Prozac* (New York: NYU Press, 2004); Charles Barber, *Comfortably Numb: How Psychiatry Medicated a Nation* (New York: Random House, 2008); Robert Whitaker, *Anatomy of an Epidemic: Magic Bullets, Psychiatric Drugs, and the Astonishing Rise of Mental Illness in America* (New York: Crown, 2010).

48. J. Lenzer, "Scandals Have Eroded US Public's Confidence in Drug Industry," *BMJ* 329, no. 7460 (July 29, 2004): 247.

49. This is still a requirement for all drugs today, with the important caveat that in some cases, companies are required to compare a new treatment against an existing one instead of against a placebo, for ethical reasons. That said, companies still prefer to use the classical placebo control in their trials because they assume it is easier to prove that a new drug is better than nothing (i.e., better than the placebo) than to prove that it is better than something (an existing treatment).

50. See, for example, Anne Harrington, ed., *The Placebo Effect: An Interdisciplinary Exploration* (Cambridge, MA: Harvard University Press, 1999).

51. Irving Kirsch, "Antidepressants and the Placebo Effect," *Zeitschrift für Psychologie* 222, no. 3 (2014): 128–34.

52. Irving Kirsch and Guy Sapirstein, "Listening to Prozac but Hearing Placebo: A Meta-Analysis of Antidepressant Medication," *Prevention and Treatment* 1, no. 2 (June 1998).

53. Donald F. Klein, "Listening to Meta-Analysis but Hearing Bias," *Prevention and Treatment* 1, no. 2 (June 1998), doi.org/10.1037/1522–3736.1.1.16c.

54. Irving Kirsch et al., "The Emperor's New Drugs: An Analysis of Antidepressant Medication Data Submitted to the U.S. Food and Drug Administration," *Prevention and Treatment* 5, no. 1 (July 2002), doi.org/10.1037/1522–3736.5.1.523a.

55. Kirsch, "Antidepressants and Placebo Effect."

56. Kirsch et al., "Emperor's New Drugs."

57. Arif Khan, H. A. Warner, and Walter A. Brown, "Symptom Reduction and Suicide Risk in Patients Treated with Placebo in Antidepressant Clinical Trials: An Analysis of the Food and Drug Administration Database," *Archives of General Psychiatry* 57, no. 4 (April 2000): 311–17; and Arif Khan and Walter A. Brown, "Antidepressants Versus Placebo in Major Depression: An Overview," *World Psychiatry* 14, no. 3 (October 2015): 294–300.

58. Steve Silberman, "Placebos Are Getting More Effective: Drugmakers Are Desperate to Know Why," *Wired*, August 24, 2009; "Merck Disappointment as Highly-Touted Antidepressant Stalls," *Pharma Letter*, January 26, 1999.

59. Silberman, "Placebos Are Getting More Effective."

60. Christopher Lane, "Listening to Placebo, Especially in the U.S." (blogpost),

Psychology Today, October 23, 2015; Jo Marchant, "Placebo Effect Grows in U.S., Thwarting Development of Painkillers," *Scientific American,* October 7, 2015.

61. Silberman, "Placebos Are Getting More Effective."

62. Andrew Gelman and Kaiser Fung, "How Drug Companies Game the Placebo Effect," *Daily Beast,* November 3, 2015.

63. While clinicians have been aware for some time of the heterogeneity of patient responses to antidepressants, I have found limited published discussion of the role it was discovered to have played in industry-sponsored failed clinical trials. One exception is B. A. Arnow et al., "Depression Subtypes in Predicting Anti-depressant Response: A Report from the iSPOT-D trial," *American Journal of Psychiatry* 172, no. 8 (2015): 743–50. I owe my own initial awareness of the problem to Steven Hyman, especially a long and thoughtful email he sent me on May 2, 2018.

64. Eiko I. Fried, "Moving Forward: How Depression Heterogeneity Hinders Progress in Treatment and Research," *Expert Review of Neurotherapeutics* 17, no. 5 (2017): 423–25; and Eiko I. Fried, "The 52 Symptoms of Major Depression: Lack of Content Overlap Among Seven Common Depression Scales," *Journal of Affective Disorders* 208 (January 15, 2017): 191–97. For a review of the frustrated and frustrating effort to identify biomarkers, see Rebecca Strawbridge, Allan Young, and Anthony J. Cleare, "Biomarkers for Depression: Recent Insights, Current Challenges and Future Prospects," *Neuropsychiatric Disease and Treatment* 13 (2017): 1245–62.

65. Thomas Insel et al., "Research Domain Criteria (RDoC): Toward a New Classification Framework for Research on Mental Disorders," *American Journal of Psychiatry* 167, no. 7 (2010): 748–51.

66. Committee for Medicinal Products for Human Use, "Reflection Paper on the Need for Active Control in Therapeutic Areas Where Use of Placebo Is Deemed Ethical and One or More Established Medicines Are Available," European Medicines Agency, www.ema.europa.eu/docs/en_GB/document_library/Scientific_guideline/2011/01/WC500100710.pdf.

67. Steven Hyman to author, May 2, 2018.

68. Steven E. Hyman, "Revolution Stalled," *Science Translational Medicine* 4, no. 155 (October 10, 2012): 1. Hyman made these points as early as 2008, when he bluntly admitted that "no new drug targets or therapeutic mechanisms of real significance have been identified for more than four decades." He suggested at the time that nevertheless some hope could be found—"glimmers of light"—in modern developments in genomics, and he continues to be a leading figure in this field. See Steven E. Hyman, "A Glimmer of Light for Neuropsychiatric Disorders," *Nature* 455, no. 7215 (October 15, 2008).

69. Greg Miller, "Is Pharma Running Out of Brainy Ideas?" *Science* 329, no. 5991 (July 30, 2010): 502–4; and Daniel Cressey, "Psychopharmacology in Crisis," *Nature* 10 (2011).

70. The single significant exception to this trend is growing industry interest in the potential of ketamine—currently an illegal party drug—to act as a new kind of antidepressant. Ketamine does not target the catecholamine systems but instead acts on the glutaminergic system. For a sense of the

growing excitement, see Alex Matthews-King, "Remarkable Secrets of Ketamine's Antidepressant Effect Unlocked by Scientists," *Independent*, February 15, 2018.

71. Olivia Meadowcrot, "The End of the Prozac Era: Why Pharma Is Abandoning Psychiatry," *Medicine.co.uk*, July 28, 2017, http://medicine.co.uk/?p=856.

72. Thomas Insel, "Transforming Diagnosis," *NIMH Director's BlogPosts from 2013* (blog), April 29, 2013.

73. Cited in Gary Greenberg, *Manufacturing Depression: The Secret History of a Modern Disease* (New York: Simon and Schuster, 2010), p. 316.

74. Quoted in Pam Belluck and Benedict Carey, "Psychiatry's New Guide Falls Short, Experts Say," *New York Times*, May 6, 2013.

75. Herb Kutchins, *Making Us Crazy. DSM. The Psychiatric Bible and the Creation of Mental Disorders* (New York: Free Press, 1997).

76. For such a critique, see Eve Leeman, "Driven Crazy by DSM Criteria," *Lancet* 351, no. 9105 (March 14, 1998): 842–43.

77. Nancy C. Andreasen, "DSM and the Death of Phenomenology in America: An Example of Unintended Consequences," *Schizophrenia Bulletin* 33, no. 1 (January 1, 2007): 108–12, doi.org/10.1093/schbul/sbl054.

78. Allen Frances, "Whither DSM-V?" *British Journal of Psychiatry* 195, no. 5 (November 1, 2009): 391–92, esp. 391.

79. Allen J. Frances, "DSM 5 Is Guide Not Bible—Ignore Its Ten Worst Changes" (blogpost), *Psychology Today*, December 2, 2012.

80. Steven Hyman, interview by author, November 24, 2010.

81. "DSM-5 Overview: The Future Manual," American Psychiatric Association, DSM-5 Development, available at www.edscuola.eu/wordpress/wp-content/uploads/2013/11/Relazione-sui-lavori-del-Gruppo-di-studio-sul-DSM-V.pdf. See also David J. Kupfer, "DSM-5: The Future of Psychiatric Diagnosis," American Psychiatric Association, n.d., www.dsm5.org/pages/default.aspx.

82. Frances, "Whither DSM–V?" p. 392.

83. Bob Roehr, "American Psychiatric Association explains DSM-5," *BMJ* 346 (June 6, 2013), doi.org/10.1136/bmj.f3591.

84. Belluck and Carey, "Psychiatry's New Guide Falls Short."

85. Antonio Regalado, "Q&A with Tom Insel on His Decision to Join Alphabet," *MIT Technology Review*, September 21, 2015. See also David Dobbs, "The Smart Phone Psychiatrist," *Atlantic*, July–August 2017.

86. Courtney Humphries, "Probing Psychoses," *Harvard Magazine*, August 2017.

Afterthoughts

1. Ironically, recent campaigns to promote the view that mental disorders are diseases no different from any other have in some cases exacerbated the stigma, not reduced it. See Patrick W. Corrigan and Amy C. Watson, "At Issue: Stop the Stigma: Call Mental Illness a Brain Disease," *Schizophrenia Bulletin* 30, no. 3 (January 1, 2004): 477–79; and Jason Schnittker, "An Uncertain Revolution: Why the Rise of a Genetic Model of Mental Illness Has Not Increased Tolerance," *Social Science and Medicine* 67, no. 9 (2008): 1370–81.

2. Karen J. Coleman et al., "Racial-Ethnic Differences in Psychiatric Diagnoses

and Treatment Across 11 Health Care Systems in the Mental Health Research Network," *Psychiatric Services* 67, no. 7 (2016): 749–57.

3. Barbara Sicherman, "The Uses of a Diagnosis: Doctors, Patients, and Neurasthenia," *Journal of the History of Medicine and Allied Sciences* 32, no. 1, (January 1977): 33–54.

4. Quoted in David Dobbs, "The Touch of Madness," *Pacific Standard Magazine*, October 3, 2017, p. 5, https://psmag.com/magazine/the-touch-of-madness-mental-health-schizophrenia.

5. S. Button et al. (2012), "Power Failure: Why Small Sample Size Undermines the Reliability of Neuroscience," *Nature Reviews Neuroscience* 14 (2012): 365–76; S. Kapur, A. G. Phillips, and T.R. Insel, "Why Has It Taken So Long for Biological Psychiatry to Develop Clinical Tests and What to Do About It?" *Molecular Psychiatry* 17 (December 2012): 1174–79; Steven E. Hyman, "The Daunting Polygenicity of Mental Illness: Making a New Map," *Philosophical Transactions of the Royal Society: Biological Sciences,* January 19, 2018.

6. Charles Scott Sherrington, *Man on His Nature* (New York: C. Scribner's Sons, 1955), p. 191.

GUIDE TO FURTHER READING

Nineteenth-Century Brain Psychiatry and Neurology

Boller, François, and Daniel Birnbaum. "Silas Weir Mitchell: Neurologists and Neurology During the American Civil War." *Frontiers of Neurology and Neuroscience* 38 (2016): 93–106.

Decker, Hannah S. "The Psychiatric Works of Emil Kraepelin: A Many-Faceted Story of Modern Medicine." *Journal of the History of the Neurosciences* 13, no. 3 (September 2004): 248–76.

Engstrom, Eric J. "'On the Question of Degeneration' by Emil Kraepelin (1908)." *History of Psychiatry* 18, no. 3 (September 1, 2007): 389–98.

———. *Clinical Psychiatry in Imperial Germany: A History of Psychiatric Practice.* Ithaca, NY: Cornell University Press, 2003.

Engstrom, Eric J., and Kenneth S. Kendler. "Emil Kraepelin: Icon and Reality." *American Journal of Psychiatry* 172, no. 12 (September 11, 2015): 1190–96.

Goetz, Christopher G., Michel Bonduelle, and Toby Gelfand. *Charcot: Constructing Neurology.* New York: Oxford University Press, 1995.

Guenther, Katja. *Localization and Its Discontents: A Genealogy of Psychoanalysis and the Neuro Disciplines.* Chicago: University of Chicago Press, 2015.

Hagner, Michael. "Cultivating the Cortex in German Neuroanatomy." *Science in Context* 14, no. 4 (December 2001): 541–63.

———. "The Electrical Excitability of the Brain: Toward the Emergence of an Experiment." *Journal of the History of the Neurosciences* 21, no. 3 (July 2012): 237–49.

Hakosalo, Heini. "The Brain Under the Knife: Serial Sectioning and the Development of Late Nineteenth-Century Neuroanatomy." *Studies in History and Philosophy of Science Part C: Studies in History and Philosophy of Biological and Biomedical Sciences* 37, no. 2 (June 2006): 172–202.

Hirschmüller, Albrecht, and Magda Whitrow. "The Development of Psychiatry and Neurology in the Nineteenth Century." *History of Psychiatry* 10, no. 40 (1999): 395–423.

Koehler, Peter J. "Eduard Hitzig's Experiences in the Franco-Prussian War (1870–1871): The Case of Joseph Masseau." *Journal of the History of the Neurosciences* 21, no. 3 (July 2012): 250–62.

Pick, Daniel. *Faces of Degeneration: A European Disorder, c.1848–1918.* Cambridge, UK: Cambridge University Press, 1993.

Torrey, Edwin Fuller. "The Year Neurology Almost Took Over Psychiatry." *Psychiatric Times*, 2002.

Weiss, Kenneth J. "Asylum Reform and the Great Comeuppance of 1894—Or Was It?" *Journal of Nervous and Mental Disease* 199, no. 9 (September 2011): 631–38.

Hysteria, Nervousness, Psychotherapy, and Psychoanalysis

Barke, Megan, Rebecca Fribush, and Peter N. Stearns. "Nervous Breakdown in 20th-Century American Culture." *Journal of Social History* 33, no. 3 (2000): 565–84.

Beels, C. Christian. "Notes for a Cultural History of Family Therapy." *Family Process* 41, no. 1 (March 2002): 67–82.

Brown, Edward M. "Neurology's Influence on American Psychiatry, 1865–1915." In *History of Psychiatry and Medical Psychology*, edited by Edwin R. Wallace IV and John Gach. New York: Springer, 2010.

Burnham, John, ed. *After Freud Left: A Century of Psychoanalysis in America.* Chicago: University of Chicago Press, 2012.

Caplan, Eric. *Mind Games: American Culture and the Birth of Psychotherapy.* Berkeley: University of California Press, 1998.

Cushman, Philip. *Constructing the Self, Constructing America: A Cultural History of Psychotherapy.* New York: Da Capo Press, 1996.

Didi-Huberman, Georges. *Invention of Hysteria: Charcot and the Photographic Iconography of the Salpetrière.* Cambridge, MA: MIT Press, 2004.

Forrester, John. "'A Whole Climate of Opinion': Rewriting the History of Psychoanalysis." In *Discovering the History of Psychiatry*, edited by Mark Micale and Roy Porter. New York: Oxford University Press, 1994.

———. *Dispatches from the Freud Wars: Psychoanalysis and Its Passions.* Cambridge, MA: Harvard University Press, 1998.

Gijswijt-Hofstra, Marijke, and Roy Porter, eds. *Cultures of Neurasthenia: From Beard to the First World War.* New York: Rodopi, 2001.

Hale, Nathan G., Jr. *The Rise and Crisis of Psychoanalysis in the United States: Freud and the Americans, 1917–1985.* New York: Oxford University Press, 1995.

Makari, George. *Revolution in Mind: The Creation of Psychoanalysis.* New York: HarperCollins, 2008.

Mental Hygiene, Eugenics, and the Interwar Years

Cohen, Sol. "The Mental Hygiene Movement, the Development of Personality and the School: The Medicalization of American Education." *History of Education Quarterly* 23, no. 2 (Summer 1983): 123–49.

Dowbiggin, Ian Robert. *Keeping America Sane: Psychiatry and Eugenics in the United States and Canada, 1880–1940*. Ithaca, NY: Cornell University Press, 1997.

Jones, Kathleen W. *Taming the Troublesome Child: American Families, Child Guidance, and the Limits of Psychiatric Authority*. Cambridge, MA: Harvard University Press, 1999.

Ladd-Taylor, Molly. "Child Guidance and the Democratization of Mother-Blaming." *Reviews in American History* 28, no. 4 (2000): 593–600.

Lamb, S. D. *Pathologist of the Mind: Adolf Meyer and the Origins of American Psychiatry*. Baltimore: Johns Hopkins University Press, 2014.

Lombardo, Paul A. *Three Generations, No Imbeciles: Eugenics, the Supreme Court, and Buck V. Bell*. Baltimore: Johns Hopkins University Press, 2008.

Lunbeck, Elizabeth. *The Psychiatric Persuasion: Knowledge, Gender, and Power in Modern America*. Princeton, NJ: Princeton University Press, 1995.

Pols, Hans. "Beyond the Clinical Frontiers": The American Mental Hygiene Movement, 1910–1945." In *International Relations in Psychiatry: Britain, Germany, and the United States to World War II*, edited by Volker Roelcke, Paul J. Weindling, and Louise Westwood. Rochester, NY: University of Rochester Press, 2010.

———. "Divergences in American Psychiatry During the Depression: Somatic Psychiatry, Community Mental Hygiene, and Social Reconstruction." *Journal of the History of the Behavioral Sciences* 37 (2001): 369–88.

Richardson, Theresa R. *The Century of the Child: The Mental Hygiene Movement and Social Policy in the United States and Canada*. Albany: SUNY Press, 1989.

Biological Treatments Before Drugs

Aruta, Alessandro. "Shocking Waves at the Museum: The Bini-Cerletti Electro-Shock Apparatus." *Medical History* 55, no. 3 (July 2011): 407–12.

Braslow, Joel. "History and Evidence-Based Medicine: Lessons from the History of Somatic Treatments from the 1900s to the 1950s." *Mental Health Services Research* 1, no. 4 (1999): 231–40.

———. *Mental Ills and Bodily Cures: Psychiatric Treatment in the First Half of the Twentieth Century*. Berkeley: University of California Press, 1997.

Brown, Edward M. "Why Wagner-Jauregg Won the Nobel Prize for Discovering Malaria Therapy for General Paresis of the Insane." *History of Psychiatry* 11 (2000): 371–82.

Doroshow, Deborah Blythe. "Performing a Cure for Schizophrenia: Insulin Coma Therapy on the Wards." *Journal of the History of Medicine and Allied Sciences* 62, no. 2 (April 1, 2007): 213–43.

Noll, Richard. "The Blood of the Insane." *History of Psychiatry* 17, no. 4 (December 1, 2006): 395–418.

———. "Historical Review: Autointoxication and Focal Infection Theories of Dementia Praecox." *World Journal of Biological Psychiatry* 5, no. 2 (January 2004): 66–72.

———. "Infectious Insanities, Surgical Solutions: Bayard Taylor Holmes, Dementia Praecox and Laboratory Science in Early 20th-Century America. Part 2." *History of Psychiatry* 17, no. 67, pt. 3 (September 2006): 299–311.

———. "Kraepelin's 'Lost Biological Psychiatry'? Autointoxication, Organotherapy and Surgery for Dementia Praecox." *History of Psychiatry* 18, no. 3 (2007): 301–20.

Pressman, Jack D. *Last Resort: Psychosurgery and the Limits of Medicine*. Cambridge, MA: Cambridge University Press, 2002.

Scull, Andrew T. *Madhouse: A Tragic Tale of Megalomania and Modern Medicine*. New Haven: Yale University Press, 2005.

Shorter, Edward, and David Healy. *Shock Therapy: A History of Electroconvulsive Treatment in Mental Illness*. New Brunswick, NJ: Rutgers University Press, 2007.

Valenstein, Elliot S. *Great and Desperate Cures: The Rise and Decline of Psychosurgery & Other Radical Treatments for Mental Illness*. New York: Perseus Books, 1987.

Drugs and Psychopharmacology

Acker, Caroline Jean, and Sarah W. Tracy. *Altering American Consciousness: The History of Alcohol and Drug Use in the United States, 1800–2000*. Amherst: University of Massachusetts Press, 2004.

Ban, Thomas A. "Fifty Years of Chlorpromazine: A Historical Perspective." *Neuropsychiatric Disease and Treatment* 3, no. 4 (August 2007): 495–500.

Callard, Felicity. "The Intimate Geographies of Panic Disorder: Parsing Anxiety through Psychopharmacological Dissection." *Osiris* 31, no. 1 (2016): 203–26.

Dyck, Erika. *Psychedelic Psychiatry: LSD from Clinic to Campus*. Baltimore: Johns Hopkins University Press, 2008.

Green, A. R. "Gaddum and LSD: The Birth and Growth of Experimental and Clinical Neuropharmacology Research on 5-HT in the UK." *British Journal of Pharmacology* 154, no. 8 (August 1, 2008): 1583–99.

Healy, David. *The Creation of Psychopharmacology*. Cambridge, MA: Harvard University Press, 2002.

——. *Let Them Eat Prozac: The Unhealthy Relationship Between the Pharmaceutical Industry and Depression*. New York: NYU Press, 2004.

Hewitt, Kim. "Rehabilitating LSD History in Postwar America: Dilworth Wayne Woolley and the Serotonin Hypothesis of Mental Illness." *History of Science* 54, no. 3 (September 1, 2016): 307–30.

Mills, John A. "Hallucinogens as Hard Science: The Adrenochrome Hypothesis for the Biogenesis of Schizophrenia." *History of Psychology* 13, no. 2 (May 2010): 178–95.

Moncrieff, Joanna. "Magic Bullets for Mental Disorders: The Emergence of the Concept of an 'Antipsychotic' Drug." *Journal of the History of the Neurosciences* 22, no. 1 (January 2013): 30–46.

Mulinari, Shai. "Monoamine Theories of Depression: Historical Impact on Biomedical Research." *Journal of the History of the Neurosciences* 21, no. 4 (2012): 366–92.

Novak, Steven J. "LSD Before Leary: Sidney Cohen's Critique of 1950s Psychedelic Drug Research." *Isis* 88, no. 1 (1997): 87–110.

Rasmussen, Nicolas. "Making the First Anti-Depressant: Amphetamine in American Medicine, 1929–1950." *Journal of the History of Medicine and Allied Sciences* 61, no. 3 (February 21, 2006): 288–323.

——. *On Speed: From Benzedrine to Adderall*. New York: NYU Press, 2009.

Schioldann, Johan. "From Guinea Pigs to Manic Patients: Cade's 'Story of Lithium.'" *Australian and New Zealand Journal of Psychiatry* 47, no. 5 (2013): 484–86.

————. History of the Introduction of Lithium into Medicine and Psychiatry: Birth of Modern Psychopharmacology 1949. Australia: Brascoe Publishing, 2009.

Slater, Lauren. Blue Dreams: The Science and the Story of the Drugs That Changed Our Minds. Boston: Little, Brown, 2018.

Tone, Andrea. The Age of Anxiety: A History of America's Turbulent Affair with Tranquilizers. New York: Basic Books, 2009.

Valenstein, Elliot S. Blaming the Brain: The Truth about Drugs and Mental Health. New York: Free Press, 1998.

————. The War of the Soups and the Sparks: The Discovery of Neurotransmitters and the Dispute over How Nerves Communicate. New York: Columbia University Press, 2005.

Weiss, Nicholas. "No One Listened to Imipramine." In Altering American Consciousness: The History of Alcohol and Drug Use in the United States, 1800–2000, edited by Caroline Jean Acker and Sarah W. Tracy. Amherst: University of Massachusetts Press, 2004.

Post–World War II Professional Relations and Political Agendas

Brunner, José, and Orna Ophir. "'In Good Times and in Bad': Boundary Relations of Psychoanalysis in Post-War USA." History of Psychiatry 22, no. 2 (2011): 215–31.

Gitre, Edward J. K. "The Great Escape: World War II, Neo-Freudianism, and the Origins of U.S. Psychocultural Analysis." Journal of the History of the Behavioral Sciences 47, no. 1 (December 1, 2011): 18–43.

Grob, Gerald N. The Mad Among Us: A History of the Care of America's Mentally Ill. New York: Free Press, 1994.

Herman, Ellen. The Romance of American Psychology: Political Culture in the Age of Experts. Berkeley. University of California Press, 1995.

Menninger, Roy, and John C. Nemiah, eds. American Psychiatry After World War II, 1944–1994. Washington DC: American Psychiatric Press, 2000.

Plant, Rebecca Jo. "William Menninger and American Psychoanalysis, 1946–48." History of Psychiatry 16, no. 2 (June 1, 2005): 181–202.

Raz, Mical. "Between the Ego and the Icepick: Psychosurgery, Psychoanalysis, and Psychiatric Discourse." Bulletin of the History of Medicine 82, no. 2 (Summer 2008): 387–420.

Sadowsky, Jonathan Hal. "Beyond the Metaphor of the Pendulum: Electroconvulsive Therapy, Psychoanalysis, and the Styles of American Psychiatry." Journal of the History of Medicine and Allied Sciences 61, no. 1 (2006): 1–25.

Scull, Andrew. "Contested Jurisdictions: Psychiatry, Psychoanalysis, and Clinical Psychology in the United States, 1940–2010." Medical History 55, no. 3 (July 2011): 401–6.

————. "The Mental Health Sector and the Social Sciences in Post–World War II USA," parts 1 and 2. History of Psychiatry 22, no. 1 (2011): 3–19, and no. 3 (2011): 268–84.

Tomes, Nancy. "Beyond the 'Two Psychiatries': Jack Pressman's Last Resort and the History of Twentieth-Century American Psychiatry: Introduction." Bulletin of the History of Medicine 74, no. 4 (2000): 773–77.

Weinstein, Deborah F. "Culture at Work: Family Therapy and the Culture Concept in Post–World War II America." Journal of the History of the Behavioral Sciences 40, no. 1 (December 1, 2004): 23–46.

Deinstitutionalization and Its Aftermath

English, J. T. "Early Models of Community Mental Health Programs: The Vision of Robert Felix and the Example of Alan Kraft." *Psychiatric Quarterly* 62, no. 3 (1991): 257–65.

Grob, Gerald N. "Historical Origins of Deinstitutionalization." *New Directions for Mental Health Services* 17 (1983): 15–29.

Johnson, Ann Braden. *Out of Bedlam: The Truth About Deinstitutionalization*. New York: Basic Books, 1992.

Parsons, Anne E. *From Asylum to Prison: Deinstitutionalization and the Rise of Mass Incarceration After 1945*. Chapel Hill: University of North Carolina Press, 2018.

Rochefort, David A. "Origins of the 'Third Psychiatric Revolution': The Community Mental Health Centers Act of 1963." *Journal of Health Politics Policy and Law* 9, no. 1 (April 1, 1984): 1–30.

Roth, Alisa. *Insane: America's Criminal Treatment of Mental Illness*. New York: Basic Books, 2018.

Gender, Mothers, and Families

Cuordileone, K. A. "'Politics in an Age of Anxiety': Cold War Political Culture and the Crisis in American Masculinity, 1949–1960." *Journal of American History* 87, no. 2 (September 2000): 515–45.

Cuordileone, Kyle A. *Manhood and American Political Culture in the Cold War*. London: Routledge, 2005.

Dolnick, Edward. *Madness on the Couch: Blaming the Victim in the Heyday of Psychoanalysis*. New York: Simon and Schuster, 1998.

Harrington, Anne. "Mother Love and Mental Illness: An Emotional History." *Osiris* 31, no. 1 (2016): 94–115.

Hirshbein, Laura D. "Science, Gender, and the Emergence of Depression in American Psychiatry, 1952–1980." *Journal of the History of Medicine and Allied Sciences* 61, no. 2 (January 5, 2006): 187–216.

May, Elaine Tyler. *Homeward Bound: American Families in the Cold War Era*. New York: Basic Books, 2008.

Metzl, Jonathan M. "'Mother's Little Helper': The Crisis of Psychoanalysis and the Miltown Resolution." *Gender and History* 15, no. 2 (August 2003): 228–55.

Metzl, Jonathan Michel. *Prozac on the Couch: Prescribing Gender in the Era of Wonder Drugs*. Durham, NC: Duke University Press, 2003.

Plant, Rebecca Jo. *Mom: The Transformation of Motherhood in Modern America*. Chicago: University of Chicago Press, 2010.

Weinstein, Deborah. *The Pathological Family: Postwar America and the Rise of Family Therapy*. Ithaca, NY: Cornell University Press, 2013.

Race

Adriaens, Pieter R., Andreas De Block, and Dennis Doyle. "'Racial Differences Have to Be Considered': Lauretta Bender, Bellevue Hospital, and the African American Psyche, 1936–52." *History of Psychiatry* 21, no. 2 (June 1, 2010): 206–23.

Bailey, Zinzi D., et al. "Structural Racism and Health Inequities in the USA: Evidence and Interventions." *Lancet* 389, no. 10077 (April 2017): 1453–63.

Deutsch, Albert. "The First US Census of the Insane (1840) and Its Use as Pro-Slavery Propaganda." *Bulletin of the History of Medicine* 15, no. 5 (1944): 469–82.

Doyle, Dennis. "'Where the Need Is Greatest': Social Psychiatry and Race-Blind Universalism in Harlem's Lafargue Clinic, 1946–1958." *Bulletin of the History of Medicine* 83, no. 4 (2009): 746–74.

Doyle, Dennis A. *Psychiatry and Racial Liberalism in Harlem, 1936–1968.* Suffolk, England: Boydell and Brewer, 2016.

Feldstein, Ruth. *Motherhood in Black and White: Race and Sex in American Liberalism, 1930–1965.* Ithaca, NY: Cornell University Press, 2000.

Gambino, Matthew. "Fevered Decisions: Race, Ethics, and Clinical Vulnerability in the Malarial Treatment of Neurosyphilis, 1922–1953." *Hastings Center Report* 45, no. 4 (2015): 39–50.

———. "'These Strangers within Our Gates': Race, Psychiatry and Mental Illness among Black Americans at St. Elizabeths Hospital in Washington, DC, 1900–40." *History of Psychiatry* 19, no. 4 (December 1, 2008): 387–408.

Gilman, Sander L., and James M. Thomas. *Are Racists Crazy? How Prejudice, Racism, and Antisemitism Became Markers of Insanity.* New York: NYU Press, 2016.

Hughes, John S. "Labeling and Treating Black Mental Illness in Alabama, 1861–1910." *Journal of Southern History* 58, no. 3 (1992): 435–60.

Jackson, Vanessa. "In Our Own Voice: African-American Stories of Oppression, Survival and Recovery in Mental Health Systems." *International Journal of Narrative Therapy and Community Work* 2002, no. 2 (2002): 11–31.

Lowe, Tony B. "Nineteenth Century Review of Mental Health Care for African Americans: A Legacy of Service and Policy Barriers." *Journal of Sociology and Social Welfare* 33, no. 4 (December 2006): 29–50.

Markowitz, Gerald, and David Rosner. *Children, Race, and Power: Kenneth and Mamie Clark's Northside Center.* New York: Routledge, 2013.

Mendes, Gabriel. *Under the Strain of Color: Harlem's Lafargue Clinic and the Promise of an Antiracist Psychiatry.* Ithaca, NY: Cornell University Press, 2015.

Metzl, Jonathan M. "Living in Mental Health: Guns, Race, and the History of Schizophrenic Violence." In *Living and Dying in the Contemporary World: A Compendium*, edited by Veena Das et al. Berkeley: University of California Press, 2015.

———. *The Protest Psychosis: How Schizophrenia Became a Black Disease.* Boston: Beacon Press, 2010.

Parsons, Anne E. *From Asylum to Prison: Deinstitutionalization and the Rise of Mass Incarceration after 1945.* Chapel Hill: University of North Carolina Press, 2018.

Antipsychiatry and Protest

Buhle, Mari Jo. *Feminism and Its Discontents: A Century of Struggle with Psychoanalysis.* Cambridge, MA: Harvard University Press, 2009.

Dain, Norman. "Antipsychiatry." In *American Psychiatry After World War II, 1944–*

1994, edited by Roy Menninger and John C. Nemiah. Washington DC: American Psychiatric Press, 2000.

McLean, Athena Helen. "From Ex-Patient Alternatives to Consumer Options: Consequences of Consumerism and the Ex-Patient Movement." *International Journal of Health Services* 30, no. 4 (2000): 821–47.

Minton, Henry L. *Departing from Deviance: A History of Homosexual Rights and Emancipatory Science in America*. Chicago: University of Chicago Press, 2002.

Morrison, Linda, J. *Talking Back to Psychiatry: The Psychiatric Consumer/Survivor/ Ex-Patient Movement*. London: Taylor and Francis, 2009.

Oliver, Jeffrey. "The Myth of Thomas Szasz." *New Atlantis: A Journal of Technology and Society*, Summer 2006, 68–84.

Rissmiller, David J., and Joshua H Rissmiller. "Evolution of the Antipsychiatry Movement into Mental Health Consumerism." *Psychiatric Services* 57, no. 6 (June 2006): 863–66.

Sedgwick, Peter. *Psycho Politics: Laing, Foucault, Goffman, Szasz, and the Future of Mass Psychiatry*. New York: Harper and Row, 1982.

Staub, Michael E. *Madness Is Civilization: When the Diagnosis Was Social, 1948–1980*. Chicago: University of Chicago Press, 2011.

Tomes, Nancy. "The Patient as a Policy Factor: A Historical Case Study of the Consumer/Survivor Movement in Mental Health." *Health Affairs* 25 (2006): 720–29.

Diagnostics and the DSM

Bayer, Ronald. *Homosexuality and American Psychiatry: The Politics of Diagnosis*. Princeton: Princeton University Press, 1981.

Bayer, Ronald, and R. L. Spitzer. "Neurosis, Psychodynamics, and DSM-III: A History of the Controversy." *Archives of General Psychiatry* 42, no. 2 (February 1, 1985): 187–96.

Blashfield, Roger K. "Feighner et al., Invisible Colleges, and the Matthew Effect." *Schizophrenia Bulletin* 8, no. 1 (1982): 1–6.

Decker, Hannah S. *The Making of DSM-III: A Diagnostic Manual's Conquest of American Psychiatry*. New York: Oxford University Press, 2013.

Greenberg, Gary. *The Book of Woe: The DSM and the Unmaking of Psychiatry*. New York: Penguin, 2013.

Grob, Gerald N. "Origins of DSM-I: A Study in Appearance and Reality." *American Journal of Psychiatry* 148, no. 4 (1991): 421.

Kendler, K. S., R. A. Munoz, and G. Murphy. "The Development of the Feighner Criteria: A Historical Perspective." *American Journal of Psychiatry* 167 (December 15, 2009): 134–42.

Kutchins, Herb, and Stuart A. Kirk. *Making Us Crazy: DSM: The Psychiatric Bible and the Creation of Mental Disorders*. New York: Free Press, 1997.

Mayes, Rick, and Allan V. Horwitz. "DSM-III and the Revolution in the Classification of Mental Illness." *Journal of the History of the Behavioral Sciences* 41 (2005): 249–67.

Paris, Joel, and James Phillips. *Making the DSM-5: Concepts and Controversies*. New York: Springer, 2013.

Pichot, Pierre. "Tracing the Origins of Bipolar Disorder: From Falret to DSM-IV and ICD-10." *Journal of Affective Disorders* 96, no. 3 (2006): 145–48.

Shorter, Edward. *What Psychiatry Left Out of the DSM-5: Historical Mental Disorders Today*. London: Routledge, 2015.

Strand, Michael. "Where Do Classifications Come From? The DSM-III, the Transformation of American Psychiatry, and the Problem of Origins in the Sociology of Knowledge." *Theory and Society* 40, no. 3 (2011): 273–313.

Wilson, M. "DSM-III and the Transformation of American Psychiatry: A History." *American Journal of Psychiatry* 150, no. 3 (1993): 399.

Disease Histories

Donvan, John Joseph, and Caren Brenda Zucker. *In a Different Key: The Story of Autism*. New York: Crown Publishers, 2017.

Eyal, Gil, et al. *The Autism Matrix*. Malden, MA: Polity, 2010.

Greenberg, Gary. *Manufacturing Depression: The Secret History of a Modern Disease*. New York: Simon and Schuster, 2010.

Healy, David. *Mania: A Short History of Bipolar Disorder*. Baltimore: Johns Hopkins University Press, 2011.

Hirshbein, Laura D. *American Melancholy: Constructions of Depression in the Twentieth Century*. New Brunswick, NJ: Rutgers University Press, 2009.

Hurn, Juliet D. "The History of General Paralysis of the Insane in Britain, 1830 to 1950." London: University of London, 1998.

Lawlor, Clark. *From Melancholia to Prozac: A History of Depression*. New York: Oxford University Press, 2012.

Lutz, Tom. *American Nervousness, 1903: An Anecdotal History*. Ithaca, NY: Cornell University Press, 1991.

Martin, Emily. *Bipolar Expeditions: Mania and Depression in American Culture*. Princeton, NJ: Princeton University Press, 2009.

McNally, Kieran. *A Critical History of Schizophrenia*. New York: Palgrave Macmillan, 2016.

Micale, Mark. *Approaching Hysteria: Disease and Its Interpretations*. Princeton, NJ: Princeton University Press, 1995.

Noll, Richard. *American Madness: The Rise and Fall of Dementia Praecox*. Cambridge, MA: Harvard University Press, 2011. Silberman, Steve. *Neurotribes: The Legacy of Autism and the Future of Neurodiversity*. New York: Penguin, 2015.

Memoirs

Danquah, Meri Nana-Ama. *Willow Weep for Me: A Black Woman's Journey Through Depression*. New York: W. W. Norton, 1998.

Dully, Howard, and Charles Fleming. *My Lobotomy: A Memoir*. New York: Broadway Books, 2007.

Forney, Ellen. *Marbles: Mania, Depression, Michelangelo, and Me: A Graphic Memoir*. New York: Gotham Books, 2012.

Jamison, Kay Redfield. *An Unquiet Mind: A Memoir of Moods and Madness*. New York: Vintage, 1996.

Orr, Jackie. *Panic Diaries: A Genealogy of Panic Disorder*. Durham, NC: Duke University Press, 2006.

Saks, Elyn. *The Center Cannot Hold: My Journey through Madness*. New York: Hyperion, 2007.

Slater, Lauren. *Prozac Diary*. Harmondsworth, UK: Penguin, 2000.

Solomon, Andrew. *The Noonday Demon: An Atlas of Depression*. New York: Scribner, 2002.

Styron, William. *Darkness Visible: A Memoir of Madness*. New York: Vintage, 1992.

Wagner, Pamela Spiro, and Carolyn Spiro. *Divided Minds: Twin Sisters and Their Journey Through Schizophrenia*. New York: St. Martin's Griffin, 2006.

Wurtzel, Elizabeth. *Prozac Nation: Young and Depressed in America*. Boston: Houghton Mifflin Harcourt, 2014.

Influential Critiques

Angell, Marcia. *The Truth About Drug Companies: How They Deceive Us and What to Do About it*. New York: Random House, 2004.

Frances, Allen. *Saving Normal: An Insider's Revolt Against Out-of-Control Psychiatric Diagnosis, DSM-5, Big Pharma, and the Medicalization of Ordinary Life*. New York: HarperCollins, 2013.

Greenberg, Gary. *The Book of Woe: The DSM and the Unmaking of Psychiatry*. New York: Scribe Publications, 2013.

Moncrieff, Joanna. *The Myth of the Chemical Cure: A Critique of Psychiatric Drug Treatment*. New York: Palgrave Macmillan, 2008.

Rose, Nikolas, and Joelle M. Abi-Rached. *Neuro: The New Brain Sciences and the Management of the Mind*. Princeton, NJ: Princeton University Press, 2013.

Watters, Ethan. *Crazy Like Us: The Globalization of the American Psyche*. New York: Free Press, 2011.

Whitaker, Robert. *Anatomy of an Epidemic: Magic Bullets, Psychiatric Drugs, and the Astonishing Rise of Mental Illness in America*. New York: Crown Publishers, 2010.

INDEX

Note: Page numbers in *italics* indicate figures.